D1192232

First published 1973 by
Pluto Press Limited
Unit 10, Spencer Court, 7 Chalcot Road, London NW1 8LH

© Copyright Pluto Press, 1973

ISBN 0 902818 90 2

Made and printed in Great Britain
by Love and Malcomson Ltd (TU)
Brighton Road, Redhill, Surrey

Designed by Richard Hollis, GrR

The Hazards of Work: How to Fight Them.

Patrick Kinnersly

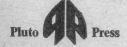

Pluto Press

Contents

Foreword:

'Health is a state of complete physical, mental, and social well-being, not merely an absence of disease and infirmity.' *World Health Organisation*

By this entirely reasonable definition millions of workers are clearly not enjoying good health.

They will not be able to achieve it until a massive and concerted attack is made on the conditions of work that cause not only disease but also increasing mental stress and disruption to social and family life.

I hope this book will provide a little inspiration and a lot of facts for the coming struggle. I apologise in advance for its many shortcomings and omissions, but I think the problem is too urgent to delay publication, yet again, for further improvement and additions. I hope that the experience and criticism of workers can be incorporated in a more serviceable second edition.

Although every word has passed through my typewriter this is not my book alone. Many people have contributed to it in many ways and I would like to be able to thank them all, particularly those who wrote the original material on which so many of the chapters are based. I cannot do this in every case, not because there is no space but because some of them have asked me not to mention them or to hide them behind a pseudonym. It is a sad reflection on supposedly humanitarian professions like medicine and sociology when their members can still fear for their jobs if they are seen to side too obviously with those their skills are designed to serve.

The inspiration for this book came from a handbook produced in the United States for the Oil Chemical and Atomic Workers union by Dr Susan Daum and a committee of scientists dedicated to making their knowledge available to workers. I am grateful to Susan Daum for her advice and for letting me see parts of the manuscript of her new book when she was last in England.

Inspiration also came from the leaflets produced by Urban Planning Aid in Massachusetts, USA, whose direct approach to information for workers was an invaluable lesson. Many ideas and much useful information came also from the British Society for Social Responsibility in Science who trustingly lent me the tapes of their lively conference on community health.

For all the inspiration this project would have been impossible without the financial support provided by Pluto Press during the first few months, and the generous backing of the Society of Graphical and Allied Trades. For their money, their encouragement and their patience I am deeply grateful to SoGAT and in particular to Vincent Flynn.

Among those who contributed written material on their special subjects I would like to single out for special thanks Dr Bill Fakes who wrote most of the chapter on disease; Jamie Ritchie for his heroic attempt at making the law of injury benefits intelligible to ordinary people; Dr Bob Hider and Dick Ranson for compiling the Directory of Toxic Substances; Dr Charles Wackstein for most of the section on noise.

Other contributors deserve my apologies as well as my thanks for I have chopped their work around or melted it into my own. I hope their ideas have not been lost in the process: I would like to thank Jake Bharier for his work on chemical hazards; Bill Kaye for work on accidents; Frank Clifford for material on the law; Kit Ryan for much work and advice on trade union organisation; George Ross for a wealth of material on patterns of work; Dr Robert MacGibbon for notes on medical services and my brother Richard for a review of machine shop design faults.

Finally I am indebted to Anthony Woolf, Dr Robert Murray, Dr Bill Jones and Dr John Steel for reading and commenting on parts of the draft manuscript; to Mike Kidron of Pluto Press for advice, criticism and encouragement throughout the project; and to Richard Hollis for taking so much trouble with the design.

1.

Introduction

David and the foam on the floor

The operator was away at lunch when foam was found leaking from a pipe beneath the insulation plant at the Frigidaire factory in North London.

The foreman gave David Adair a paint scraper and told him to go in and scrape it off the floor before it hardened. He had to go right in under the machinery. The smell was so strong that the foreman went off to look for a respirator. He came back with one from the paint shop; it was covered in paint and the air came in round the edge. David wore it for the rest of the job which took him an hour and a half in all.

A few days later he began to feel chesty, wheezed a lot and had great difficulty in breathing.

The works doctor said his throat was infected. In the middle of the following night he had to get up and go outside to get enough air to breathe. The doctor said he had a cold but when his 'cold' got no better it was finally realised that he was suffering from severe asthma.

His condition was caused entirely by exposure to toluene di-isocyanate (TDI), one of the chemicals used in making the polyurethane foam he scraped off the floor. Even if it had been brand-new the respirator he wore would not have stopped the vapour. It was not the right type.

TDI is so powerful that one teaspoonful of vapour mixed into the air of a large room would make the air very dangerous to breathe. Under the machine where David worked the vapour was so concentrated that he could hardly stand it. By the time the respirator arrived, 20 minutes after he started, it probably didn't matter what type it was: irreversible damage had already been done to his lungs.

The specialist who later tested his lungs concluded that he was 30 percent disabled, could never be cured and might get worse as he got older.

David had already got older. The damage to his lungs had turned him into an old man at the age of 36.

Labouring was out of the question: the best job he could get was as a lavatory attendant. Light sweeping was about all he could manage and that left him too exhausted at the end of the day to do anything but sit watching TV. His nights were often a gasping agony.

o *David sued Frigidaire for negligence. They denied that the accident had even happened and resisted all attempts to uncover the truth. When he had told his story in the High Court, Frigidaire finally admitted their negligence. David was awarded just over £4,000 for his ruined life.*

We could have started this book with more horrifying examples of physical injury or callous neglect. What happened to David is not spectacular by the standards of a society in which you have to die suddenly before you can earn the headlines reserved for a minor case of mugging.

A simple little task on an ordinary day in an ordinary factory owned by a 'respectable' employer quietly stole half a man's life.

It could have happened to any worker and that is why it is so important. In theory many safeguards stood between David and the TDI. One by one they failed him.

1. The employer:

Frigidaire, a division of General Motors, largest company in the world, was as negligent as any one of the thousands of back street slum factories which provide the backdrop for such 'stars' of capitalism.

The firm knew the dangers of TDI; the manufacturers had issued a warning and several other workers had fallen victim to it. David was not told of the danger.

2. The foreman:

Did not appear to have understood the danger, which reflects more on the employer than him.

3. The works medical officer:

He could have educated management about the dangers, ensured that everyone was given the right information and warnings and raised the general level of awareness and concern. Instead he diagnosed a throat infection in a man who had been handling one of the most potent and best-known causes of industrial asthma.

4. The safety officer:

He ought to have been in the front line in publicising the risks and precautions and insisting on safe working practices. Instead he was more concerned to cover up the incident—perhaps to maintain his plant's chances in the company's annual international safety league contest and, at the same time, to save the insurers from having to pay compensation.

5. The plant:

It leaked but that need not have developed into an 'accident' if:

    a. The failure had triggered an automatic shutdown or alarm.

    b. Warning notices all round the area made it clear even to outsiders – firemen for example – that any leak was an emergency requiring evacuation or breathing apparatus.

6. Protection:

A suitable respirator, either breathing apparatus or air line, was not located close to the plant and labelled so that anyone could find it in an emergency.

7. The law:

The law was broken. The Factories Act lays down the minimum conditions for safety in manufacturing establishments and one of its requirements is that everything possible must be done to protect you from 'injurious or offensive' substances. The law has not caught up with TDI as a specific hazard so it is not yet written into any special regulations under the Factories Act. But the Factory Inspectorate, the puny enforcement agency for this branch of criminal law, had publicised its dangers – not of course in publications usually read by workers.

The Factories Act provides no deterrent because firms do not expect to be prosecuted. The average factory is inspected once every four years. The maximum fine for each offence is only £300 (average fine £40) and the factory inspectors rarely use their powers to have unsafe plant closed down. (See Section 10, Safety law.)

Claims for compensation provide no deterrent because the insurance company picks up the bill. (See Section 11, Winning damages.)

8. Public opinion:

Public opinion provides no deterrent because much of what goes on is concealed from the public. The law placed no obligation on the employer to report this incident. David was not off work more than the three days which makes an accident reportable and asthma is not among the diseases which have to be reported. (See Section 5, Disease and Section 7, Accidents.)

The case therefore joins thousands of others which never appear in the national statistics of occupational in-injury and disease.

This is one of the ways in which the scandalous industrial health problem is made to look smaller than it is so that the demand for a clean-up is minimised. (See figures later in this section.)

The case only came to light because Frigidaire took the unusual step of maintaining its denial of liability to the end, forcing the case into the High Court. Most employers would have settled quietly (and cheaply) out of court and many workers would have given up in despair at ever winning proper compensation.

9. The unions:

Obviously no worker should rely totally on safe-guards provided by his employer or the law. But you should be able to rely on your shop steward to warn you of any hazards known to have affected other workers. Only militant action at shop floor level can bring occupational hazards under control. (See Section 13, Organising.)

Nine Safeguards Failed.

When David took the paint scraper he was down to the last line of defence – his own knowledge of the hazards in his place of work. Unfortunately for him and his family, he didn't know about TDI.

Would you have known?

Do you know what chemical and other hazards you may encounter at work? (See Sections 2 to 5.) Do you know what the employer should be doing to protect you? (See Section 6, Prevention.)

This book is intended to help you find out so that you can begin to control the level of risk in your job. That is only the first step towards real health for all workers. Hazards at work are not just isolated failures in an otherwise humane system. They are caused by the same social, political and economic priorities which ensure the worst health for workers.

Unhealthy working conditions, low wages, rotten housing and poor nutrition continue to undermine the health of millions. Yet under the supposedly egalitarian National Health Service, the areas of greatest need receive the worst medical care.

o Twice as many children of the poor die in the first week of life as do babies of the well-to-do.

o In 1970 six boys and three girls were rejected for factory employment because pre-employment medical checks showed them to be suffering from malnutrition. Seven boys and four girls were rejected in 1971.

Once you have been accepted as suitable material by industry, your life expectancy already shortened by being born into the working class may be further reduced by the work you do.

The class way of death covers every occupation. The Registrar General's report recognises this by dividing deaths into five social classes ranging from professional at the top to unskilled at the bottom. The report calculates its statistics by establishing the total number of deaths in all occupations and then applying the national average to each of the 340 occupational groups that it studies. This average is called a 100. Where less than the average number of deaths for all workers is found the figure is below a 100 and where more above. On this scientific basis which takes years to compile, averages are found for deaths from all causes and certain diseases and illnesses. Some examples from the report are shown opposite.

o When at work your earnings fall as your strength and speed decline once you are past the age of 40 – the age when the professional classes are moving into their most lucrative phase.

o By the age of 65, ten per cent of workers are already retired through ill health.

o One in three workers over the age of 60 has bronchitis. (See also the table of occupations, page 147.)

o Each winter about 10,000 old people die of hypothermia, a combination of malnutrition and exposure to cold.

These are the hazards not of work but of belonging to the working class. They belong in this book because disease and your position in society are closely linked.

By organising to control the hazards of work – and then demanding that work be made fit for human beings – you are on the way to changing a society that puts profits before human needs.

Occupations	Death from all causes	Tuberculosis	Lung Cancer	Bronchitis
Workers				
Coal face miners	180	294	140	293
Construction riggers	142	138	152	149
Engineering labourers	139	169	151	217
Furnacemen	108	106	168	151
Fishermen	144	171	188	148
Textile process workers	133	111	116	161
Dockers	136	180	171	220
Kitchen hands	130	410	88	165
Professional Classes				
Mine managers	66	18	56	33
Contracting managers	50	33	66	21
Engineering managers	70	17	68	25
Personnel managers	67	40	44	64
Ministers, MPs	75	29	69	28
Judges, solicitors	76	33	40	24
Clergymen	62	9	17	17
Teachers	60	23	34	23

Conflict:

The disablement of David Adair is one example of the conflict of interest between workers and employers when it comes to health and safety. The conflict exists because safety is paid for out of profits.

Both literally – in the case of machines – and figuratively – in the case of industry as a whole – it is an extra that the employer may or may not decide to purchase rather than an integral part of the way work is done.

Many employers argue that there is no longer a con-

flict in this area – though they do not say at what point between the industrial revolution and the present day it disappeared. **The report of the Robens committee on safety
and health at work, published in 1972, claimed that 'there
is a greater natural identity of interest between the two
sides of industry in relation to safety and health problems
than in most other matters.' This convenient theory lies at
the heart of the Robens conclusion that better control of
industrial hazards will be achieved not by more law but
through 'voluntary self-regulation' by industry itself.** (For
more detailed summary of the report, see page 228.)

**Identity of interest is a dangerous myth which
dovetails with the fiction that most accidents are caused
by carelessness and can therefore be eliminated if
everyone 'pulls together' and remembers their safety
slogans. (See Section 7, Accidents).**

o The fantasy cannot be sustained when it comes to
industrial disease Each year more than one thousand workers are officially diagnosed as suffering from various forms
of pneumoconiosis, caused by coal dust in mines, silica
dust in foundries and potteries and cotton dust in the mills.
Was it careless of them to breathe? Or is it simply that employers do not want to pay the 'crippling' cost of installing
proper exhaust ventilation to extract the dust at source?

The conflict shows through in all its ugliness.

**By no stretch of the imagination could the statistics
which follow be said to represent an identity of interest.**

Statistics:

**Each year the figures for occupational injuries and
disease are washed and shrunk in the statistical laundries
of industry and government and then delivered in
separate bundles.**

**It is hard to believe that the system is not designed to
conceal the truth.**

It is certainly not designed to reveal it.

You need to obtain four different annual reports to collect the figures for factories, mines, farms, and offices and shops. Numerous other sources must be consulted and quite a few guesses made to obtain figures for other jobs.

If you complete this mammoth task the result will be meaningless unless you make substantial adjustments. Under the Factories Act, for example, factory owners report only about 60 per cent of the injuries they are required to report by law; construction industry employers report only about half theirs. Only 70 firms were prosecuted for this offence in 1971. The unadjusted figures are the ones quoted in the report and in Parliamentary debates.

It is not known how many cases of industrial disease go unreported but there is no reason to suppose that the proportion is much different. The figures for farms and for offices and shops are probably even less reliable.

Employers do not have to report injury or death of self-employed workers. In the construction industry 100 deaths and more than 20,000 injuries may therefore be going unrecorded each year – with the full approval of the law.

In 1970 about 1.5 million workers were known to be self-employed and the 'Freeze' is accelerating this trend, particularly in white collar areas.

The reporting system for industrial diseases produces grossly misleading figures.

The 1970 report of the Factory Inspectorate, for example, lists just over 300 cases of industrial disease, among about eight million workers, which might make you think that industrial disease was a relatively small problem. But these are only the **notifiable** diseases. **Pneumoconiosis, the most important industrial disease of all, is not notifiable and was therefore not included in the total.** Other omissions are dermatitis, which costs workers more lost days than any other disease, and poisoning by substances which are not notifiable – for example the TDI that disabled David Adair.

All these irregularities and omissions should be ironed out in the annual report of the Department of Health and Social Security. This records the totals for industrial injury, disablement and death benefits, whether or not a claimant's case has found its way into any of the other catalogues. Here again the whole truth is not revealed.

o Self-employed people do not qualify for injury benefit (in spite of paying a higher contribution) so their injuries and deaths again go unrecorded.

o The figures for death benefits paid to widows or other dependents can indicate only the number of *married* workers killed by injury or disease.

o Victims of occupational diseases only get into these statistics if their condition *and* occupation are 'prescribed' – in other words on the list of diseases which are recognised as being caused by work. The asthma suffered by David Adair and thousands of others is not prescribed. Many other conditions caused by or aggravated by work are not on the list.

Miners, foundrymen, steelworkers and others in dusty trades are known to suffer more bronchitis than other workers; those in outdoor jobs get more rheumatism and arthritis; people who use vibrating tools get 'whitefinger', a painful condition caused by damage to the blood circulation in their hands; over 100,000 have been robbed of some of their hearing by working in dangerous levels of noise.

Many more victims are conveniently hidden from view when industry's debt to society is reckoned up each year.

So most people have no idea how large a toll of life and health is taken by work.

Asked to put figures to it they usually come out with 600 dead and 300,000 injured. These are the uncorrected totals given by the Chief Inspector of Factories in a typical annual report.

Significantly, this is the only one of the annual safety reports which press and television cover in any detail. **The mass media can be counted as the last stage in the statistical laundering.**

To arrive at realistic annual figures involves some guessing but these are probably near the truth:

Killed at work or dying from injuries	2,000
Killed by recognised industrial diseases	1,000

Injured or off work with industrial disease for at least three days	nearly 1,000,000
Injured – needing first aid	10,000,000

Even the most honest annual reckoning tends to shrink the problem by omitting the disabled and bereaved left behind by previous years of profitable production.

o At the present time more than 200,000 workers are receiving industrial disability pensions and the working class contains nearly 30,000 women who have been widowed by industry.

Most firms totally ignore the law that requires them to employ three per cent disabled workers wherever there is a workforce of more than 19. Many firms would exceed this quota if they just employed those people disabled in their employment.

Prosecutions for ignoring this law are unheard of.

Industry's performance:

The employers' commitment to safety can be judged from their unwillingness to set up joint safety committees.

They have resisted ever since 1927, when the first proposals for compulsory safety committees were put forward, claiming that industry would introduce them voluntarily. Successive governments have fallen in with this line and the Robens committee, with its commitment to the voluntary principle also rejected the idea of compulsory committees. The result is as follows:

Number of factories: about 250,000

Number with safety committees: 9,487 (1969 figure)

This is only 3.79 per cent.

The first figure contains thousands of small workplaces. The situation is said to be better among the large companies but in 1970 less than half of all factories employing more than 50 had any form of joint safety committee.

Even among firms employing more than 500 workers, one in five had no such arrangement.

Resistance to joint safety committees has been ably led by Mr Albert Costain, Conservative MP for Folkestone and Hythe. In a debate on the Employed Persons (Health and Safety) Bill which would have given workers' safety representatives certain rights of inspection after accidents, he voiced the employers old fear that committees would interfere with production.

He said the bill would be 'a sea-lawyers paradise, giving a wonderful opportunity to those who want to make trouble and disrupt our industries, where all strikes have failed. Under the guise of safety it will be possible to delay matters while an inspection is made.'

He did not mention the wonderful opportunity to reduce the disruption to life caused by accidents, such as the bridge collapse on a Costain construction site near Dartford, Kent, in March 1971 which killed a man.

The health and safety Bill died with the Labour Government in 1970 and the Conservatives naturally made no attempt to revive it.

The employment of safety officers is another test of industry's willingness to invest in safety. The national statistics for factories speak for themselves: in the 20,000 factories employing more than 50 workers an official survey found only 1,261 full time safety officers. Another 3,598 firms had part-time or shared safety officers. Eighty per cent of firms had no safety service of any kind, and even among companies employing more than 500 people, only 35 per cent had full time safety officers.

If all the thousands of small factories were taken into consideration these figures would be even more diluted. Even then they would not give any idea of the neglect in other jobs, so often ignored in public statements and statistics on occupational safety. Millions of workers in agriculture, hospitals, deep sea fishing, transport, offices, shops and warehouses have no safety committees or safety officers of any kind.

Employers are even more sparing in their use of doctors. The whole of industry employs only about 500. In the one area where you would think medical supervision could be easily achieved, the hospital service, there has been no occupational health service for the 850,000 workers until very recently. Some hospitals are now setting up their own schemes but these do not have to meet any nationally-agreed standard.

So:

The conclusions which emerge from these facts are:
1. Employers do not care about your health and safety enough to spend more than an absolute minimum on it.
2. There is no 'natural identity of interest' between employers and workers on this subject. Just the opposite.
3. The law is not going to intervene in this conflict.
4. You are on your own – unless there is an effective shop floor organisation keeping a constant watch for hazards and prepared to take militant action in answering any threat to health with a threat to profits.

Not even the most ardent capitalist denies that the shameful conditions of the industrial revolution were a direct product of the conflict between profits and health. For example machines needed frequent oiling but it cost money to stop them for this to be done. Therefore they were oiled in motion. It was difficult for a man to reach all the oiling points; children are smaller. Therefore children oiled machines in motion. Therefore children were maimed and killed.

Workers today are often amazed that their forebears did not rise against this merciless logic. It is hard to understand until you realise that the threat of starvation was more immediate than the threat of violent death from a machine. The first was a certainty if you did not work; the second was a gamble you might get away with. The mouse goes to the trap for his cheese, the fish to the hook for a worm, the worker to the mill for his bread.

The Sheffield grinder's a terrible beade
    Tally hi-o, the grinder!
He sets his little 'uns down to trade
    Tally hi-o, the grinder!
He turns his baby to grind in the hull
Till his body is stunted and his eyes are dull
And the brains are dizzy and dazed in his skull
    Tally hi-o, the grinder!

He shortens his life and he hastens his death
    Tally hi-o, the grinder!
Will drink steel dust in every breath
    Tally hi-o, the grinder!
Won't use a fan as he turns his wheel
Won't wash his hands ere he eats his meal
But dies as he lives, as hard as steel
    Tally hi-o, the grinder!

These Sheffield grinders of whom we speak
    Tally hi-o, the grinder!
Are men who earn a pound a week
    Tally hi-o, the grinder!
But of Sheffield grinders another sort
Methinks ought to be called in court
And that is the grinding Government Board
    Tally hi-o, the grinder!

At whose door lies the blacker blame?
    Tally hi-o, the grinder!
Where rests the heavier weight of shame?
    Tally hi-o, the grinder!
On the famine-price contractor's head
Or the workman's under-taught and fed
Who grinds his own bones and his child's for bread?
    Tally hi-o, the grinder!

From Folk Songs in England, A.L.Lloyd, Panther Arts.

    The Sheffield grinders who sang this song in the 1860s recognised the hazards of their work and of the system that exploited them.

Identity of interest: 1

o 'Ideally the company would have liked to have had an arrangement whereby the whole length would have been scaffolded. But this was out of the question because of the expense which would have been involved.'

Mr Green of Babcock and Wilcox, giving evidence after the death of a welder on its Baglan Bay chemical plant site in December 1970. The company's decision to skimp on provision of safe access and a proper guard rail cost it a fine of just £600.

In 1970 Babcock and Wilcox made a profit of more than £3 millions.

Identity of interest: 2

o In January 1968 two British deep-sea trawlers operating off the coast of Iceland froze over. The weight of ice in masts and rigging caused them to capsize. Thirty-eight fishermen were killed.

Throughout that year research scientists and development engineers worked at Palmer Aero Products in Leyland, Lancashire to develop a simple de-icing system.

By January 1969 they had the answer and the equipment was fitted to the deep-sea trawler Boston Phantom. Tested in the Icelandic fishing grounds it was highly successful.

The company made sure that every trawler company knew about it. They did not get a single order and to this day the Boston Phantom is the only trawler fitted with the de-icing system.

One ship can be equipped for £2,000: with a crew of 20 that represents an investment of about £100 to protect the life of each man. Over the life of the system it would come to a few pounds per man per year.

o 'I have often asked the representatives of the trawler companies what price they put on men's lives. I find it rather difficult to get an answer to this question.'

Campbell Thomas of Palmer Aero

Identity of Interest: 3

o 'We have the knowledge and apparatus for absorbing gases, arresting grit, dust and fumes and preventing smoke *formation. The only reason we still permit the escape of pollutants is because economics play such an important part in the word "practicable" in the expression "best practicable means", and most of our problems are cheque-book rather than technical.'*

Chief Alkali Inspector addressing International Air Pollution Conference, Washington, December 1970

Identity of interest: 4

o *An engineering firm employed labourers on Saturday mornings to change the cutting oil in the machine tools. As part of an economy drive this overtime working was ended and the sumps were not cleaned out for nine months. The result was an outbreak of dermatitis which cost many workers weeks of lost wages.*

Identity of interest: 5

Mr E Peel, for the company (W and C French) said that if the regulations regarding shoring-up of trenches were rigidly enforced there would be a thousand such prosecutions a day. There would have been no prosecution now had there not been an accident.
He added that contractors would find many jobs economically impractical if they shored earth works as thoroughly as the regulations demanded.
Report in Colchester Evening Gazette of magistrates court case after a man was injured in a trench collapse. The company was fined £50.

2

Patterns of Work

This section is about different patterns of work and their effects on your health.

Some of these effects, like inflammation of the tendons in fast repetitive work, are purely physical. But a more serious hazard is present in all intensive work patterns – mental stress. This is now one of the most urgent issues in the struggle for workers' health because the productivity deal you sign today may be an order form for illness.

This section deals with the effects of :

o Rising productivity
o Increasing stress
o Patterns of work:

Prod deals; work measurement; MDW; piecework; the Lump; automation; speed-up; shift-work; job enrichment; flextime.

Rising productivity :

Since the war Britain's Gross National Product has increased fourfold. In the period between 1957 and 1968 the productivity of the average worker increased by almost 20 per cent. That average worker puts in only two hours less a week than 20 years ago. More than a third regularly work overtime to make up a decent wage and the amount of extra time they clock up has remained constant at around eight hours a week since 1960.

In the ten years to 1964 the proportion of industrial workers on shifts grew by more than half, from 12 to 18 per cent. By 1973 the proportion had nearly doubled – more than a third of all industrial workers are now on shifts. The trend is continuing.

No job is safe from the employers' drive to extract more production.

Manual jobs are mechanised, machine jobs are automated, automated jobs are speeded up. All kinds of work, from filling forms to mending roads, are measured and linked to bonus or productivity payments. One third of all industrial workers are now governed by productivity deals.

Employers have paid for each change with pay rises that have been swallowed up by the rising cost of living. Workers have paid in redundancies, disruption of social life and an increasing burden of stress.

There is no end to productivity bargaining.

When the effects of the last deal have worn off you can get more money only by selling something else: tea breaks or a few more jobs in the early stages, weekends or any semblance of convenient working hours as you get deeper in.

Work becomes more and more attuned to the needs of machines and less and less to the needs of human beings.

'Equal sharing':

o Towards the end of 1972 the Union of Post Office Workers called a halt to further productivity deals until the benefits were equally shared: the Post Office had been getting 60 per cent of productivity savings and workers only 40 per cent.

o The union leadership was not against the proposed work measurement and mechanisation changes that would have affected almost every sector of the service – only against the unequal shareout.

o They forgot that there can be no equality when only the workers suffer the harmful effects of more intensive working.

Increasing stress:

Machines must be operated within certain limits of speed and stress or they break.

Humans are more adaptable.

Few of us know the limits to our own physical and mental resources, let alone those of other people, and in any case the limits are not fixed like those of a machine.

The man who can dig a trench for hours without getting too tired might be exhausted if he had to put straws in boxes all day. In his case, monotony and the feeling that he was doing something unworthy of his strength and skill could cause enough stress to drain his energy. A group of housewives doing the same job, perhaps on a part time basis, might actually find it relaxing to get away from their homes to meet other women and talk while they worked. But if the pace of their work was speeded up, requiring full concentration all the time, and new equipment made it too noisy to talk, they too might come under stress.

It is impossible to measure stress like other hazards because it is an individual human reaction to a given situation.

Whether the 'dose' of stress in any situation is likely to be harmful depends on the individual and is very difficult to predict.

All you can do is learn to recognise the type of situation that causes stress and, individually and collectively do everything in your power to avoid it.

The urgency of this warning is shown by the statistics.

In the 15 years up to 1970, working days lost from the effects of severe mental stress increased by 152 per cent for men and 302 per cent for women.

o In the year ending June 1970, 37 million working days were lost and in the following year the figure rose to 38.5 million (compare with 28.5 million for accidents, 10 million from colds and flu and about 11 million for strikes).

o At any one time some four million people are taking tranquillisers prescribed by their doctors.

o Millions more depend on cigarettes, alcohol and other drugs to fight or release stress.

By no means all of the blame can be laid on working conditions.

Many of the causes lie deep in the present organisation of society and will not be eliminated until people believe that society can be changed for the benefit of all. Meanwhile it is vital that the situation over which workers already have some control, the organisation of their work, should be kept to the lowest possible levels of stress.

Some causes of stress:	Some effects:
Overwork, long hours, poor diet	
Pace of work too fast	
Too much responsibility, over-promotion	
Unsatisfying, monotonous, boring or meaningless work	Fatigue
	Accidents
Isolation from workmates, lack of release from tension in talk or organising	Ulcers
	Indigestion
	High blood pressure
Lack of control over pace of production and conditions of work	Heart attack
	Skin rash
Insecurity and anxiety about job, redundancies, takeovers, retraining, money, retirement, pension	Backache
	Depression
	Anxiety neurosis
Environment– noise, vibration, heat, cold, poor lighting	Headaches
	Migraine
Narcotic and other chemicals affecting nervous system	Asthma
Fear of hazards, disease and injury	
Domestic problems resulting from shiftwork or excessive overtime	

NB: These factors are additive. For example if you are getting too much noise you will have less energy to resist other stresses.

Warning signs:
Change in behaviour: eg quiet man becomes aggressive, loudmouth sulks and doesn't seem to care
Sharp swings in mood: 'You don't know whether you're coming or going with that bugger'

Patterns of work:

Productivity deals:

These deals introduce many different patterns of work that can attack health and welfare.

A common feature is the removal of 'restrictive practices' and 'non-productive' workers. The craftsman's mate is a favourite target for the axe: without his mate the tradesman has to get through more work and often finds himself working in isolation. This is a bad combination not only from the point of view of stress but also as a potential cause of accidents – there's no-one to foot a ladder, pass a tool or, if anything goes wrong, go for help.

Anything that breaks the flow of production, particularly when expensive assembly lines or continuous plants have to be stopped, will be scrapped if workers allow it. Traditional ten-minute tea-breaks in the morning and afternoon are the first to go, often replaced by vending machines from which you can get 'instant' – often nasty – 'tea' at any time or within periods set by management. Lunch periods are shortened or staggered so that lines can be kept running. Vending canteens with microwave ovens are introduced to speed up the 'eat period'.

Tea breaks are important for a number of reasons. The tea is stimulating. The breaks provide opportunities to talk to friends, fix small details of union business, shut down machines so that ear muffs can be taken off in noisy places, or to get right out of the workroom. It all helps to recharge your mind and body. It has been shown for example that the highest accident rate among train drivers is two hours after breakfast – the cause: low blood sugar.

All this may seem very obvious but workers are still selling tea breaks, regretting it and finding out that it takes a lot of struggling to get them back.

o Workers in a small chemical plant were asked to give up not only tea breaks but the paid washing and changing periods at the beginning and end of each shift as part of a deal that would have brought in £10 a week extra. This should never happen. Washing periods help protect against poisoning and disease. They should never find their way onto the bargaining table – except as a demand that they be introduced.

Productivity deals tend to demand even more fundamental concessions from workers. This is what Rolls-Royce hoped to get from AUEW (TASS) workers in Bristol:

> The acceptance of shift work in order to exploit high capital equipment, the acceptance of work measurement techniques, the division of work into basic elements, and the setting of times for these elements, such time spent to be compared with actual performance.

Deals like this are being peddled in areas where labour or equipment costs are rising. Many white collar workers are at risk.

o In a West London electronics factory 17 draughtsmen got involved in a productivity deal which meant doing the work of twice their number. The pace of work caused so much stress that four of them had nervous breakdowns in the space of 18 months. (Reported in *DATA News*, April 1969).

Work measurement:

This is now at the centre of many productivity deals and managements are prepared to pay high prices for acceptance. The threat is greatest where high-output and automated equipment is being introduced: employers find that the old piecework and bonus systems of payment which still work to their advantage in labour-intensive situations backfire in a highly automated plant. If they are to reap the full benefit from this type of investment they need to establish absolute control over your hourly pace of work rather than just being able to induce you to turn out a certain amount by the end of the day. Secondly, they need to regain control of wages so that the labour content of the job can be precisely costed and kept stable.

That is what measured day work *(MDW)* is all about. For the worker it means an unrelenting pressure to keep up with a rate of production over which you have no control.

This is how MDW was defined by the Coventry engineering employers' association:
A fixed hourly rate payment system based upon quan-
tified performance standards which have been established by work measurement techniques. When operators fail to meet standards through their own fault,
this becomes a question for discipline or re-training.

The daily carrot of the bonus system is replaced by
one big carrot to get you to accept the deal. After that
there is just the stick hanging over your performance hour
after hour.

There are variations on the system but all start with
work study, a procedure that involves timing each operation in a particular job, using a stop watch, and then by
various pseudo-scientific adjustments, arriving at a 'standard time' for the job.

o For a good description of work study which clearly
shows that it is just guessing dressed up as science, see
Colin Barker, **The Power Game**, Pluto Press, especially
p 57, where he deals with the inaccuracy of 'effort rat-
ing'. The leaderships of the four unions representing
electricity supply workers actually called for faster introduction of work study. As a result output rose and
the number of industrial workers was cut by nearly 19
per cent between 1967 and 1970.

Getting everybody working to the discipline of standard timings is not good enough for some managements.
The more advanced plants use closed circuit television, or
electronic 'production monitors' built into your machine, to
relay your performance back to a central control panel
where it is compared with target figures.

Measured day work is a formula for stress. Workers
lose individual and collective control of their pace of production; there is less time for the social elements in work
which provide relief from stress – and less chance to make
time for an unofficial break by putting on a spurt of work.
Only selected workers are timed by the work study man
and the slower ones may be constantly worried about keeping up. Unfair timings cause resentment which worsens the
stress, as does the fear of redundancies.

Piecework:

Workers fighting the introduction of *MDW* find themselves defending the piecework bonus system as the lesser of two evils.

Given that a choice has to be made between two forms of work intensification, this is the right course to follow because of the stress risk in MDW. But there should not be any illusions about the safety of piecework. It is a dangerous system because it transfers to the worker part of management's financial stake in unsafe working methods. To earn a reasonable bonus, particularly when rates are low, it becomes a common practice to remove or modify machine guards which slow production.

The answer of course is to do away with the incentive, let everyone work at their own natural safe speed and pay a good wage for an (unmeasured) day's work. But that would not be so profitable.

MDW does remove the personal incentive to cut corners on safety, but management's is still there in the way that job timings are pared to the bone.

This kind of contradiction is inevitable under the twisted priorities of profit. You can reduce its harmful effects in various ways:

1. Hang onto the bonus system and fight for decent rates so that people do not have to cut corners.
2. Attack all hazards.
3. Don't give in to the pressure for MDW unless strong safeguards are written into the agreement to reduce the risk of accidents and stress:

o *every timing to be subject to approval by safety stewards*
o *every possible safeguard to be built into each timing – the best possible tools, safety devices and test procedures*
o *maximum personal relief time*

o In May 1973 workers at Rubery Owen, Darlaston, Staffs, succeeded in defeating proposals for MDW after a five-week strike. The company conceded wage rises based on piecework earnings, the biggest rises going to the lowest earners.

Construction piecework:

In construction the dangers caused by piecework are in a class by themselves and the system is indefensible by any standards.

The risks are generally greater than in most factory jobs, and much more elaborate safeguards must be built in as part of the work.

Yet on piecework you are paid for the 'square' of scaffolding (not the number and security of ties holding it back to the building or the inclusion of toeboards and guard rails), the length of the trench (not the quality of the shoring), and so on.

o The significant thing about this accident (failure of a riveter's staging which sent the worker in it 180 ft to his death) which would not be considered in a Factory Inspector's investigation is that riveters are paid on this job by the hundred rivets, not for the time it takes them to put up the staging. Needless to say they try to get the staging put up in the shortest possible time, so that they can start earning. Many accidents like this are caused not by the nature of the work but by the speed at which the work is expected to be done.

James Tye, Director General of the British Safety Council, in **Safety Uncensored,** Corgi Books.

The Lump:

For construction employers the Lump is the ultimate in piecework systems.

Gangs of self-employed workers are induced to work at an astounding pace for a lump sum payment. The gang is thus welded into the nearest thing to a machine that the employer can get for jobs that can't be mechanised. The lump user gets almost total control of output and costs.

The lump endangers its members and everyone else on sites where it gets a hold. Neither the unions nor the law can see that safety standards are enforced, the unions because membership is diluted by the non-union lumpies

B

and the law because self-employed workers are not covered. (See page 247.)

All the dangers of piecework are magnified and the shaky temporary works that result can threaten the safety of other workers and the general public.

o As the lump grows towards one third of the labour force, even committed trade unionists are sometimes forced to take lump jobs to get work. This is how Don Quinn, convenor, and John Fontaine, bricklayer's steward, on the World's End housing contract in Chelsea, described it:

o *'On the lump you couldn't straighten your back from one end of the day to the other. You had to get a sub every day for a drink just to get the sweat back into your body.*

o *It was pure slavery. You have no right to notice, they can sack you on the spot. And if you have an accident on the lump you get nothing. Instead of getting benefit, they probably discover you haven't been paying tax or stamps and you get prosecuted.*

o *When you work, you have a pacemaker in front of you who gets £4 more than you, and you have to keep up with him. You look for bricklayers' jobs in the Evening News and it will say "greyhounds only", meaning speed merchants. But we're not dogs, we're human beings.*

o *It increases unemployment fantastically. Four men do 20 men's work. And when you're over 45 you're finished completely.*

o *There's a non-union site next to us. There are no proper eating facilities, no washing facilities, nowhere to change your clothes. Men have to keep a change of clothes in cardboard boxes, in the middle of the site, where the rain can get at them.'* Quoted in *Socialist Worker*, 19 August 1972.

Automation:

Automation should be a boon, taking over the hard, dirty and boring jobs, allowing us to concentrate on the interesting and worthwhile tasks (and giving us more time for activities that make us more human).

In practice, machines are expensive and employers only automate where it is profitable.

Dirty jobs like refuse collection, which can be completely automated, are retained (often with 'cheap' imported labour) and satisfying craft jobs that carry a high wage are automated into boring repetitive tasks where the worker is paced by the machine.

> o Every operation has been simplified so much that the Americans say even monkeys could build Avengers.
> o Some new starters have said that they have sleepless nights, dreaming about Avengers coming down the track at them, for the first few weeks.
> Eddie Tomlinson, National Union of Sheet Metal Workers shop steward at Chrysler Ryton, writing in Socialist Worker, 23 June 1973.

The highly-automated production line condenses all the worst stress-producing conditions into one situation.

It reaches its peak in a car plant on MDW. The work is monotonous, repetitive, fast and noisy.

It requires concentration and responsibility and yet is increasingly beyond the control of individuals and stewards.

The combination is not good for anyone's health and is particularly hard on older workers. Not only is their skill and experience of less and less value to management but also they find they cannot keep up with new, less skilled but faster jobs.

Old age begins early on the tracks:

> o In Standard Triumph in Coventry, it is reckoned that a man is burned up in ten years on the main production line. Clearly the employer wishes those years to be as early as possible, in order that the operator in question is active enough to exploit the plant at the highest rate possible. The company recently attempted to get some of the manual workers to agree that only workers of up to 30 years would be recruited for this high tempo work.
> M.J.E.Cooley in Computer Aided Design.

What does it mean to be 'burned up' in ten years? Ford for one would rather you did not know.

Dr James Allardice, a senior medical officer with the company, was going to speak at a London conference on industrial stress in May 1973. In March the firm's public relations department told him some of the statistics in his paper were unacceptable and he should not present it to the conference. Dr Allardice is believed to have found a high incidence of stress disorders among workers including stomach ulcers, high blood pressure and skin diseases.

The conference organiser told the *Guardian* that Ford's problems were no worse than those in similar organisations.

The stress of car production line working was recognised in an unusual American court case.

○ A man with mental problems collapsed after 10 days on the line and was admitted to hospital suffering from paranoid schizophrenia. The employer was held responsible for his illness.

Office automation:

A French report on the automation of a large number of office jobs came to the conclusion that routine and uninteresting work

> . . . became more frequent as the machines took over more and more of the mental operations of the clerks, leaving them the purely routine jobs or auxiliary operations such as classifying and preparing the data for the machines to work on.

Machine pacing then becomes just as inevitable in offices as it is on the shop floor:

> When technical staff work in a highly synchronised computerised environment, the employer will seek to ensure that each element of their work is ready to feed in to the process at the precise time at which it is required. A mathematician will find that he has to have his work ready in the same way as a Ford worker has to have the wheel ready for the car as it passes on the production line.
> M.J.E.Cooley, **Computer Aided Design, its Nature and Implications,** published by AUEW (Technical and Supervisory Section).

○ A survey of office workers in mechanised jobs found that 40 per cent reported symptoms of nervous tensions, depression, digestive and heart troubles, insomnia, nervousness and irritability.

Speed-up:

There is nothing very new in the idea of speed-up. Employers have been pushing it since before the Industrial Revolution by the simple method of lowering rates on piecework.

Speed-up takes on a new quality with automated production lines where the employer can actually increase your pace of work by moving a lever.

In the long term, line speeds increase with automation.

Some workers are safe from the assembly line, but not from speed up. Studies of London bus drivers and conductors in 1958 and 1959 found they had much more than the expected amount of sickness for all age groups, particularly diseases of the stomach and duodenum (the part of the small intestine immediately below your stomach), and nervous disorders. Irregular meals and the stress of dealing with London traffic and passengers are thought to be the causes.

In spite of this health warning, one-man buses are being introduced into town services all over the country. The driver is on his own with the bus, the traffic and the passengers *and* he's got another job to do – collecting fares.

A conductress said that several of the older drivers operating one-man buses from her depot in South East London had been laid off with heart attacks.

This may not be the kind of evidence that satisfies medical researchers but it is exactly what you would expect in this situation. An American study of patients with coronary heart disease found that 91 per cent gave a history of severe occupational strain. This factor appeared to outweigh other causes like smoking, lack of exercise and obesity.

Most car plants operate at speeds of between 50 and 80 cars an hour – about one a minute. The new General Motors plant at Lordstown, Ohio, has the fastest line in the world: a car comes at you every 35 to 40 seconds.

Much of the speed-up is taken by faster machines, but this removes even more interest from the job and leaves the operators with the mental and physical strain of doing the same task every 35 seconds for the whole day.

Warning:
Wilbur Haddock, a production worker in a US Ford plant described speed-up:

o *At the beginning of the year on one operation there might be four workers doing the same operation. By the middle of that year, it's cut down to two men, and there's no way in the world that two men can do that job. So instead of putting in six screws, a man might put in two, or he might put in six but turn them just enough to get them in there and let it go down the line . . .*

o *And the worker, he does just enough to keep up with the line and keep the man off his back. He can't worry about who's going to buy the car, because he's got to make money. So the poor slob who buys it, he can go out there and the steering wheel can fall off – and people wonder how can the steering wheel fall off or how can the brakes be bad when this car is a brand new car?*

o *Most of the things we have to deal with are just ridiculous, like even going to the bathroom. You're a grown man. You might have diarrhoea or something. They want you to stand there and work until you can get the foreman or the supervisor to find somebody to relieve you while you go to the bathroom. Now if you walk off the line and go to the bathroom, then you can be disciplined, you can be sent home, you can lose pay, because you had to go to the bathroom.* Quoted in *Safety Kit* published by the Industrial Safety Group of Urban Planning Aid, Massachusetts.

Shiftwork:

In terms of damage to physical, mental and social wellbeing shift work is probably the worst of all work patterns, especially when MDW and other intensification methods are part of the routine.

Recently we've heard a lot about what is fashionably called 'jet lag', the disturbance to physical and mental performance caused by flying across time-zones.

In experimental simulations of the London to Japan time shift, subjects lost seven per cent of their muscular strength and five per cent in central nervous system efficiency.

o After a London to San Francisco experiment 14 human guinea pigs took four to five days to recover full mental performance. After the flight out it took four days for sleep patterns to settle down and after the flight back, six days.

Jet-lag is just a short taste of what it's like to be on night shift, but without the dreary surroundings of a factory at night and in circumstances when mistakes can cost only money – not life or limb. Shift-lag is an altogether more serious condition. It affects you every day, every week, every year for the rest of your working life – if you can stick it.

Although it involves millions of people instead of a few thousands, shift-lag has not attracted the same publicity as the fashionable executive's complaint. Research findings have mostly remained embalmed in the pages of management papers and learned journals (under the headings of 'efficiency' and 'productivity' rather than 'health' and 'wellbeing'). They show the same short term effects of disturbing your body's natural rhythms, *plus* actual physical disorders, *plus* disruption of social and family life.

o In a survey carried out by Hilda Brown, 75 per cent of the men interviewed said they felt physically below par. They blamed this mainly on the fact that they found it difficult to sleep during the day and lost their appetites.

Your body clock is the key to most of the harmful effects of shift work. It is set to a certain programme when you are a child and you cannot reset it completely unless you change to a different living/sleeping routine *and stick to it.* On shiftwork the only way to achieve this would be to work nights right through the week and the weekend. Because no employer has achieved this highly beneficial system, all shift routines fool around with your *body's* routines.

You probably feel tired and lethargic, perhaps with dangerously slow reactions by the time you are a few hours into the night shift. (A Vauxhall survey found the highest accident rates were after midnight). By day, on the other hand, your body clock has got everything set for action when you need to sleep.

Not surprisingly researchers have found that you don't get as much sleep as you need and it's not as deep as it should be. An American study of rotating shift workers found they got an average of only five and a half hours sleep when they were working the night segment.

Permanent tiredness, irritability and constipation are among the 'minor' effects reported in these surveys. Shift systems that have you changing from day to night work and back on a regular basis are more disruptive than continuous nights. The constantly changing 'continental' system is most disruptive of all – your body cannot begin to settle into a new routine. **See table opposite.**

o In a five year study of workers in the Norwegian electro-chemical industry Dr A.Aanonsen was able to include people who had given up shift working. He found that shift workers were much more likely to suffer from nervous disorders and ulcers than day workers, as shown in the table below.

Some medical investigators have come to the conclusion that shift work does not cause any serious damage to health. This is probably because those who can't take it are at present able to get back onto days; there is certainly a high rate of labour turnover on shifts. Those who remain are mostly people who can make some kind of physical and social adjustment to the routine and those who actually like the arrangement. **See facing table.**

40 hour week rota: 21 shifts

Working cycle

M=mornings 6–2; A=afternoons 2–10; N=nights 10–6

Week no.	S	M	T	W	Th	F	S	Shifts worked
1	A	—	—	M	M	M	M	5
2	M	—	N	N	N	N	—	5
3	—	A	A	A	A	A	—	5
4	—	M	M	M	M	—	N	5
5	N	N	N	N	—	—	A	5
6	A	A	A	—	—	M	M	5
7	M	M	—	—	N	N	N	5
8	N	—	—	A	A	A	A	5
9	A	—	M	M	M	M	—	5
10	—	N	N	N	N	—	—	5
11	—	A	A	A	A	—	M	5
12	M	M	M	M	—	—	N	5
13	N	N	N	—	—	A	A	5
14	A	A	—	—	M	M	M	5
15	M	—	—	N	N	N	N	5
16	N	—	A	A	A	A	—	5
17	—	M	M	M	M	M	—	5
18	—	N	N	N	N	—	A	5
19	A	A	A	A	—	—	M	5
20	M	M	M	—	—	N	N	5
21	N	N	—	—	A	A	A	5

Based on private and confidential document produced by the Iron and Steel Employers' Federation, ref S/26, 854

Day work and shift work sufferers, per cent:

	345 continuous day workers	731 continuous and former shift workers	Increase for shift workers
Nervous disorders	13	19	40
Peptic symptoms (but no peptic ulcers)	7	12	81
Peptic ulcers	7	10	36

A German survey found that the ulcer rate among rotating shift workers was eight times as high as for the fixed shift group.

It seems that about one third of workers in any group can adjust their eating and sleeping habits within a few days of any shift change. At the other extreme a large proportion – 38 per cent in one survey – just cannot get used to it. In between, the adjustment period varies widely, but for many it is too long to be able to get used to a rapidly changing routine.

The implications for workers' health are important. If shiftwork is allowed to spread, more and more people who cannot adjust will be unable to find alternative jobs. They will be forced to work shifts and their health will suffer.

Social disruption:

Shift work can put a heavy strain on your family and social life.

One of the basic contradictions of the shift system is that the regime which causes least physical disturbance – continuous night work – is the most socially disruptive. You have to go off to work just at the time when life for most people is just beginning, when families and communities are getting together after the divisions of the day, when the stresses of work, school and home are relaxed.

Rotating shifts give you a chance to enjoy this period on a regular basis – though the shift pattern may roll right across weekends and give you days off at other times instead. Family and friends may find it hard to keep up with your routine and it becomes difficult to arrange meetings – particularly union meetings.

Loss of contact between workers can undermine solidarity and union organisation in a situation when they need to be at their strongest – particularly in the struggle for health and safety.

Action:

After years of happy prod-dealing, union leaders are at last waking up to the cost that is being paid by the members they have sold into the shift system.

In April 1973 a TUC guide to union negotiators at last urged them to consider the social and health disadvantages of shift working.

The warning came a bit late for the delivery drivers at the ABC bakery, Camden, North London. In January, 80 drivers were locked out after protesting against long weekend shifts which made a normal sex life almost impossible. They refused to take out deliveries later than 8.30 on Saturday mornings.

o *'You just can't get in the mood when you get home from a 14-hour night shift on Saturday. You're just whacked for the whole weekend,' Mr Barry Jefferies, one of the drivers, told the* Guardian.

o *'My family look at me as if I'm the lodger or the wife's fancy man. A fat lot of good I'd be to her if I was.'*

Such protests will become more common as workers realise that the promise of a higher standard of living is meaningless when the *quality* of life is lowered.

Once shiftwork is firmly established it will be difficult to scrap but much can be done to reduce its harmful effects. Companies are now laying down strict rules to protect their precious executives from the effects of jet-lag. One authority recommends them to take 24 hours off to recover from a five-hour time change and 48 hours for a change of 10 hours or more.

Demands:

If you demanded equal protection from shift-lag most shift systems would rapidly collapse – every time you went back on nights you'd have to come off for a rest period.

More realistically, you could demand shorter hours, extra days off, and longer holidays. From the health point of view the four-day week for shift workers is an entirely reasonable demand: it would do a lot to reduce fatigue and stress. (Many systems make you work only four night shifts a week, at the expense of bumping each shift up to 10 hours, which is not the same thing at all.)

Safety, health and welfare facilities should be up to the same standard on all shifts, which means that safety officers, first aid rooms, emergency arrangements and canteens should all operate fully at night.

Stewards from different shifts should have a right to meet regularly in the firm's time rather than struggling to get a meeting together in their own time.

If management want to meet stewards from the night shift they should come in at night instead of expecting stewards to come in during sleeping or leisure hours.

Stress-producing incentives or production targets backed by discipline should be replaced by a high flat-rate for nights – a fair night's pay for a fair night's work, and no messing.

The struggle for improvement in existing shiftwork conditions will be a long one. Nothing can make them both an acceptable way of working for workers and profitable to employers. Any extension of shiftwork to new areas should be resisted unless the purpose is to meet some real human need that cannot be satisfied any other way. Even then, the best possible health protection must be built into the system.

Overtime:

o Cuts into family and social time.
o Increases exposure time to chemicals, noise, stress and other hazards.
o Reduces the body's 'recovery time', lowering your resistance to occupational diseases, particularly dermatitis.
o Increases your chances of an accident.
o Can cause chronic fatigue if you regularly work long hours (you begin to feel tired not just at the end of the day but all the time; life becomes a

**routine centred on work, you become more
vulnerable to accidents and less concerned to do
anything about the risks of the job – or about
anything else except getting through the day).**
o **Contributes to unemployment and low wages**

Job enrichment:

Many employers are finding that their intensive methods do not always pay off as well as expected.

Labour turnover, absenteeism, reject rates and supervision costs rise as the pace of work hots up and jobs get even more boring. They are now looking around for ways to put interest back and stop people jacking it in. Job enrichment and job enlargement are two terms for this process. It can certainly make things better but it needs to be approached with caution. It is not done for your good but for the good of the company. Its limits are those of profitability.

> o 'If we had the answer which would make the job greater for everybody we would do it . . . but we can't eliminate the production line because we can't build to the right price without it.'
> Frank Schotters, director of personnel development for General Motors.

Smaller firms are trying to get away from the production line into a method of assembly which goes under the fancy name of 'group technology'. In Sweden in the 1960s the Volvo car company found it increasingly difficult to get Swedes to work on a production line. Labour turnover was as high as 50 per cent a year and absenteeism went up to 15 per cent. Their answer is a new plant where people work in teams of 15 or 20 to assemble a whole car.

The workers decide who is to lead the group and how the work is to be shared. They must work to an average overall rate but they can vary the pace so as to create their own breaks.

This method of working is likely to cause less physical and mental stress than the deadening routine of the production line. The individual and the group regain some control over their work, and get more satisfaction from actually *making* something. The group can break down the isolation of workers, so reducing the build-up of stress and developing a social unit more able to challenge management control.

Volvo and Saab, which is trying the same thing in an engine plant, have not achieved any more productivity by this method and apparently did not expect it. The system does not of course give you any protection from speed-up.

It would be foolish to think that job enrichment can resolve all the contradictions between what is good for people and what is good for profits. Upstream of the assembly workers, someone has still got to work the power presses and the automatic machine tools, jobs that are almost impossible to enrich. They can be fully automated but in the present set-up that means redundancies.

Group technology requires a heavier investment in floor space and equipment and the big car manufacturers, with their huge stake in automated assembly lines, are approaching it with caution.

o General Motors, whose plant at Lordstown alone has twice the capacity of the whole Volvo company, is said to be experimenting with the idea at a secret plant somewhere in the US but has made no commitment to attack the assembly line. Fiat is the only mass car producer to go that far: new plants in Italy will try out group assembly of engines and a 'half-way' solution involving four assembly lines in place of one. Instead of a minute to do one small operation you would have four minutes to do something more constructive – perhaps putting in a whole brake system. Industrial psychologists apparently do not agree on whether this limited job enlargement will:

a. make you less tired, because the bigger job is more satisfying.

b. make you more tired, because you have to concentrate harder and can't let your mind wander.

Some kinds of manufacturing do not lend themselves to the group method. The idea of workers all crowding round to 'assemble' biscuits is obviously ridiculous. o For

United Biscuits at Isleworth the answer to high labour turn-over was not to change the structure of the job but to dress it up so that it seems richer. Disc jockeys play record requests interspersed with hygiene and safety jingles, you get time off to visit the firm's hairdresser and there's a company shop. Things are a bit better, accidents have been reduced and people seem to like it.

This kind of job enrichment is not done for workers and it should not be mistaken for benevolence. When UB introduced a day nursery at Isleworth to attract married women workers, none of the existing staff was allowed to bring their children.

Anything that makes work more interesting or pleasant is a good idea but it is important to test management motives carefully before such schemes get under way. If the aim is just to cut labour turnover and absenteeism and not to bring in productivity under the cloak of enrichment then management will not object to signing a no-redundancy agreement beforehand.

o When a group technology scheme was introduced at Serck Valves, 150 jobs were scrapped straight away. An agreement on equal sharing of any productivity benefits would be an additional precaution.

You can call management's bluff by demanding things that really enrich the job – nurseries for all, equal pay, paid maternity leave, full medical services.

Flextime:

Flextime is a system of flexible working hours which can make life a bit easier for you. It is often presented as a big 'concession' to workers but in fact management stands to gain a great deal from it.

Under flextime you have to work a core time – typically from 9.30 am to 3.30 pm or 10 to 4 – and outside this period you clock on and clock off at times which suit your domestic and travel arrangements. To ensure that they are not short-handed at any period management may want individual start and finish times to be pre-arranged – to their advantage, they hope. Hours are not shortened: they are averaged out over a four-week period and you can carry forward a debit or credit of up to 10 hours.

Clive Jenkins, general secretary of the Association of Scientific, Technical and Managerial Staffs, has described this as 'liberation' for the office worker. Undoubtedly it has many attractions but TASS, the technical and supervisory section of the AUEW, sounded a warning in December 1972.

Describing flextime as 'the thin end of a wedge which might broaden out in time to an attack on fundamental conditions,' the union advised its members 'not to readily involve themselves in this system, if at all.'

TASS believes that flexible hours are just another way to squeeze more work out of you without paying for it. Productivity can go up by five or 10 per cent and by stretching the day at each end *'the unscrupulous employer could use flextime to slide members towards full shift working . . . there is little doubt that such attempts are part of the present effort to introduce intensification of labour at work.'*

That's certainly how it looked to *Business Administration* magazine which described it as 'a valuable productivity and efficiency booster' giving employers 'much more extensive and profitable use of plant and machinery.'

Workers are prepared, according to a management consultant's handbook on the system, 'to work longer hours when the demand is there. In this way the company saves on overtime payments and employees get more satisfaction from their work.'

o Lufthansa, the German airline has cut its overtime bill by 80 per cent with flextime.

o Messerschmidt got more productivity and halved the number of days lost through illness and personal reasons.

What this means is that you have to make up all time lost through uncertified illness or family problems where previously these reasons might have justified absence with or without pay.

Ultimately the real argument against flextime is that personal deals between boss and worker weaken the collective struggle for real improvements in the structure of work, notably the four-day week. Whether flextime turns out to be a liberator or the thin end of another wedge depends on the strength of organisation in the workplace and the vigour with which conditions for real health and well-being are pursued.

If you decide the attractions of flextime are worth the risk of work intensification, the minimum safeguard is an agreement on redundancies and equal sharing of productivity gains.

Conclusion:

More intensive patterns of work provide one of the most important and difficult challenges in the struggle for health.

Their roots go even deeper into the profit system than the causes of industrial injuries or occupational disease. Nobody tells you that *they* are good for the country, yet politicians, businessmen and even trade unionists join hands to sing the praises of productivity without counting (perhaps without recognising) the human cost.

Millions of individual workers know the price they are paying for more intensive work but it is difficult to challenge a situation which is endorsed by union leaders. Improvements will not come by waiting for these leaders to recognise work intensification as an occupational hazard or for employers to bring in job enrichment. They will come when workers organise to challenge all the conditions that undermine their health and safety.

3.

Physical Hazards

This part of the book deals with hazards caused by different kinds of physical energy – noise, vibration, radiation, abnormal temperatures and pressures.

All can damage your body directly in different ways but they also add to physical and mental stress, making you tired and more likely to have accidents or develop physical disorders apparently unrelated to the hazard itself.

Stress effects are additive. If you are exposed to too much heat you may be less able to deal with noise or vibration and so on.

The important thing is to judge your working conditions in terms of comfort as well as hazard: if you're not comfortable it's probably not doing you any good. Any improvement in physical conditions will help: if you can't make any progress on, say, noise reduction, have a go at the lighting or ventilation. It won't help your hearing but it'll help to make people less tired and less prone to accidents.

Ionising radiation may be the most frightening of all these hazards but noise is now the most widespread cause of concern. That is why it is dealt with first and in the greatest detail.

This section is about the hazards of:

Noise
Vibration
Radiation
Temperature
Pressure

Noise:

Most people are frightened by chemical risks, but not by noise, yet noise can kill the delicate cells in the depths of your ear so that you have the hearing ability of an old person before you even reach retirement.

It's not only loud bangs that damage hearing. Most hearing damage is caused by long exposure to noise that is loud but not so loud that you can't get used to it.

Such noise is very common in industry. A million workers are thought to be at risk in factories alone; and there are probably 150,000 who have lost so much hearing that they could claim compensation from their employers.

In the heavily industrialised North of England, amplifiers in cinemas are set at a higher level than they are in the South.

o In America a recent government report estimated that as many as 16 million workers may already have hearing loss. In Australia a survey of 5,000 workers in all trades found that one third of them had suffered hearing loss. A survey of 743 steelworkers in Italy showed all had hearing damage. In an Italian shipyard every riveter and caulker was affected. In France nearly half of the forge workers studied had had their hearing damaged by noise.

How does it happen?

You would think that people who work in forge shops, say – or at least their families – would realise that their hearing was going. But the loss is usually too gradual for you or anyone else to realise it's happening.

One day though someone says: 'Didn't you really hear what I said? I think you must be getting a bit deaf.' He or she might even say: 'That's right, your father was getting a bit hard of hearing at your age: perhaps it's in the family.' Perhaps the job was in the family as well.

Naturally, employers do not go out of their way to dispel such convenient illusions, in spite of the fact that the connection between noise and deafness has been known for a very long time and was officially recognised as an industrial problem in the Report of the Chief Inspector of Factories for 1908.

Noise has since spread with mechanisation to many more jobs, and workers are beginning the offensive against it. Union-backed legal actions against employers have shown that, even if there is still no written law against exposing workers to excessive noise, claims for compensation can be won.

o In December 1971 Frank Berry became the first worker to win damages for loss of hearing. He was awarded £1,250 against Stone Manganese Marine because of their failure to protect him from the noise of his job, dressing large bronze ship propellers with a pneumatic chipping hammer.

Mr Berry and the GMWU have prised open the doors of the civil courts. The publicity generated by this case and by the publication a few months later of the Department of Employment's *Code of Practice* on noise exposure mean that employers can no longer claim in their defence that they were unaware of noise risks. Mr Berry's damages were lower than they might have been if he had claimed earlier. Other victims of noise are expected to win very much more.

o *In June 1972 a professional engineer was awarded £27,000 for damage to his hearing against the Ministry of Aviation Supply who failed to protect him fully from the noise of an anti-tank missile.*

Even at only £2,000 per case, if all the 'noise-disabled' were to bring a successful action, industry would face a bill for £300 millions.

Compensation is important but the vital thing is to make it clear that your hearing is not for sale, whether the payments are weekly, as danger money, or in a lump sum as damages.

First find out if your job is a threat to your hearing.

Risky jobs and machines are listed in Table 3, on p 57. It is not a complete list.

If you know the noise level you work in you can use tables 1 and 2 on page 56 to check the risk you are running.

What is noise?

Noise is often thought of as unwanted sound. This is fine for environmental noise. The sound of someone's motor-bike may be music to him and noise to you, but it doesn't convey the idea that noise can be dangerous. Sound that is unwanted or damages health might be a better description.

Frequency:

Sound gets to your ear by a kind of shunting action in the particles of air between the source and you. The particles don't move from the source to you but they are alternately compressed and decompressed, rather like the individual trucks in a train that's just been shunted.

The number of times the air is compressed and decompressed in a given time, usually a second, is the frequency of the sound. The measurement is given in cycles per second (cps), or Hertz (Hz).

Frequency is what gives a sound its character. Low notes like the buzz of a fluorescent tube have a low frequency; high notes have a high frequency.

We can distinguish these different characteristics because our ear drums move with each cycle. They respond to frequencies as low as 15 cycles a second (the longest pipe in a church organ) and as high as 20,000 (the whistle from a TV set has a frequency of about 15,000 cycles per second).

Outside this range of frequencies, sound cannot be heard. Lower frequencies come into the range of *infrasound* and higher ones into the range of *ultrasound*. Both are dangerous. (*See* p 60.)

A tuning fork produces a tone of only one frequency – a pure tone– but most other sounds are made up of more than one frequency. The roar of a factory is composed of a very large number of tones completely covering a wide range of frequencies. Which tones are present and how powerful each one is gives each sound its own *spectrum*. The spectrum of a sound is important in determining how harmful it will be to hearing. (*See* p 69.)

Intensity:

This is the amount of energy that the 'shunted' air particles can deliver to your ear. Intensity falls off with distance (if you are leaning against a rail wagon when the loco hits the other end, you'll be sent flying; if you are leaning against the last of a hundred wagons when the loco hits the first one, with the same force, most of the energy will have been spent by the time it reaches you.

It may be hard to think of sound in terms of energy but very loud noise can burn your skin and the world's armies are busy developing noise weapons that can kill you.

The range of intensities between the smallest sound you can hear and the loudest you are likely to meet is so great that most ordinary scales of measurement would show the smallest sound at zero and the noise that deafened Mr Berry at one billion. To avoid the inconvenience of writing such large numbers they are shrunk to manageable size by a kind of mathematical shorthand – the **decibel** (dB).

The decibel scale tells you how many times bigger the intensity of a particular sound is than the intensity of the reference sound at the bottom of the scale.

The scale is based on powers of ten (it is logarithmic) so that when you see the figure 10dB you know it is ten times as intense as the reference sound ; 20dB is a hundred times as intense as the reference sound; 30dB is a thousand times, and so on.

If you go on doing this you will eventually get to 120dB – the sound in the dressing shop where Frank Berry collected his hearing loss – a billion times as intense as the smallest audible sound.

o Thomas Down had the hearing in his right ear completely destroyed by two weeks work with a cartridge stud driver on a building site. The sound in each bang reached a peak level of 160dB. That's 40dB more than the dressing shop, or four tenfold increases in intensity ($10 \times 10 \times 10 \times 10$) or 10,000 times as intense.

As long as you remember that 10 more dB always means a tenfold increase in sound intensity you won't be

taken in by the managers who talk about 'a few more decibels' as if they are counting out apples. In fact each increase
of 3dB on the scale represents a doubling of sound intensity
– so 93 decibels is not 'just over 90'. It is twice as much
sound energy going into your ears.

It is difficult to measure the intensity of a sound
directly but very easy to measure the pressure fluctuations it
generates – the sound pressure level – and get a reading in
decibels. This is what the sound level meter does.

Most meters now give a reading in dBA, which means
simply that a bias has been built in which makes it respond
more like the human ear. Like your ear, it is less sensitive
to sounds in the higher and lower frequencies than in the
middle range.

A dBA reading therefore gives a good idea of how loud a
noise will seem and also how much damage it may do.
See table on next page.

What is hearing damage?

Pressure fluctuations in the air set the ear drum in
motion. A linkage of tiny bones transmit this movement to
a window in the end of the *cochlea*, a snail-shaped organ
filled with liquid. When this window moves the motion is
carried through the liquid and is picked up by tiny *hair cells*.
These convert it into electrical impulses which travel to the
brain and are interpreted as sounds.

These hair cells can take just so much energy – and
they should last you the best part of a lifetime at the noise
loads for which they were intended. But too much noise
wears them out before their time. **The damage cannot be repaired** and a hearing aid is unlikely to make up for the loss.
It may make it more difficult to hear clearly.

**Any loss caused by noise will be added on to whatever
you are going to suffer anyway as you get older. Even a
small loss now will make you hard of hearing much sooner.**

Hearing damage makes your ears less sensitive; sounds
have to be louder before you can hear them, which means
that you miss some sounds. What matters is which ones you
miss. Things don't just get 'softer'; they are **distorted.**

Decibels and sounds

Sound pressure level dB	Some sounds and their relative intensity
0	Most sensitive hearing threshold; reference sound for dB scale
10	Leaves rustling
20	Quiet country lane
30	Tick of watch, rustle of paper; hearing threshold for disabled; one thousand times intensity of reference sound
40	Quiet office, quiet conversation
50	Quiet street; inside average home
60	Normal conversation at 3ft; one million times intensity of reference sound
70	Busy street; large shop
80	Hearing damage begins here
90	Official safe level; most factories; one thousand million times the intensity of reference sound
100	Food blender at 2ft; circular saw; construction plant
110	Earthmoving motor scraper, woodworking shop
120	The noise that deafened Mr Berry One billion times intensity of reference sound
130	Threshold of pain; jet engine at 100ft; riveting steel plates; pneumatic press at 5ft; Absolute limit without ear muffs
140	Jet with afterburner at 50ft
150	Sound at speech frequencies can burn the skin; unsafe without acoustic helmet
160	The cartridge stud gun that deafened Mr Down
180	The anti-tank rocket that deafened Mr Darby
200	Noise weapon

The parts of your ear that pick up high frequencies are damaged first. When your hearing is tested the threshold of hearing (the quietest sound you can hear) at different frequencies is marked on a chart (an audiogram). The first and clearest indication that your hearing is being damaged by noise is a 'notch' in the audiogram at 4,000Hz.

Speech has a large high frequency content. In general, consonants have higher frequencies and are quieter than vowels. As hearing damage gets worse you stop being able to hear consonants. At first you can't hear plurals, then you can't distinguish 'fifteen' from 'sixteen' and finally you can't understand what is being said, even though you can hear that talk is going on. Sentences are stripped of meaning, as in the following example:

'Kiss me sweetheart' becomes (k)i(ss) me (s)wee(the)-ar(t). You might be able to guess that one, but normally the effect is to cut you off from other people.

o This isolation has been described well by Dr J.Sataloff in his book, *Hearing Loss*.

> o A hearing impairment may cause no handicap to a chipper or a riveter while he is at work. His deafness may even seem to be to his advantage, since the noise of his work is not as loud to him as it is to his fellow workers with normal hearing. Because there is little or no verbal communication in most jobs that produce intense noise, a hearing loss will not be made apparent by inability to understand complicated verbal directions. However, when such a workman returns to his family at night or goes on his vacation, the situation assumes a completely different perspective. He has trouble understanding what his wife is saying, especially if he is reading the paper, and his wife is talking while she is making noise in the kitchen. This kind of situation frequently leads at first to a mild dispute and later to serious family tension.
>
> The wife accuses the husband of inattention, which he denies, while he complains in rebuttal that she mumbles. Actually, he eventually does become inattentive when he realizes how frustrating and fatiguing it is to strain to hear. When the same individual tries to attend meetings, to visit with friends, or to go to church services and finds he cannot hear what is going on or is laughed at for giving an answer unrelated to the subject under discussion, he soon, but very reluctantly, realizes that something really is wrong with him. He stops going to places where he feels pilloried by his handicap. He stops

going to the movies, the theatre or concerts, for the voices and the music are not only far away, but frequently distorted. Little by little his whole family life may be undermined, and a cloud overhangs his future and that of his dependents.

In addition, loss of all the little sounds that remind you of the world around you can lead to a feeling that the world seems dead. This is very depressing – and it can lead to serious psychological difficulties. You can't tell in advance whether it will have that effect on you.

○ **Sounds you would no longer hear:**
Leaves rustling ○ *Pens on paper* ○ *Water boiling* ○ *Gas escaping* ○ *Clocks ticking* ○ *Bacon frying* ○ *Rain* ○ *Cars approaching* ○ *Nylons and tights, etc* ○ *Coal fires burning* ○ *Waves* ○ *Birds in distance* ○ *Whispering* ○ *Wind in the trees* ○ *Birds flying overhead* ○ *Matches* ○ *Cutting bread* ○ *Sugar pouring* ○ *Fizzy drinks* ○ *Paper rustling* ○ *Pages turning.*

Not only do you miss the sounds you want to hear, you get a lot you don't want. First you will have *ringing* in the ears. In some cases it is always there and can be more disabling than the loss of hearing. Secondly you may suffer from *loudness recruitment* which means that things grow louder very suddenly. The person with noise-damaged hearing will say: 'Louder, I can't hear you,' and, when the speaker does talk louder, 'Not so loud – don't shout.'

Hearing aids may have the same effect and in addition they amplify all the other signals reaching your ear so that background noise comes crashing in on top of the conversation you are trying to follow.

Risk:

All this could happen to you as a result of exposure to noise at your job – the process may have started already – and you cannot tell in advance how bad it will be. In any group of people exposed to the same level of noise, there will be an average amount of hearing damage after a given time. A minority will be affected earlier and more seriously (just as another minority at the other extreme will be affected less).

Since you can't tell which group you will be in and scientific tests can't predict individual damage from a particular noise level, you have to look at the risk in terms of the odds. If one in 50 workers in a factory will collect a hearing disability are the odds acceptable? Such decisions can only be made by the people at risk, but 'acceptable' levels of noise and deafness are settled by experts and committees without reference to workers.

Deafness:

There is no simple unit of deafness. The experts have to decide how much hearing loss constitutes a disability and this tends to be a political and economic decision.

The commonest method, developed by the American Academy of Opthalmology and Otolaryngology (AAOO) involves measuring your threshold of hearing for pure tones in the 'speech frequencies' of 500, 1,000 and 2,000 Hz, and comparing them with normal hearing levels. When the average increase in these three frequencies exceeds 25dB the AAOO says you have a disability. For every dB over 25 you are considered to have lost $1\frac{1}{2}$ per cent of your hearing.

Under the AAOO method 'the ability to hear sentences and repeat them correctly in a quiet environment is taken as satisfactory evidence of correct hearing for everyday speech. The American expert Karl Kryter has described this as 'a highly questionable definition of everyday speech and everyday conditions'. He went on:

o 'Everyday speech includes single words or phrase messages (which are generally less easily correctly understood than sentences), distortion due to such things as the talker having a cold, poor pronunciation, speaking from a distance, using a telephone, etc. and often, some ambient noise or competing music or speech from other persons. All of these conditions much more severely degrade the understanding of speech in the partially deafened person than in the person with normal hearing. *In short AAOO defined a type of speech material and listening condition that would be least likely to show any impairment in the deafened person.*' (our italics.)

It is easy to forget that this 'expert' bickering is about *your* hearing, and, possibly, *your* deafness, *your* compensation. The condition of your inner ear remains the same whether its performance is assessed by the AAOO method or by Kryter's. But the diagnosis, and therefore the amount of compensation you might be able to get, will be different.

Why should the AAOO use a definition that seems biased against the victim? One American ear specialist has suggested that the US insurance companies used their influence because they did not want to have to pay the enormous amount of compensation that would be demanded if all workers who had already suffered hearing damage brought a claim.

Both methods are given later in the tables that enable you to work out the risk in your job; we suggest you use the Kryter method.

'Safe' levels:

Deafness is a matter of opinion. The same is true of the levels of noise that cause it. You don't have to be a scientist to decide how risky a life you want to have – providing the risks are fully explained and you have a chance to decide. At present they aren't and you don't.

'Safe levels' for noise in industry are a compromise between what's good for you and what's good for business.

> o At the end of the Johnson administration in the US the Labour Department recommended the noise standard should be reduced from 90-85dBA. Nixon got in and gave in to business pressure for keeping the standard at 90.
> o 'We are suggesting to the government that it makes 80-dBA the maximum for industrial exposure. The employers are asking for 95 and hoping to get away with 90.'
> Mr John Connell, Chairman of Noise Abatement Society, September 1972.
> o In Holland the recommended limit is 80dBA.

There is no legal limit for industrial noise in Britain. Employers are supposed to follow the Department of Employment Code of Practice which recommends 90dBA as the maximum level for eight-hour a day exposure without ear protection. 90dBA is the equivalent of working all day within 20 yards of a pneumatic drill going full blast.

Research work sponsored by the Government itself demonstrates that this is by no means a safe level.

The research, by Dr Burns and Dr Robinson, makes it possible for the first time to predict the average amount of damage that will be done by different noise exposures and what the odds are that the damage will be worse.

There are only three pieces of information you need to feed into the Burns and Robinson procedure to find out what extent of hearing damage you are risking:

1. The noise level in dBA
2. The period of exposure
3. The odds you want to take that you will acquire more than the average hearing damage

The method is based on the amount of sound energy that goes into your ears. Remembering that each step of 10dB represents a *tenfold* increase in sound energy, it is easy to see why working in say 105dBA for 10 years will do the same amount of damage as 115dBA for one year or 125dBA for one tenth of a year – or about a month.

To make the calculation just as easy for all combinations of dBA and exposure time a series of factors has been developed. These are given in Table 1 on the next page. To work out the 'dose' you are getting at your work just add (or subtract) the appropriate factor to (or from) the dBA sound level for your workplace.

The next stage is to decide what odds you want to take that your hearing loss will be more serious than average. (The average loss in any exposed group does not help you to work out your own risk: you might be the one in the group who is going to get really bad hearing damage).

Table 2 enables you to do this. It is worked out by two different methods, the notorious AAOO scheme and the fairer one proposed by Kryter. The odds assumed in constructing the top half of the table are one in 10; in other words one in 10 people will lose a greater percentage of their hearing for speech than the amount shown. The bottom half of the table assumes odds of one in 50.

Table 1

Calculating the immission or 'dose'

Time	Approximate amount to be added to the A-scale noise level to obtain figure for your 'dose'
1 week	−17
1 month	−10
3 months	−6
6 months	−3
1 year	−0
2 years	+3
5 years	+7
10 years	+10
20 years	+13
40 years	+16
50 years	+17

Table 2

Loss of hearing for speech for different noise doses

Odds: one in ten that you will lose more

Dose (dBA level plus factor from Table 1)	Approx. % loss by AAOO method (sentences in quiet)	Approx. % loss by Kryter method (weak conversational speech)
100	0	16
105	0	28
110	0	44
115	0	60
120	21	74

Odds: one in fifty that you will lose more

100	0	32
105	3	48
110	21	64
115	26	80
120	38	92

We can use the tables to check up on the protection given by the *Code of Practice*. The 'dose' for 90dBA and a working lifetime of 40 years is 106 (90 plus 16 which is the factor for 40 years in Table 1). Using Table 2 you can see that one in 10 workers will lose at least 30 per cent of their hearing for speech as assessed by the Kryter method. One in 50 will lose at least 50 per cent. For one worker in four (not shown) the loss is at least 12 per cent.

A code that allows 10 per cent of workers to lose a third of their hearing is not giving much protection. It is easy to see why the Dutch authorities have recommended a limit of 80dBA – *one tenth* as harmful as the British code.

It will be a long time before 80dBA is officially accepted as a maximum noise level, and backed by law, and actually enforced. In fact all three are unlikely to be achieved. Workers must decide what level is acceptable to them and fight for it. Mr Connell of the Noise Abatement Society says that the engineering union in Australia is doing just that: 'If the union has complaints from workers of noise above 80dBA they go to management and say: "put it right or we'll be out".'

Levels above 90dBA carry quite unacceptable risks. At a dose of 120 (eg 110dBA for 10 years) the odds are one in 10 that you will lose at least 75 per cent of your hearing and one in 50 that you will lose at least 94 per cent.

It is important to realise that even brief exposure to very high noise levels can really ruin your hearing. The same dose (120) could be collected from an exposure of only three minutes a day to 126dBA during a working life.

Table 3

Jobs where the noise level may be dangerous to your hearing:

Food – sugar refining: packaging of sugar and syrup filling
Iron and steel: dressing and fettling castings, grinding and tagging. Rolling mills
Boiler making: boiler erection, caulking, chipping, riveting
Ball and roller bearings: machine operations

Bolts, nuts, screws and rivets: auto heading and screw turning machines and allied processes

Cans and metal boxes: press machines, can lines, body making and wrapping

Sparking plugs: auto machines, tamping and assembly

Bottle fasteners: pressing, assembly of crown corks

Motor industry: foundry, moulding, core dressing, fettling, presswork

Textiles: spinning, weaving and other processes

Stationery and printing: continuous stationery, letterpress and gravure printing

Chemicals: especially compressor plant

Shipbuilding: see boiler making, above

Timber and joinery: circular saws, bandsaws, moulding machines

Forestry: chainsaws

Mining: face work

Tunnelling: drilling, blasting, pneumatic tools, tunnelling machines

Construction: all classes of plant: breakers, vibrators, dumpers, diggers, cranes, heavy earthmoving.

Quarrying: drilling, blasting, mobile plant

Agriculture: tractors, combines

Transport: heavy trucks, work near aircraft, ships' engine rooms

---

Obviously there is an urgent need to find out what the noise levels are in your workplace. If they are very high you may already have lost a lot of hearing and what's left may be seriously threatened.

Finding out:

There are some checks you can do to see if your job is jeopardising your hearing, but they are by no means foolproof:

1. Is your industry or machine mentioned in Table 3, above?

2. Does anyone get ringing in their ears after a day's work? The best test is to ask young workers after their first

day. (If anyone gets a tickling sensation in the ears, or actual pain, the noise level is dangerously high.)

3. Do you have to talk very loudly or shout at someone only a few feet away?

4. Does the bus, car, television, husband, wife, sound quieter after the shift than before?

5. Do quite a few of the older, long-serving workers seem hard of hearing?

If the answer to any of these is positive, further investigation is needed. If the answers are all negative don't take it as an 'all clear' unless there are no sources of noise other than people.

In most industrial workplaces there is likely to be some area or machine that turns out dangerous noise. The safest thing to do is to press management for a proper survey of the whole place by someone qualified in noise measurement techniques.

If the management dismisses your fears, you may be able to prove the point by taking your own readings. The Noise Abatement Society, see organisations, p 326, sells its own 'Noise Torch', a simple sound level meter which lights up when a preset sound level is exceeded. The most suitable one can be set at 80, 85 or 90dBA; it costs around £10 which should not be beyond the reach of a shop floor whip-round. (In the long term, this is the kind of equipment shop stewards should have anyway to keep a constant check that sound levels don't creep up with new machines or speed-up. A typical noise increase is 2dB per 15 per cent increase in machine speed.)

Ultimately a professional noise survey must be carried out because simple equipment cannot evaluate the risk from the following:

Impact noise:

Power presses, pile drivers, cartridge guns, etc. More dangerous than continuous noise.

Pure tones:

A characteristic high-pitched whine from a machine may mean that some pure tone is dominant in the sound. This will be more dangerous than a flatter spectrum.

C

Low frequency sound:

Inaudible and audible low frequency sound *can* produce very unpleasant symptoms, like nausea, giddiness, headache, coughing, choking, reduced visual acuity and fatigue after exposures lasting only a few minutes. Exposure to intense low frequencies should be flatly rejected.

Ultrasound:

Inaudible high frequency sound. Sources like jet engines, dental drills and ultrasonic cleaning or welding equipment can give you headaches, dizziness and nausea. Young workers, particularly girls, will have these symptoms more often because their hearing is better.

Action:

If conditions are really bad and management refuses to order a noise survey, a call to the Factory Inspectorate might get things moving. (See Using the Inspectorate, page 248.)

o Workers at British Steel's Lackenby Works on Teesside had been arguing with management about noise in the Universal Beam Mill for more than 10 years when the draft of the Department of Employment Code was was circulated. The code recommends that managements should survey all areas where levels above 90dBA are suspected and this provided the opportunity to step up the campaign.
'The most difficult part of the exercise was pressuring management into measuring noise levels,' said Arthur Affleck, Chairman of the Shop Stewards Committee. After several months of pressure, levels were checked against the code and found to be well over the limit in the majority of locations.
'After that it was straightforward tactics – work to rule, overtime bans and eventually a 24-hour stoppage.'
'The management then accepted a rates revision for several hundred men and agreed to 45p per shift on bonus rates. This usually amounts to 60p per shift.'
The extra payment for 'environmental conditions' is only the first stage in the campaign; pressure is still being applied on the main demand, that noise be cut.
Whether the acceptance of danger money strengthens or weakens this pressure is a matter of opinion.

Noise control:

Engineering controls to quieten machines at source are the only acceptable answer to excessive noise. Managements may say this cannot be done but in the vast majority of cases it can. Often what they mean is that the cost will be too high. They are often wrong on this too; acoustical engineers will tell you that most managements have little idea of noise control and assume it will be expensive even when the solution is simple.

Whatever the cost, workers must make it clear that in the long run it is going to be even more expensive to ignore their health and comfort.

> o On another occasion the proprietor of a factory ordered that microphones be installed throughout the works, and be connected to amplifiers and loudspeakers on a patch of waste land outside so that the noise in the works could be sucked up by the microphones and blown out by the loudspeakers!
> Rupert Taylor, Noise, Pelican

Protection:

While noise is being reduced to acceptable levels your hearing must be protected from any further damage. One approach is to reduce your daily dose. For every three dB added to the sound level, your exposure time must be halved, as follows:

90dBA – 8 hours
93dBA – 4 hours
96dBA – 2 hours
etc.

You can do this calculation for all exposures throughout the day and arrive at what is called an 'equivalent continuous sound level', known as the Leq. Using the DE Code, four hours at 93 and four hours at 87dBA would give the same Leq as eight hours at 90. (This is an example, not a safe exposure.)

If the method were based on a safe level of 80dBA it might be acceptable as a way to protect your hearing.

It ignores the unpleasantness of working in higher noise levels.

Many jobs cannot be made safe by this method. A lot of construction machinery, for example, would be standing idle most of the day.

Ear protection:

Often there is no alternative, in the short term, but ear protection – cotton wool is virtually useless but mouldable *waxed* cotton wool and glass down are both effective. Many managements seem to think that all they have to do is pass round a box of ear plugs in the morning break and the job is done. In fact the type and make of ear protection can only be specified after a very thorough analysis of the sound intensity at different frequencies.

Once the class of protection has been decided workers should have a choice of types so that they can pick the most comfortable.

Ear muffs give most protection and many people find them the least uncomfortable and most convenient method. On the other hand many find they are too tight against the head. They may make your ears hot and sweaty or produce a skin rash.

Ear plugs should be a tight fit in the ear. They can also be uncomfortable, and can cause irritation and infection. If you have any history of ear trouble your ears should be checked by a doctor before you start wearing plugs. Disposable plugs that you mould from waxed cotton wool or glass down tend to lose efficiency because of jaw movements. They can be less hygienic than manufactured plugs if you don't wash your hands before moulding and inserting them

Ear protectors must be issued to each worker personally and checked for fit by someone who knows about ear protection. This is particularly important with ear plugs – the wrong size may be almost useless.

At the same time the risk must be explained to each worker so that he or she really knows that hearing damage will result from not using the protection and what hearing loss will be like. Borrow a pair of ear muffs and wear them for a time at home; they will probably give you a 'hearing loss' of about 30dB in the speech frequencies and a horrible feeling of being cut off from the world.

Real hearing loss is much worse because you get distortion as well. And you can't take it off when you've had enough.

No ear protection devices are comfortable or pleasant to wear and although they may sometimes improve communication in noise people often get a feeling of isolation and oppression.

They should be regarded only as a short-term measure to be used while your working environment is being made quieter.

Management should be made to set a firm programme for noise reduction, with firm dates for achieving levels acceptable to workers. Meanwhile all areas and machines producing more than 90dBA should be labelled with the yellow warning sign 'Use Ear Protectors', as recommended in the DE Code.

Hearing tests:

Any programme for protecting your hearing in dangerous noise levels should include regular hearing tests so that the smallest deterioration can be detected before it begins to erode the speech frequencies. You should be given a copy of your audiogram.

Until 'noise induced hearing loss' is made a prescribed disease the only way to get compensation is to sue your employer. So if you don't have your hearing checked regularly it may be difficult to beat the old employer's defence that your hearing was bad when you started working for him.

Audiograms can give misleading results and it is probably best if the tests are done by an independent specialist under proper conditions and at a time when your ears are as near normal as possible – eg after the weekend and before they have started to pick up the week's noise dose.

If you don't wear ear protection when it is provided your chances of a successful claim will be greatly reduced.

Other kinds of noise risk:

The risk of deafness is not the only reason why noise levels must be cut.

It stops you hearing warnings. When the Loddon motorway viaduct near Reading collapsed during construction on 24 October 1972, killing three men and seriously injuring seven, eye-witnesses who scrambled clear said that their warning shouts were drowned by the noise of concrete pumps and vibrators.

> o Many researchers have shown that you make more mistakes, and produce less, in noisy conditions.
> In one example, 110 electronics assembly workers made 60 mistakes per 24 hours with a noisy background and only seven in the same period when noise was reduced. If your work involves dangerous situations the mistakes could turn into accidents.

It produces irritability and stress which lead to disease, mental illness and more accidents:

o The French researcher J.Bourgoin examined several hundred men working pneumatic drills. He found noise and vibration caused nervous and digestive disorders. o An Italian researcher, A.Tarantola reported on medical examinations of 73 workers employed on fixed grinding machines; in the majority of cases there was marked deterioration of the digestive tract after one or two years. o In Russia researchers have shown that noise produces abnormally high levels of activity in the nerves controlling heart and other organs, causing a faster heartbeat and liability to ulcers. And high pitched sound around 85dB, which could be produced by a lathe, has been found to cause deterioration of muscular performance and disturbances of nervous functions. For example noise may cause dilation of the pupils of your eyes so that it's difficult to focus on detailed close work and you get eye strain. Dilation of the blood vessels in your brain may help to cause headaches.

Doctors are still arguing about the importance of – and even the existence of – these effects. More research must be done but workers do not have to wait for the result and for the setting, no doubt, of yet another *maximum* 'safe level'.

As with so many other unnecessary work hazards, if maximum levels were set for comfort, as defined by workers, there would be no hazard.

Vibration:

Like noise, vibration can cause anything from annoyance to physical damage, though scientists are less certain where to set exposure limits for different levels of vibration and the parts of your body they affect.

It will be a long time before they agree, and even longer before protection is written into the law. Meanwhile trade unionists are in the best position to lead the fight against the hazard by recognising that nearly all vibration exposure is unnecessary, a product of cheap or thoughtless design. Most of it can be eliminated or isolated if workers put a price on dangerous or uncomfortable equipment.

Vibration can harm you only if some part of your body is in direct contact with a vibrating surface, typically the seat of a vehicle or the handle of a power tool.

The level of risk depends on the characteristics of the vibration:

1. Frequency:

How often the surface moves back and forth in a given time. As with noise, frequency is measured in cycles per second (cps) or Hertz (Hz). Frequencies that coincide with the body's own resonances tend to be the most uncomfortable; these are mostly in the range from 2-30Hz.

2. Amplitude:

How far the surface moves each time it vibrates, measured in thousandths of an inch or microns (millionths of a metre). Medical standards now tend to express amplitude in terms of *acceleration*, given in metres per second per second (m/s^2), or 'g'.

3. Duration:

How long it goes on. The longer your exposure the higher the risk.

The table below shows some different combinations of frequency and amplitude and the sensations they cause.

Freq.Hz	Amplitude in thousandths of an inch				
3	0.7 – 2.0	2.0 – 6.0	6.0 – 30	–	–
5	0.4 – 1.1	1.1 – 3.2	3.2 – 16	16 – 43	43
10	0.2 – 0.6	0.6 – 1.6	1.6 – 5.0	5 – 13	13
20	0.1 – 0.3	0.3 – 0.8	0.8 – 1.8	1.8 – 3.1	3.1
50	0.4 – 0.1	0.1 – 0.3	0.3 – 0.5	0.5 – 0.6	0.6
sensation	just perceptible	clearly perceptible	annoying	unpleasant	painful

Source: Colin G.Gordon (Institute of Sound and Vibration Research)
at Symposium on Structural Insulation, London, March 1971.

You can see that it gets painful as amplitude rises at
each frequency. The levels of vibration that cause pain also
cause damage. Less intense vibration that is annoying or unpleasant may not harm you directly but it is tiring and can
make you liable to accidents.

The range of potentially hazardous frequencies extends beyond those shown in the table, to an upper limit of
2,000Hz.

What vibration does to you:

1. Whole Body Effects:
Most of these occur below 30Hz when you sit or stand
on a vibrating surface. You can feel disorientated, giddy or
sick; you may not be able to focus properly or perform
simple manual tasks. In a dangerous situation these effects
can be fatal: helicopter crashes are thought to have been
caused by disorientation and inability to read instruments.

Whole body vibration can also cause permanent damage to your body. Drivers of tractors and other heavy equipment suffer abdominal, spinal and bone damage. If you
drive a tractor and have a persistent pain low down in your
back, vibration may be causing it. Get proper medical attention; make sure the doctor knows what job you do and that
he takes this into consideration when making a diagnosis.

2. Vibration-induced White Finger (VWF).
More commonly known as whitefinger or dead hand.

Its medical name is Raynaud's Phenomenon. The blood vessels and nerves in your fingers are damaged by using vibrating power tools, usually for long periods each day for several years.

The first sign of the disease you are likely to notice is when one or more fingers turns white and stays like that for anything up to an hour. You can't feel the affected finger and your hand movements are clumsy. As the circulation returns it may hurt.

The shorter the period of exposure before symptoms appear the more severe the condition is likely to be if you go on using vibrating tools.

With more exposure to vibration, all fingers of both hands are affected from finger tip to base. Attacks are rare during vibration. They usually start in the early morning when the weather is cold or damp. Touching the cold steering wheel of a car coming to work may set off an attack. They get more frequent as the disease progresses.

After long-term exposure – perhaps 10 or 15 years working six to seven hours a day with vibrating tools – the blood vessels in the fingers may become permanently damaged. With severe damage your hands may become bluish in colour. Prolonged exposure to high energy vibration has resulted in a few cases of gangrene requiring amputation.

If you stop using vibrating tools soon enough the condition *may* get better. It is more likely to stay with you for the rest of your life and may get worse even without further exposure, especially if you work in cold or damp conditions, for example in construction, farming and forestry.

Whitefinger is an unpleasant disease which can not only make it more difficult to earn a living but also spoil many leisure activities. Swimming, gardening, going for a walk, or watching football can all bring on an attack.

There is no medical remedy for whitefinger: pills designed to dilate the blood vessels of the fingers have been disappointing ; surgery has been unsuccessful.

Other effects:

Power tools may cause pain in the wrists, elbows and shoulders but it is not clear whether this is due to vibration or the weight of the tools.

All vibration, whether it involves your whole body or just your hands, can make you tired or irritable. Since noise and vibration often go together you may be exposed to a double stress.

Who is at risk?

Whole body vibration is likely to be experienced by anyone sitting or standing on a vibrating surface. Drivers of agricultural tractors and a wide range of construction machines, pilots, and people who work in ships' engine rooms may all be at risk from vibration which the designers have failed to eliminate or isolate.

But vibration is increasingly used for its own sake, particularly to speed the handling or consolidation of materials, and this may put more people at risk.

For example, workers making precast concrete beams have to stand for long periods on top of large steel moulds which are vibrated to compact the concrete. They are exposed to intense whole-body vibration and there is a possibility, as yet not investigated, that they might get Raynaud's of the feet.

Not much research has been done to identify potentially dangerous situations of this kind and it is best to assume that **if it vibrates and you're on it, you're at risk.**

In the case of the precast concrete works, the measures needed to create a safe place of work – walkways with guard rails alongside the moulds – would isolate the workers from vibration.

Whitefinger: Most of the risk comes from 'accidental' vibration but, again, higher vibrational energy is being deliberately introduced into an increasing number of hand-held tools, such as poker vibrators for concrete and small soil compactors.

Pneumatic, electric and petrol-powered tools have all been found to cause whitefinger. The list of hazardous equipment includes *pneumatic roadbreakers, hammers, chisels,* and their variants ; *rotary rock drills* used in mining, quarrying and construction ; *air tools* used in manufacturing ; *rotary/percussive electric drills* ; *riveting hammers and electric grinders.* Grinding of small castings against carborundum wheels, where vibration enters your hands from the workpiece and not the tool, is also hazardous.

One of the biggest risks is the *petrol-powered chain-saw* (also a dangerous noise source). Introduced to Britain in the mid-Fifties it was not recognised as a hazard until the Sixties when reports of whitefinger among forestry workers came from Japan, Australia and Scandinavia. A Japanese survey published in 1966 found that more than half the tree fellers examined had whitefinger.

o *In Britain a study carried out by the Department of Occupational Medicine of the University of Dundee found symptoms of the condition in 65 per cent of forestry workers who used power saws continuously.*

o *There do not appear to have been any investigations of whitefinger among workers in other industries in Britain but the Japanese survey found that 30 per cent of metal miners and 37 per cent of workers in limestone quarries suffered from it.*

Prevention:

Clearly a very large number of workers is at risk from vibration. Individual and collective action by workers is vital if manufacturers, employers, researchers and government departments are to treat the problem with the urgency it deserves.

At present there are no statutory limits for vibration exposure. Research is unco-ordinated and the experts do not agree on methods for calculating a safe 'dose' of vibration in different situations.

Standards for whole body vibration are being developed on the basis of 'fatigue-decreased proficiency' (FDP) – the point at which fatigue produced by vibration causes you to start making mistakes. Different methods of assessing the same exposure can lead to very different ideas about 'safe' limits.

In the case of a tractor driving over ploughed fields one method would give a safe exposure of almost eight hours ; another, stricter, method would give only 3.7 hours. Both conclusions are based on the same data from tests with a *suspension* seat. A rigidly-mounted seat would definitely give you an overdose of vibration in a very short time, whichever way you interpret the figures.

Proposed standards for hand vibration are designed to protect you from whitefinger, not necessarily from discomfort or fatigue. Because it is believed that regular breaks in a shift greatly reduce your effective dose the standards may make allowances for rest periods in setting safe exposures.

Limits from two proposed safety standards are given in the tables at the end of this section. It is not known if either gives adequate protection from whitefinger. The stricter Czech limits are probably the minimum standards with which to start a safety campaign.

Action against vibration:

Assurances that a particular vibration exposure is safe are meaningless unless management can produce figures that fall within one of the proposed standards. As with any other hazard, the employer must be able to tell you what risk he is exposing you to. That means he will have to get vibration levels measured by an independent consultant or one of the university departments specialising in this field. Present equipment and work patterns may be safe or they may have to be modified.

With or without measurement, some precautions should be taken as a matter of principle.

1. Reduce vibration to the lowest possible levels. The ideal solution is to eliminate it at source, which may be a long term engineering problem. This doesn't mean you can't be protected: it should always be possible to isolate the source so that vibration reaching your body is reduced to acceptable levels.

Hand tools should be fitted with special vibration-absorbing handles (not just rubber grips, though these are better than bare metal). Spring grips introduced on chain saws around 1970 were probably the main factor in halting the epidemic of whitefinger among forestry workers.

Tractor-type vehicles should be fitted with suspension seats.

2. Reduce exposure time: Forestry workers on chain saws are given a 10 minute break in every working hour and you could legitimately press for this arrangement if you work continuously with any of the hazardous hand tools. The working day should be as short as possible: if you have been on a pneumatic breaker all day, don't take on another three hours overtime. Don't take on chain saw work at weekends as well as the working week. Rotate hazardous jobs so that individual exposure is shortened.

If you drive off-road tractor-type vehicles try to keep below 8 hours a day 'in the saddle', even if you have a suspension type seat.

3. Protect hands from cold: This is important in the prevention of whitefinger. Pneumatic tools should be designed or modified to direct exhaust air away from the hands. For indoor work, good heating is important; outdoors, windbreaks and temporary shelters can be erected for some kinds of work and there should be a warm messroom in which you can spend rest periods.

Personal precautions:

1. If your fingers normally go white on exposure to cold – a fairly definite reaction that you will have noticed since your early teens – you may have 'constitutional cold finger' and you should not work with vibrating tools.

2. If a tool makes your fingers tingle, or the tip of a finger turns white, vibration is excessive and steps must be taken to reduce it.

3. Equipment should be held in a normal, comfortable position, with as loose a grip as possible. Gloves will help to damp high frequency vibration and to keep your hands warm. If you work outdoors, two or three pairs are recommended, mainly so that you can have a dry set at all times. As essential protective clothing, gloves should be provided by the employer.

4. Watch for symptoms: If you start getting tingling fingers followed by numbness it may mean that the condition will progress. The sooner you can stop exposing your hands to vibration the less chance there will be of permanent damage.

5. If you have to continue with vibrating tools, take the precautions advised above and keep checking with the union for any new safety standards. See that the employer applies them. Get medical attention.

Compensation for whitefinger:

Whitefinger is often belittled by medical authorities, particularly those responsible for deciding which diseases should qualify for industrial injury benefits.

Since 1950 two separate committees have spent a total of nearly seven years considering whether whitefinger should be put on the 'prescribed' list and both have decided that it shouldn't. The main reason seems to be what the first committee called the 'triviality' of the disablement which 'only rarely interfered to any marked extent with work'. Aside from the fact that many victims would disagree strongly with both opinions, this is a classic example of the way in which establishment medicine judges the health of workers by their ability to work.

Another reason for official caution is that 8 – 10 per cent of the general population suffers from Raynaud's *disease* without having anything to do with vibrating tools. The idea that one or two non-occupational cases might slip through to claim disability benefit is abhorrent to those who guard the Industrial Injuries Fund.

Even in their terms it must be a tiny risk because 90 per cent of non-occupational victims are women and few women clock up the long exposures needed to cause whitefinger. Many of the 'constitutional' cases also have the condition in their feet, an improbable effect of using hand tools.

Eventually the medical bureaucrats will overcome these taxing problems– as they have done in other countries – and whitefinger will be prescribed. Victims will be able to draw a small disablement allowance.

There is little hope that damage done by whole body vibration will be prescribed.

In the meantime your only hope of compensation is to sue your employer for damages. (See Section 11.)

○ *In May 1973 Mr James Lambert, was awarded £1,500 damages and costs in the High Court after Vauxhall admitted liability for his whitefinger, caused by a pneumatic hammer he used for sheet metal work on the assembly line. Many similar cases are on their way to the courts.*

The table below shows proposed limits for vibration exposure to the hands, submitted to the International Standards Organisation by the Czechs. The limits are specified in terms of 'rms' acceleration measured by octave filters centred on seven frequencies. If the level in any octave band exceeds the limit then vibration is excessive. (The letters 'rms' stand for root-mean-square, the *effective* value of a fluctuating quantity. The values of a quantity are squared, averaged and then the square root is extracted.)

The figures in the right hand column are the less stringent limits proposed in a draft British Standard yet to be published.

Table 1:

Frequency (HZ) Octave centres	Max. rms acceleration (m/s^2) for 8-hr exposure Czech proposal	Max. rms acceleration 400 min in 8-hr day BS draft
4	*	1
8	1	1
16	1	1
31.5	1	2
63	3.16	4
125	5.63	8
250	5.63	16
500	5.63	32
1000	*	64
2000	*	128

*Not covered in Czech proposal

Table 2:

Correction factors for Czech limits – work continuous or not interrupted on regular pattern

Exposure time during shift	Multiply limit by –
Up to 30 minutes	10.00
30 min – 1hr	3.16
1 – 2hrs	1.78
Over 2hrs	No correction

Table 3:

Correction factors for Czech limits – regular rest periods

Rest period Length	Number in 8hr shift	Multiply limit by
0 – 2min	any number	no correction
2 – 10min	1 – 5	no correction
	5 – 10	1.78
	10 or more	3.16
Longer than 10min	1 – 2	1.78
	2 – 5	3.16
	5 – 10	5.63
	10 or more	10.00

NB: The employer cannot use correction factors from both tables to adjust the same exposure limit. He must choose one or the other.

Radiation:

You are reading this book with the help of one form of electromagnetic radiation, light.

Light waves of different lengths register in your eye as different colours: at one end of the spectrum there is red, the longest visible wave and at the other there is violet, the shortest.

Ordinary light is not a hazard in itself though poor lighting is a common cause of eyestrain, headaches and accidents. Miners suffer from nystagmus, rapid oscillation of the eyeballs resulting from working in near-darkness.

The rest of this section is about the forms of electro-magnetic radiation which exist outside the familiar spectrum of visible light. The table shows how this larger spectrum extends from the longest, radio, waves at one extreme to the shortest, gamma rays, at the other. The section will deal with them in the same sequence.

Longer wavelength

Radio waves
    Microwave radiation
        Infra-red radiation
            – Visible light –
                Ultra violet radiation
                    X-rays
                        Gamma rays
                        higher frequency

Radio waves:

Despite the fears of earlier generations ordinary radio waves are apparently harmless, but they may lead to secondary hazards:

1. Voltage may build up in metal structures close to high-powered transmitters, eg, crane jibs. Construction workers in America have been burned on touching crane hooks in this situation. It seems a charge may also be induced in ship's rigging by new radar installations on the East Coast, but reports have been confused, perhaps for reasons of defence secrecy.

2. Walkie-talkie sets may accidentally trigger detonators when explosive blasting is being controlled by radio.

3. High powered electronic equipment can generate X-rays. These are dealt with later.

Microwaves:

Very short length radio waves (wavelengths between 3

and 300mm), are being used increasingly in industry, communications and catering – typically the microwave oven which cooks meals in a few seconds. The obvious risk is that you will 'cook' any part of your body exposed, so good maintenance of safety devices is important. Less obvious is the possibility that exposure to this form of radiation may cause cataracts to form in your eye – the lens becomes opaque and you begin to go blind.

Infra-red radiation:

Any red-hot material gives out infra-red radiation so it is a common industrial hazard. Strong radiation produces burns similar to the various stages of sunburn.

Long-term exposure can give you cataracts (see above under Microwaves). The damage can be done by much lower levels of radiation than those which affect the skin and you get no warning that it is happening.

Persistent reddening of the skin from working near infra-red sources is a sign that you are probably getting too much. Levels of this kind of radiation can be easily tested; you should wear safety glasses with special filter lenses and your eyes should be examined regularly.

Ultra violet radiation:

We are now at the other end of the visible light spectrum – literally beyond violet. For most people the sun provides the biggest source of UV radiation: if you get enough the skin tries to defend itself by developing brown pigmentation – a sun tan. There are good reasons for the reaction because this kind of radiation can have various harmful effects on your skin:

1. It gets dry and wrinkled. Not serious, but a warning that you may be vulnerable to more harmful conditions.

2. Localised skin sores. See a doctor if these develop.

3. Skin cancers. Can result from many years work in the open air, typically on farms and construction sites. (See page 127.)

4. Coal tar and other chemicals react with the skin and make it more sensitive to UV, causing an exaggerated form of sunburn, often with blistering. This is a particular problem for pipewrappers on pipeline contracts where the hot 'dope' gives off dense clouds of fumes. Get the employer to provide a choice of hats, face visors and protective creams so that everyone can find a comfortable form of protection.

If you have a light skin you will probably be more vulnerable to all these conditions. If you get persistent skin irritation, see a doctor.

The commonest industrial sources are arc welding and ultra-violet sterilising units. Protective gear used by welders should protect all skin from exposure anyway: bare arms are vulnerable to ordinary burns and a mask (in preference to goggles) helps deflect fumes away from mouth and nose.

Eyes must always be protected from the UV radiation produced by arc welding. Even a moment's exposure can cause 'arc eye' or 'welder's flash', a condition that comes on some hours later and feels as if sand has been thrown in your eyes. It is not believed to cause any long-term damage. Welding operations should be screened to protect other workers. If this can't be done they should be issued with safety spectacles which filter UV light.

Ionising radiation:

This is radiation as most people understand it – one of the most dangerous of all occupation hazards and probably the only form of electromagnetic radiation which really scares people. It is a healthy reaction, linked in many minds with the devastation of Hiroshima and Nagasaki, and responsible for much tighter standards of control than are applied to other hazards.

But control is not so good that you can leave your safety entirely in the hands of the experts.

About 75,000 people are estimated to be working in regular contact with equipment or substances which give out ionising radiation. Many thousands more will become involved as these techniques become more widely used in industry and the risks will grow if familiarity and commercial pressure are allowed to undermine safety precautions. As with most of its other hazards, the construction industry has already become a leader in safeguard-stripping.

Except in the case of severe over-exposure, you can neither see nor feel ionising radiation. You can feel perfectly fit after receiving a dose that will later cause serious damage to your body.

Types of damage	1. Burns, dermatitis, cataract 2. Cancers, leukaemia 3. Damage to reproductive cells, causing sterility, infertility, abnormalities in later generations
Types of radiation	
Alpha particles —given off by some radioactive substances, eg plutonium, radium	Not much range or penetrating power. Produce intense ionisation in short distances. Therefore substances which emit alpha particles are not very dangerous outside the body and very dangerous if you get them inside, eg by inhaling or swallowing. Anaemia, leukaemia, bone cancer, lung cancer
Beta particles —streams of fast-moving electrons	More penetrating than alpha particles but mainly affect skin unless you inhale or swallow beta emitter. Burns, dermatitis, warts which may lead to skin cancer. Cataract
X-radiation —generated by X-ray and other electronic equipment. Can be turned off	X- and Gamma radiation can be dealt with together. Both are very penetrating electromagnetic radiations that can go right through you, and can cause all the effects listed above
Gamma radiation —given off by many radioactive substances. Cannot be turned off, only shielded	Gamma rays are more penetrating than X-rays but the more concentrated beam from most X-ray equipment causes a greater risk from skin burns

Radiography is the most widespread radiation hazard.

Originally found only in hospitals X-ray machines are now commonly used in industry for examining castings, welds and many other components. Because X-ray equipment tends to be cumbersome and inflexible, gamma radiography has replaced it for many applications, particularly on pipeline sites and other construction projects.

In gamma radiography the source of radiation is a small metal capsule inside which radioactive material, for example Iridium-192, is sealed. The capsule is kept in a larger container and only exposed when the radiographer wants to pass the penetrating radiation through an object in order to take a picture, just as X-ray equipment is turned on so that a doctor can get a picture of your chest.

The important difference is that the gamma source is never fully 'turned off' until its radioactivity dies. Even when closed, the exposure containers used on site are seldom as heavily shielded as they would be if built for protection instead of portability.

Some exposure containers are safer than others:

1. Remote-controlled containers which stick the source out and then retract it, are the safest because you can get well away during exposure. The main danger is that the source may not retract properly. Maintenance must be very good.

2. Shutter types require you to be near the container and are not so safe as **1**.

3. Torch type containers. Again you have to be near the container but your dose rate is likely to be at least five times higher than with the shutter type.

Insist that the employer uses only the first or second type.

Construction sites are a particular hazard because the subcontractors who do this work are often under pressure not to hold up the next stage of the job. The heavy labyrinth walls which usually shield other workers from gamma radiography in factories do not suit the pace or economics of site work. Areas are just cordoned off, sometimes without proper warning notices.

o *Out of 70 reported overexposures to all forms of radiation in 1971, no less than 48 came from construction sites.*

Reports and court cases show that the most elementary precautions are being ignored, so it may be useful to list some of them:

1. Before any X- or gamma radiography is carried out on a new site, the Factory Inspectorate must be informed.

2. You should be issued with a film badge (see below) which you must wear at all times of possible exposure and the employer must keep an official record of all exposures. You must be given a transfer record when you leave for another job.

3. Keep as far away from radiation sources as you can. See that danger areas are cordoned off properly, allowing a wide safety margin. If you are not a radiographic worker keep well out of the area.

4. Don't ever touch a sealed source. If proper handling equipment is not available, leave the source where it is.

5. Radiation levels should be monitored frequently, each time the equipment is used where there is no permanent installation.

Safeguards are generally much better in factories, hospitals and laboratories where radiographic installations can be properly shielded, but there is often room for improvement.

Checklist:

Do all doors, etc, seal tightly?

Is there an interlock on the door?

Is there an emergency cut-out switch that can be used by anyone trapped inside?

Is there a shielded area for anyone who gets trapped?

Do alarms go off automatically before each exposure?

If the enclosure has an open top, could maintenance or other workers be exposed? Could gamma radiation be scattered down into the surrounding area?

You can do a better check if you read the Department

of Employment booklet on ionising radiations or the appropriate Code of Practice, listed at the back of this book.

'Unwanted' X-rays:

A variety of electronic equipment can give out X-rays:

Electron microscopes

Cathode tubes

Electronic valves, particularly high voltage rectifying type as used in colour TVs

Radar equipment – klystrons and magnetrons

Special regulations apply when the equipment operates at more than 5kV, or 20kV in the case of TV equipment. A lead glass screen should give sufficient protection when equipment is being tested outside its cabinet. Film badges will give a record of personal dosage from this source.

Manufacturing:

There are many situations in manufacturing where you may be exposed to radioactive materials, either as sealed sources (materials sealed in capsules and used as a radiation transmitter, as in gamma radiography) or as unsealed sources (usually when something is being made from the substance).

Sealed sources are used increasingly for gauging the thickness of materials like polyethylene during continuous manufacture, for level gauging and for sterilising. Safeguards should prevent you touching the source or putting a hand or foot across the beam. The container must be protected from accidental damage. All containers must be tested regularly for leakage.

Unsealed sources are used in the following operations:

1. Manufacturing and processing nuclear reactor fuels.

2. Luminising. (Painting luminous materials on dials, etc.)

3. Extracting thorium from various ores.

4. Making gas mantles.

5. Making electronic devices and self-luminous tubes containing radioactive gases.

6. Monitoring industrial plant using radioactive 'tracers'.

In all cases you should be protected by the highest

possible standards of industrial hygiene to prevent inhalation, swallowing or absorbtion through the skin, as for any very toxic substances (see Section 6, Prevention). Total enclosure, as in glove boxes, and very good exhaust ventilation of fume cupboards, are essential. In addition regular tests must be done for contamination of working surfaces, skin and air.

o *Plutonium. Ten per cent of Britain's electricity is now generated by nuclear power stations, all of which produce or consume plutonium. An American expert has said that one pound of plutonium is enough to cause nine billion lung cancer cases. He estimates that world plutonium production will reach 64,000 kilogrammes (140,800lb) by 1984.*

Luminising:

Tritium and promethium have replaced radium as luminising materials. They are less toxic but larger quantities have to be used and the risk remains about the same. Any contamination of a workplace is easily detected because these materials glow brightly if you turn the lights off and shine an ultra violet lamp around the room. You could do this test with a UV health lamp: if the result is positive, hygiene controls are not good enough. Demand a clean-up, better controls and regular independent measurement of conditions.

Tritium penetrates unbroken skin. Regular tests should be done on your urine to see what dose you are getting.

Demolition:

Demolition of buildings in which activities 2, 3 and 4 in the list above have been carried on could release large amounts of active material. Ordinary houses have been used by family business or sweat-shop operators and it is always a good idea to check on its history before knocking down a house. Neighbours should know. If in doubt, contact the Factory Inspectorate because it is vital that such places be decontaminated first.

Radiation dosage:

There is no level of radiation below which scientists

can honestly say that no damage is done, so it is important to get as little as you possibly can. Some scientists believe that the 'safe levels' at present used to protect workers will soon be drastically reduced.

> o Joseph Rotblat, professor of physics at St Bartholomew's Hospital, London, has said: 'Present estimates of the risk of cancer following radiation exposure are higher than when safety levels were originally established some years ago. I believe the maximum permissible safety levels for exposure to radiation should be a tenth of what they are now.'
> Sunday Times, 18 March 1973.

Exposure to radiation is measured in units called rems. The present internationally agreed limits are:

Whole body exposure	5 rem/yr
Testicles, ovaries and red bone marrow	5 rem/yr
Skin, thyroid, bone	30 rem/yr
Hands and forearms, feet and ankles	75 rem/yr
All other organs	15 rem/yr
Pregnant woman, *total* during pregnancy	1 rem

A film badge, consisting of a photographic film inside a lightproof holder, will record your individual radiation dose. A film badge or other approved dosemeter must be worn by all workers in radiation areas. This is a legal requirement under the Ionising (Sealed Sources) Regulations 1969 and the Ionising (Unsealed Radioactive Substances) Regulations 1968. These do not apply in places not covered by the Factories Acts – for example hospitals or universities, where you should see that the employer follows the appropriate code of practice.

Film badges are 'read' by the Radiological Protection Service and the employer must keep a record of your exposure and hand you a transfer record when you leave.

If you exceed the dose limits you may be taken off exposed work for weeks, months or indefinitely.

Workers must have a pre-employment medical test and subsequent tests at maximum intervals of 14 months. New workers must receive training before they start.

If you are worried that your film badge record is higher or lower than it should be, the actual dose received by your body can now be determined by counting abnormal cells in a sample of your blood. This can be done several months after any disputed or worrying exposure. **Tests are carried out by the National Radiological Protection Board at Harwell.**

Action:

1. Get the employer to agree lower exposure limits – preferably ten times lower – and engineering controls to make them workable.

2. If anyone is suspended because of an overdose, insist on a full investigation – with workers' representation – and be prepared to stop work unless you are satisfied it cannot happen again.

3. Anyone who is suspended should be given alternative employment with no loss of pay.

4. There should be full consultation before any sealed or unsealed sources are introduced into normal manufacturing processes. Don't be satisfied on safety until you have had a report from an independent authority.

Compensation:

Except in obvious cases of skin burns appearing directly after an over-exposure, it is exceedingly difficult to prove that any illness, for example leukaemia, is caused by radiation.

Although they had collected massive doses of plutonium and were suffering from typical symptoms of radiation exposure, two workers at the Windscale, Cumberland, plant of British Nuclear Fuels were unable to get an admission of liability from the employer.

o One of them, Mr Harold King, became so ill he had to retire: he has had all his teeth removed and after seven operations for cataract is now blind in his right eye and partially blind in the other. He told the Sunday Times, 18 March, '73: 'Doctors wouldn't say that plutonium caused the illness, and they wouldn't say that it didn't.'

Dermatitis, ulceration, skin cancer, damage to bones and blood, and cataract caused by the different forms of

electromagnetic radiation are all prescribed diseases.

The problem of diagnosis encountered by Mr King in trying to get compensation from his employer could cause just as much difficulty when you claim industrial injury or disablement benefits.

The only insurance against this kind of problem is a critical shop floor where you are not afraid to question management's safety performance and where every suspension is treated as a failure in the system of protection.

o *According to the* Sunday Times *report 38 BNF workers had been transferred to clean areas because of excessive plutonium exposure.*

Temperature:

o 'The Factory Act poster in a passageway was ignored, and conditions of heat and humidity were bad. Yet men didn't even bother to ask if they could have the fans on, or the windows open. If you did, "nobody took any notice". There was much satisfied comment when a factory inspector arrived and made James Shaw have all the windows open and the fans switched on. "Aye, it's about time an' all".
Brian Jackson, describing Cartwrights Mill, Huddersfield, in **Working Class Community**, Pelican.

Computers are very sensitive to temperature and tend to stop working if conditions are not right. Humans are also sensitive to temperature. They also work effectively and safely only within a narrow range of temperatures. But, unlike computers, they appear to adapt to all but the worst extremes of heat and cold. Usually they do not stop working.

Which is why many computer rooms are air-conditioned and most offices and factories are not.

It is not simply a matter of comfort, though that is important enough. It seems that people do not fully adapt to working outside the range of temperature in which they are comfortable.

As usual the main research effort has been directed at discovering the effects on productivity, but several studies have shown that accidents increase with both higher and lower temperatures. The report *2,000 Accidents* (National Institute of Industrial Psychology) found significantly more accidents at temperatures below about 20°C (68°F) in an assembly shop and a machine shop. In the first, work was mostly done sitting down ; in the second, more was done standing up. Neither involved much walking around. The NIIP observers did not find any similar upper limit, which was almost certainly because workers reduced their output in hot weather.

Other researchers have found that the chances of a factory worker having an accident increase by four per cent per degree Centigrade above 19°C (66°F).

It seems that the temperature for comfort and safety should be around 19 or 20°C where light factory work is going on.

Office workers who are not moving around a lot may need slightly higher temperatures.

People doing heavy manual work will need cooler conditions – probably between 13 – 16°C (55 – 60°F).

The important thing is to get management to install a heating and ventilating system which can be controlled to produce safe and comfortable conditions all the year round.

The Factories Act requires a 'reasonable' temperature to be maintained in each workroom. In rooms where much of the work is done sitting down, without much physical effort, temperature must not be less than 15.5°C (60°F) after the first hour.

This is not good enough. Many strains and sprains, particularly among older workers, happen first thing, when your body is not warmed up for work. All rooms should be at an acceptable temperature from the moment you start work. (It's still a good idea to do lighter jobs first, to loosen up before starting any heavy lifting).

Where the environment cannot be controlled, as in construction, farming, trawling, cold stores or kiln loading, appropriate protective clothing must be provided and a pattern of work arranged so as to reduce cold stress and heat stress to a minimum.

If these measures are not taken your body constantly

consumes energy trying to keep to its correct temperature. The short-term effects vary from individual to individual, depending on how you adapt to different degrees of heat and cold, your age and fitness, and the amount of work involved.

For most people, work in even moderately high or low temperatures – an unventilated factory in summer, an unheated warehouse in winter – is tiring. The heat can make you irritable, the cold can slow your reactions.

Extreme heat:

As temperatures rise well beyond any comfort range, the effects become more pronounced. It is difficult to give precise temperature ranges for different effects. Heavy work will bring them on at lower temperatures. Strenuous work in an impervious suit and hood – for example stripping asbestos lagging in a dockyard – can expose you to severe heat stress and exhaustion, even in winter.

Workers in steelworks, foundries, glassworks, mining, heating and generating plants and those who have to enter kilns and ovens are among those at risk. There are many other situations and it should be fairly obvious if yours is one of them.

o Workers starting on hot work for the first time may faint. They may first complain of feeling dizzy, sick or even chilly and you may notice their breathing is fast and shallow, their skin moist and clammy. Get them away from the heat (and any danger) if you notice these warning signs. They soon feel better after a rest in a cool place.

o Heat shock is a more serious reaction, caused by losing too much fluid and salt from your body. You get heat cramps, feel weak, sick, tired and dizzy. You will have to rest for some time while the fluid and salt losses are made good.

o Heat stroke is a complete failure of the body to regulate its temperature. Your body begins to overheat and instead of sweating your skin is warm and dry. It can be fatal and your body temperature must be lowered as quickly as possible, preferably in hospital, by sponging or cold baths.

These effects of heat can be prevented in most healthy

workers by giving the body time to adjust its cooling system to the conditions. This takes from four to six days according to the temperature, the work and the individual. Older workers never acclimatise completely.

If you are away from hot work you quickly lose acclimatisation – as much as two thirds of it in one week and all of it by the end of the third week. When you return you have to start all over again.

Exposure should be increased gradually each day until you are acclimatised. You should be given plenty to drink, and you may need salt tablets.

Working hours should be kept short and there should be plenty of breaks and a cool place in which to take them.

Developments are being made in protective clothing that has built-in cooling systems. They are probably suitable only for really extreme conditions but if you think they might make work more comfortable you could get management to obtain some different types for you to try – on the understanding that nobody should be expected to work for more than a few hours in special protective clothing. (See page 181.)

Cold:

Your body does not adjust physically to cold in the same way as it does to heat, though regular cold work should increase the blood circulation to your hands so that they keep warmer.

But you do get used to working in cold conditions and feel less uncomfortable after a while – **providing you have efficient protective clothing.**

Most workers in Britain are unlikely to experience the more spectacular effects of extreme cold but they should be borne in mind by divers, trawler crews and workers in cold stores. ○ As cold gets more intense, your body loses heat. As your brain is chilled you may start to behave irrationally, become unconscious and go into a coma. As blood circulation to hands and feet is reduced to conserve heat for more essential areas, you risk frostbite. ○ When your body temperature falls to 28°C (about 82°F) your heart stops.

Long-term effects:

You don't have to get locked in a cold store over the weekend for cold to be a real hazard. At least a million workers risk damage to health from work in normal winter temperatures.

In fact air temperature alone doesn't always indicate the amount of cold stress you may be experiencing. In a mine for example the air temperature at the bottom of a downcast shaft or in a main intake roadway may be just over 7°C (46°F), but with an air speed of 800ft a minute.

Working there would expose you to the same amount of stress as freezing air moving at only 20ft a minute.

This combination of moderate temperature and wind is a common experience for many outdoor workers, as well as conditions that actually are freezing. Clothing is often damp with rain so that you lose heat even faster.

o Dr Geoffrey Taylor has made two studies of workers on building sites in winter. He found that one in three had low body temperatures; that they were at risk from this condition for more than half the year and that it could have serious effects on their health. The 300 men he examined were mainly aged between 20 and 50 – his evidence suggested that older men left the construction industry because of diseases related to cold – rheumatism, bronchitis and heart disease. Low body temperatures and malnutrition among the men was linked with higher accident and illness rates; lower bonus earnings, productivity and efficiency.

'Cold conditions, with inadequate clothing and often a poor diet, turn healthy young men into old men at 50 with arthritis, rheumatism and chest complaints, unwilling and unfit to work outside,' according to Dr Taylor. He suggests that similar conditions exist among farm, municipal and road workers, seamen, shipbuilders, many electricians, post office engineers and people working in inadequately-heated factories.

Dr Taylor's report has not been published by the Government department which commissioned it and the Government refused to pay for further research. Academics have criticised the studies because of the small number of workers examined and the methods used to measure body temperature.

Earlier work by Dr Taylor, who first drew attention to the problem of hypothermia (low body temperature) in old people, was also dismissed as exaggerated. It is now recognised that thousands of old people die from it each winter.

o **In the case of construction workers, a Ministry of Social Security report in 1965 showed that they were 22 per cent more likely to get arthritis and rheumatism and 18 per cent more likely to get bronchitis than the average worker.**

Protective clothing:

Temporary enclosure of outdoor work and heated cabs on machines should be made standard practice on building sites but the answer which cuts across all the different groups at risk is proper protective clothing. More research is needed into materials which will deflect wind, keep you warm and yet prevent uncomfortable sweating. But this will be almost pointless unless employers can be forced to accept their responsibility to actually buy and issue such equipment.

The TUC Centenary Institute of Occupational Medicine has developed protective suits for trawlermen which give much better protection from the elements *and* help keep you afloat and alive if you go overboard. (Present clothing actually helps you sink.)

The suits will be expensive to make and at the time of writing no manufacturer has taken up the idea. Unless the trawler owners commit themselves to buying the new clothing it is hard to see how it will ever go into production. They will make that commitment only when workers demand it.

If you work in cold conditions and cannot get your employer to issue protective clothing, a pair of long johns under your trousers, thicker socks and several thin layers instead of one thick sweater will help keep you warm. But you can't hope to reproduce the wind and weather protection of special clothing.

o *The vitamin B and C deficiencies discovered by Dr Taylor were particularly acute in Scotland, a regional difference which he attributed to the high price and poor quality of fruit and vegetables in the shops. You could try getting the employer to issue orange juice with the tea, but a more realistic answer is to fight for an organised, decasualised building industry in which all workers can achieve steady employment, good earnings and good nutrition all the year round.*

Many of the worst problems of cold are in industries where workers have little influence on safety, like construction, farming and deep sea fishing. Better protection cannot be achieved without stronger organisation.

Organised workers can do a great deal to control the hazards of heat and cold.

Demands:

o **Effective, controllable heating and ventilating or air conditioning systems to be installed wherever possible, including all mobile equipment.**

o **Outside work in cold weather to be sheltered or screened and warmed with hot air blowers if at all practicable. Comfortable messrooms, hot meals and places to dry clothing to be provided on all sites, whatever the industry.**

o **Suitable protective clothing to be provided for all work in cold conditions and for any hot conditions where it improves comfort.**

o **Work patterns to be adjusted to allow for acclimatisation to very hot work.**

o **Shorter shifts and frequent rest periods for all working in extreme temperatures. Rest room and hot or cold drinks to be provided.**

Pressure:

Two types of work can subject your body to abnormally high pressures – underwater diving and work in shafts, tunnels and caissons where compressed air is used to keep ground water out of the workings.

There are two main hazards:

1. The bends, caisson sickness or 'pains'. These are different terms for the same condition. What happens is that nitrogen dissolved in your blood while you are breathing compressed air turns into bubbles if the pressure on your body is reduced too quickly, The effect can vary from pains in joints, muscles and other parts of the body (Type 1 bends) to more serious symptoms like loss of vision, unconscious-

D

ness, dizziness, paralysis and death (Type II bends).

2. Bone damage (bone necrosis). Thought to be caused by bubbles blocking off blood supplies near bones, it is unlikely to affect you unless you have been doing this kind of work for some time. Hip or shoulder joints become stiff and painful, as in arthritis, and you may not be able to do manual work.

Both conditions can be prevented by correct decompression procedures and other safety precautions, some of which can be found in two sets of regulations under the Factories Act:

Work in Compressed Air Special Regulations, 1958
Diving Operations Special Regulations, 1960

Both sets of regulations are out of date. Research has shown that the decompression tables in the compressed air regulations do not provide protection against bone necrosis and don't even stop Type II bends.

Much better protection is given by the 'Blackpool' decompression tables. It is thought that no workers have contracted bone necrosis on contracts where these have been applied since their introduction in 1966. The tables are now incorporated in the *Medical Code of Practice for Work in Compressed Air*, published in February 1973 by the Construction Industry Research and Information Association. The code has no legal force but workers can see that it is applied and enforced.

The diving regulations were not very good when first made, relying too much on 'qualified' divers to set their own decompression procedures and placing too few duties on the employer. There is no requirement to provide a medical lock or make emergency arrangements for getting to one.

New, more hazardous deep diving techniques developed for the offshore gas and oil boom are not of course covered, but it would make little difference if they were. Regulations made under the Factories Act do not apply to work in the North Sea, where the risks of bone necrosis are thought to be increasing as diving operations go down towards the 1,000ft level.

In the absence of statutory protection, divers can insist that the employer follows *Principles of Safe Diving Practice*, published by the Construction Industry Research and Information Association.

Divers and workers in compressed air can improve their medical protection against bone necrosis by putting their names on the **MRC Decompression Sickness Control Registry,** 21 Claremont Place, Newcastle upon Tyne NE2 4AA.

The registry arranges for you to have twice yearly X-rays to detect early signs of bone damage. **It had 10,000 civil engineering workers on its books at the beginning of 1973; of 1,700 with detailed X-ray records, 334 showed positive bone lesions.**

Out of 350 divers, 11 had positive bone lesions.

As commercial pressures, particularly in diving, force workers to operate beyond the limits of medical knowledge, the Registry provides not only a personal safeguard against disability but a collection centre for information from which real safety standards can be developed.

Precautions for compressed air:

o Check that the outside lock attendant is keeping a proper record of all men who enter and leave the lock and is following the right procedures. He should be working to the 'Blackpool Tables'.

o Decompression should never be speeded up and no-one should go out through the muck lock unless there's an emergency.

o Check with the lock attendant that the equipment is being maintained regularly and doesn't leak. Is there an emergency power supply?

o If you get any symptoms of the bends you should be recompressed without delay. Attacks usually start within one and a half hours of decompression. After working at pressures below 40 pounds per square inch, stay near the medical lock for at least an hour; above 40, stay for at least an hour and a half. This time should be paid as part of the job, and there should be somewhere comfortable to wait where you can get a hot drink or a meal.

o If you get an attack away from the site, get back to the medical lock as quickly as possible. Always wear a standard compressed air worker's label in case you collapse where people wouldn't know what was wrong with you. The label must be up to date, showing the address of the medical lock on your current job.

o If you have a cold, earache or sore throat, don't work in compressed air; you may get bad pains in the ears and head. If these come on during compression, ask to be decompressed and let out.

Medical supervision:

1. You must be passed fit for work in compressed air by a doctor before you start the job.

2. If you have been off sick or injured for more than three days you must be re-examined by the doctor before you go back into compressed air.

3. If the working pressure is over 18psi, you must be examined by the doctor at least once every four months.

These are legal requirements.

If joint pains or other symptoms persist after you have been treated in the medical lock, ask to see the doctor.

Action:

Keep a check on the number of workers who have to be recompressed. *If this rises to two per cent of all compressions, safety procedures need to be improved.*

4.

Chemical Hazards

Chemical hazards – substances that can harm your health or endanger life by fire or explosion have spread to most occupations.

All workers must regard themselves as being at risk.

This section deals with the ways in which chemicals get into the workplace. It provides some of the information needed to recognise hazards and fight for a clean-up.

The effects of the major poisons on your body are described in the next section and hundreds of dangerous substances are listed in the Directory of Toxic Substances.

In an emergency use the directory first, because it describes the treatment after exposure to each chemical.

If you are building up a list of chemicals used in your workplace, look them up in the index because a substance may be referred to in different parts of the book.

This section has:

o Introduction o Risks for all o Hazards in bulk o Erosion of health o Workers' offensive o Recognising hazards o Chemical terms o Labelling o Concentrations o 'Safe limits' – TLVs o Environment

Introduction:

Nobody knows how many different chemical substances are manufactured. There are probably half a million. According to one American estimate, a potentially harmful new chemical enters industrial use every twenty minutes.

Most of them will do nothing to improve life for ordinary people. Many will satisfy quite artificial 'needs' – just as arsenic oxide was included in Victorian bread to make it white, today's batch of chemicals may include new food additives to add to the two and a half thousand already available to Western 'food technologists'. There may be chemicals to make animals fat, and drugs to make people thin; sprays to make fruit look as smooth as plastic and substances to make plastic taste like food; deodorants to take away our human smell and synthetic odours to make us smell again; cosmetics to make crinkly hair straight and straight hair curly.

For the workers who handle it, each new substance contributes another uncertainty. No one is particularly surprised when girls bottling bubble baths – supposed to make skin soft and lovely – get dermatitis, or when women making potato crisps are made ill by an enzyme used in the process.

Such perversions of chemical knowledge are inevitable when profit comes before need, when funds are available in abundance to develop and market products that may cause cancer while those who seek a cure for the disease must scratch for every penny.

> o Methylene-bis-o-chloroaniline (Moca) is a chemical used as a hardener in the production of solid urethane, rubber, and of certain types of plastic foam. Animal experiments have indicated that Moca may be carcinogenic (cancer-causing) and until further evidence is available, firms using this material are being visited and given specific advice on the most efficient precautionary measures which can be devised at the present time. It must be emphasised however that this advice is based upon the best practicable measures known and is given in the absence of specific medical knowledge of the precise dangers of the material.
> HM Chief Inspector of Factories Annual Report 1971.

Protected by the 'best practicable measures' against an unknown hazard, the guinea pigs work on.

Moca is just one among thousands of recent additions to the backlog of substances piling up around the few scientists and doctors who unravel the health problems created by industry. None of the oldest hazards, like lead and mercury, are fully understood – let alone the newest.

Against such criticisms the chemical houses offer the antidote of progress through profit: the moneyspinners help to subsidise research into chemicals that improve the human condition.

Certainly drugs like the contraceptive pill and the Salk anti-polio vaccine can bring immeasurable benefits but profits are not the only way to pay for such advances.

New wonder drugs may cure diseases but they can never bring health for all. Not one single new drug is needed to reduce child mortality in the Rhondda to the same level as in the South East of England. The drugs for this condition are good wages, nutrition, housing and medical care – all expensive and unprofitable.

The argument that such things will be provided by mass prosperity generated by the new technologies is now threadbare.

> o 'The ruling doctrine of the time was that progress was measured by trade and profits, that popular misery could be cured only by encouraging capital; that the needs of the new industrial system must govern and limit the development of social life. No mill owner thought he could afford fair wages, especially as new machinery was paid for out of profits.'
> Donald Hunter on the Industrial Revolution, Health in Industry, Pelican.

The proliferation of new industrial chemicals reflects industry's constant search for the one that will satisfy the craving for profits by cutting materials costs, production time or labour. The irresponsibility with which it does so is often staggering.

Even when new materials offer the chance to eliminate hazards to workers and the community, no advantage is taken of this positive feature. In domestic plumbing for example, plastic can now replace lead for cold water pipes and so could eliminate one source of community lead intake. But in fact the PVC used in plastic piping contains lead compounds as fillers and it actually releases more lead when new than pipes made entirely from lead.

Lead has been eliminated from many paints and finishes but fresh hazards are built into the new mixtures – powerful solvents to make them dry quickly, or TDI resulting from the inclusion of polyurethanes to make them hard-wearing, or asbestos to stop them cracking.

The lead content in paint on children's toys is controlled, but gummed paper shapes do not count as toys, so lead-based pigments have been used freely by some manufacturers.

o In 1971, 22 workers in the **plastics** industry suffered lead poisoning.

> The situation would be instantly recognisable to Dr Turner Thackrah, of Leeds, who wrote in 1832:
> o 'I am told indeed, by an intelligent manufacturer of earthenware in Leeds, that the comparative cheapness of the leaden glaze is the chief recommendation. Surely humanity forbids that the health of workmen, and that of the poor at large, should be sacrificed to the saving of half-pence in the price of pots.'

Risks for all :

Industry's growing dependence on chemicals is clear from its consumption of raw materials. o World production of lead now amounts to about four million tons a year and is expected to double in the next 20 years. World mercury production doubled between 1950 and 1970 and is expected to reach 15,000 tons by 1975. Cadmium production has been doubling every 10 years and is expected to rise from about 20,000 tons a year to around 50,000 by 1980. o Most of the growth in these poisonous metals can be attributed to the demands of the chemical industries.

These figures may not mean much to the individual; but the fact that each year car exhausts spew 7,000 tons of lead into the air we breathe, or that 1,000 tons of metallic contaminants find their way into London's sewage sludge each year, is revealing.

There is plenty of poison for everyone. Chemicals have penetrated every activity; some, like paper making and farming have become chemical processes in their own right.

You may not think you have much contact with chemicals in your job – any more than the garage worker dispensing a thousand gallons of petrol a week thinks of himself as selling chemicals – but there are now few jobs where you don't use them.

For any one substance the occupational spread can be

enormous: miners, refiners, seamen, dockers, drivers, process workers and – 'downstream' – users, sewermen, dustmen, scrapmen, demolition men, families and whole communities.

The table shows how asbestos spreads throughout industry when it arrives in this country from the mines of South Africa and Canada.

Work where you can be exposed to asbestos:

Docks and transport: handling sacks and bales **Asbestos factories:** milling, weaving, turning **Power stations:** lagging and de-lagging **Steelworks:** lagging and de-lagging **Heavy engineering:** furnace insulation **Loco building and railway carriage building:** heat and sound insulation **Dockyards, shipbuilding, ship repairing:** lagging and de-lagging **Boiler making:** heat insulation **Paper making:** making filter papers and grinding rollers **Linoleum, floor tiles, rubber paints, plastics, adhesives, roofing compounds:** used as filler **Motor industry, garages:** grinding brake and clutch parts; repairs to same, making battery cases, car undersealing **Light engineering:** making gaskets and washers **Building materials:** asbestos cement sheets, pipes, etc **Building trades:** trimming asbestos cement sheets; insulation boards; asbestos spraying; laying asbestos asphalt mixes; insulation and repair of heating apparatus; demolition, especially de-lagging; disposal of waste (may be in hard core) **Electrical engineering:** insulation systems.

Many of those at risk are not protected by any safety laws. Lethal substances like the poison gas phosgene, for example, may be manufactured under fairly strict conditions and theoretically under the regulation of the Factories Act. They are then put in road tankers for transport to other plants without any special regulations covering the construction of tanks or the protection of drivers and public. (Compare this with the special containers and police escort involved in moving less dangerous, but politically more sensitive, CS riot gas from its factory in Cornwall.)

Some impact on official complacency was made when two acid tankers crashed in separate accidents on the M6 in December 1972 and a woman motorist died after being drenched in sulphuric acid.

But regulations on tank construction may come too late to prevent the massive disaster that would result from, say, a phosgene tanker being breached in a busy shopping street.

At the time of writing, tankers containing highly inflammable or corrosive substances have to be labelled. Labelling is to be extended to toxic loads. But apparently no substances are actually banned. 'We are concerned not with what is carried but with the labelling and identification to help police and fire brigade to deal with it,' said a Home Office spokesman.

Anyone who drives chemical tankers or lorries carrying drums should insist that the employer use the voluntary 'Tremcard' system – transport emergency cards which tell the driver and emergency services what is being carried and how to deal with it. You should also be issued with breathing apparatus, protective clothing and first aid equipment appropriate to the load, even though this is not a legal requirement.

For sewermen chemical wastes are one of the most important hazards in industrial areas. Most of them are discharged illegally. The list includes pickling acids, cyanides, paraffin, petrol, oil, alkalis, ammoniacal liquors containing phenols and tar compounds and explosive gases..

Scrapmen come across completely unexpected hazards. One worker cut up an old heat exchanger and suffered acute mercury poisoning.

o A plumber died from cadmium fumes given off while he was soldering some pipes. When you buy silver solder nobody tells you it may contain more than 20 per cent cadmium.

There are so many other examples of workers being harmed by unsuspected – or undisclosed – risks that all workers should regard themselves as being potentially at risk and find out exactly what they are working with.

Hazards in bulk:

The sheer bulk of materials involved in many processes can add a different dimension to chemical hazards. A handful of polyurethane foam is quite harmless but a storeroom full of the stuff can be a death trap if it catches fire.

Within minutes the place will be filled with a dense cloud of smoke, carbon monoxide and hydrogen cyanide. Unless exceptional precautions are taken the chances of escape will be small. Flame retardant grades may actually burn faster than untreated foam and give off just as much smoke.

Many substances, like liquefied petroleum gas, oxygen and chlorine, are now stored in such large quantities that an explosion or leakage could threaten not only an entire workforce but also the community outside.

Highly automated, sealed plants, where workers are not exposed to contamination during day-to-day operation, may be more of a danger in this respect. A thermostat failure plus a computer fault, for example, could unleash a monumental disaster.

Erosion of health:

Workers are now caught in a runaway reaction of chemistry and profits that has long since outstripped the resources of medical researchers and control agencies.

Recent legal actions against Central Asbestos, ICI and Dunlop, and the belated shutdown of Rio Tinto Zinc's leaky lead smelter at Avonmouth, have shown that when it comes to chemical hazards the forces of law and order move exceedingly slowly – if at all. When the authorities display the same zeal in stamping out abuses of industrial chemicals – the hard drugs of big business – as they put into tracking down pot smokers, workers may be able to feel that their health is taken seriously.

In the meantime there is only one safe attitude – extreme suspicion.

Workers can no longer accept bland assurances from management that all is well. Fears about chemicals are now the biggest single cause of enquiries to the AUEW's safety department.

Anxiety is growing, not just about risks of acute poisoning but about the long term threat to health from working in chemical-rich atmospheres.

o Even the most 'responsible' experts can do nothing to allay these fears. In 1958 Bryan Harvey and Robert Murray wrote that they were 'firmly of the opinion that the low vitality brought about by the absorption of industrial poisons is an important factor at the present time'. (*Industrial Health Technology*, Butterworth).

Both men were then in the Factory Inspectorate. Mr Harvey is now its chief and Dr Murray is Medical Adviser to the TUC.

In his 1970 annual report Mr Harvey wrote:

o 'The proliferation of more subtle hazards and particularly potential carcinogens must also be the subject of continuous vigilance. . . Any failure at the present time to bring these risks under control can only therefore be reaped as a bitter harvest, not by us but by the next generation.'

And again in 1971:

o 'If it is not possible to develop adequate measures of controlling the hazards which some processes create then industry may well have to take a decision not to develop a particular plant or process until the way ahead for both workers and the environment is clear. This is an uncomfortable thought which may cause a good deal of heart searching in many boardrooms.'

Dr Murray has made the same points himself but he wonders how control is to be achieved. In July 1972 he told a TUC conference on the environment:

o 'There is an industrial hygiene division of the Factory Inspectorate. The problem is that it has a staff of under 30 and I calculate that a staff of 300 is needed to tackle the problem of pollution at the workplace.'

There is no clear line between health and illness; it is easy to forget what it feels like to be really well, to get gradually used to often having a headache, feeling irritable or tired. In his book *The Toxic Metals* (Pan/Ballantine), Anthony Tucker presents evidence to show that there is an

'unrecognised proportion of the population which has been tipped over the brink into ill health by ubiquitous contaminants.'

He is referring to the daily doses of poisons taken in by the general population. For workers, getting poison both from the environment and from the workplace, the implications are frightening.

Workers' offensive:

These are formidable problems which cannot be left to 'boardroom heart searching'. By the time industry discovers that the bulge it has been probing is the wallet not the heart, it will be much too late.

This stage has already been reached in the more 'advanced' industrial economy of Japan where tens of thousands have now been disabled by mercury, cadmium and polychlorinated biphenyls.

Action is needed now if this kind of situation is to be headed off.

But official thinking has already shied away from measures that might blunt the competitive edge of industry. The Robens Committee rejected suggestions by the Medical Research Council for compulsory screening of toxic substances like that applied to new medicines.

Instead Robens recommended a standing 'advisory committee on toxic substances' to which manufacturers would notify basic details of *new* chemicals. In addition manufacturers would have a statutory duty to test for safety.

These proposals, if accepted *and enforced* would be better than nothing. But there is no suggestion in Robens for backing proposed law with the large force of hygienists, chemists, doctors and inspectors needed to investigate health risks and to check whether manufacturers' instructions for safe handling are carried out by employers.

These weaknesses are symptoms of the Robens' commitment to 'self-regulation' by industry – see page 228.

With or without Robens, workers will remain more or less on their own and will have to look to their own strength and organisation for protection. The problems may seem too complex to tackle, but you don't have to qualify as an industrial hygienist to get safe working conditions. What is needed is a recognition that, however complex the biological action of a particular poison and however little the scientists know about it, it will be a health risk only as long as there is a basic assumption that it's all right to expose you to some of it.

Pollution in the workplace and community results from the profits drive. Within the present economic and political system, it can be eliminated only when workers show managements that any threat to health will be answered by a threat to profits.

Recognising hazards:

First you need to be able to recognise chemical hazards and understand some of the jargon they are usually wrapped in. That is what the rest of this section is about.

The three types of risk to look out for are:

1. Poisons:
Industry usually refers to its poisons as 'toxic substances'. The effects of the main poisons on your body are dealt with in the next section.

2. Corrosives:
Acids and alkalis which burn whatever part of the body they touch and can blind you if they get in your eye.

3. Fire and explosion:
In spite of the enormous number of fires – 20 fire brigade calls a week in the chemical industry alone – fire is not the major killer you might expect. Smoke, fumes, and gases are more of a risk than the fire itself.

You can't tell just by looking at a substance whether it is dangerous in any of these ways. Many hazards, like dusts and vapours, are invisible.

The first consideration is whether a chemical can get into your body. Because 90 per cent of unwanted substances are found to have entered through the lungs, the most important question is: can you breathe it in?

The answer is not always obvious but its physical state should give some indication of risk:

Solids:

A solid chunk of something is unlikely to be dangerous but heat may turn it into a *liquid* and then a *gas* or *vapour*. Some substances go straight from the solid to the gaseous state – eg iodine and 'dry ice' (solid carbon dioxide). The main risk will usually be from fire, especially when the substance is stored in large quantities; many substances give off poisonous *gases* when burned. Some of the worst health risks arise when solids are turned into *dusts* or *vapour*.

Liquids:

Probably the widest range of hazards come in this form, most obviously acids, alkaline solutions and solvents. Liquids penetrate clothing (even viscous liquids like tar can work their way in) and some of them, notably phenol, easily penetrate skin. All liquids evaporate and the main health risk may be *vapour* which may be toxic, inflammable or explosive. Volatile liquids are ones that evaporate easily. They are said to have a high 'vapour pressure'. A very volatile liquid will quickly reach high concentrations in an enclosed space and because of this it may be more dangerous than more toxic materials that don't evaporate so easily. Volatility should not be confused with inflammability. Some volatile liquids, carbon tetrachloride for example, are not inflammable. Evaporation increases as more liquid is exposed to the air or its temperature is raised. In a fire it is not the liquid itself that burns but the vapour above it; the heat evaporates more vapour to feed the fire. The **flash point** of a liquid is the temperature at which its vapour is ignited by a spark. It refers to the temperature of the liquid – the air can be freezing. The lower the flash point the greater the risk and official regulations usually require special precautions when the flash point is below 73°F (23°C). The '**auto-ignition point**' is the temperature at which the chemical will ignite without the aid of a spark – perhaps 200°F higher than the flash point.

Dusts:

Dusts or powders are tiny particles of solids. Most workplaces generate dust, usually as an unwanted by-product of handling and processing materials. The main health risk comes from inhaling it. When dust is being produced by cutting, grinding or polishing you will probably be able to see it on surfaces near the machine. **But you cannot rely on being able to see it in the air.** The smallest particle visible to the naked eye is 50-100 microns in diameter while the particles most dangerous to your lungs are 5 microns or smaller (anything bigger is trapped by the lung's defences – described in the next section). The smaller particles do not even show up under an optical microscope.

When you can see dust in the air you can be sure that the smaller, breathable particles are there as well.

Chemicals in powder form can also irritate and penetrate your skin and they are easily transferred to your mouth and, on your clothes, to your home.

Dusts and powders may burn more easily than the solids they come from. A bigger risk is from explosions. A cloud of dust in the air can explode violently when ignited by a spark or flame. If there is dust on floors and ledges this can be whipped into the air by the blast and a second explosion follows. Explosions can travel right through a plant in this way.

The most notorious raw material for such explosions is coal dust in mines but many other dusts can explode, including flour, magnesium, zinc particles from metal spray.

The only sure way to prevent dust hazards is to insist on exhaust ventilation wherever dust is produced, plus regular cleaning of all surfaces. (See Section 6, Prevention.)

Normally-invisible particles may show up in a shaft of sunlight in a gloomy part of the workroom, but this won't tell you if they are harmful. A more useful check is to run your finger along a ledge; if the dust is any colour other than the grey of an ordinary household dust further investigation is needed. Many process dusts are white or cream. Deep black may be coming from oily sprays or a faulty heating device.

Vapours:

Vapours are tiny particles of liquid suspended in the air. Metals also vaporise at temperatures above melting point, as in soldering, welding and flame cutting. The metal particles quickly turn to *dust*, usually in the form of the metal's oxide – eg iron oxide when steel is being welded. Metal *fumes* are usually visible as a white plume or cloud above the process.

Vapour from liquids is usually invisible. Visible vapour may be referred to as a *mist* – eg, oil mist in engineering shops. Industrial hygienists may refer to both dust and vapour in the air as an *aerosol*.

The main health risk is from inhalation, though vapours can irritate eyes and skin.

Fire hazards are dealt with under 'liquids', above. If the mixture of air and inflammable vapour in a confined space is in the right proportions – as it is, by design, in the combustion chamber of a petrol engine – a spark will set it off and produce a violent explosion. 'Confined space' can mean anything from a gallon can to a whole workroom, so long as there is enough of the mixture to fill it in the right proportions.

Gases:

Gases are encountered as the raw materials, end products or unwanted by-products of many processes. They are often stored under pressure as *liquids* and leakage can rapidly fill the workplace with toxic or explosive gas. By-product gases are more likely to be a long-term health risk because the employer has no commercial interest in retaining them. Some are visible, eg, nitrogen dioxide (nitrous fumes) have a brownish colour and your nose gives you a good warning of others – eg, chlorine (if you can smell it you are getting too much). Others, eg, methyl bromide cannot be seen or smelt.

Because gases mix so easily with the air, exhaust ventilation must be installed wherever they are used or given off ; a fan in the wall is unlikely to be of any use. Specific health risks from the main gases are dealt with in the next section, under Lungs/gases.

Like vapours, inflammable gases need to be mixed with air (or oxygen itself) before they will burn or explode. In general industry, liquefied petroleum gas (LPG) is being used for more and more heating and burning jobs and stored in ever-increasing volumes. All tanks and cylinders should be well away from workrooms, preferably underground.

Most gases and vapours are heavier than air and will tend to 'flow' into pits and drains where concentrations can build up to dangerous levels.

Fire:

The fire risks described so far have all involved some 'trigger' like heat or a spark. Fire is really a violent chemical reaction between a substance and oxygen and the reaction can sometimes start in other ways. A number of inorganic chemicals, like the chlorates and some of the nitrates, while not themselves inflammable, can react violently with organic substances to start a fire. Particularly dangerous are the peroxides, eg hydrogen peroxide, used in dilute solution as a bleach, and organic peroxides sold as Butanox, Triganox or Lucidol, used as catalysts for curing resins in glass fibre reinforced plastics. All these could start a fire if they come into contact with paper or an organic solvent, for example in a heap of waste material. (A **catalyst** is a substance that triggers a chemical reaction in other substances without itself being changed in the reaction.)

Substances may appear in more complex forms than the ones described so far:

Mixtures:

Different substances blended together but not chemically joined.

Suspensions:

Mixtures of particles in liquids that will eventually settle out.

Solutions:

Solids or gases dissolved in a liquid. The solvent liquid may evaporate, leaving the solid behind – glyceril trinitrate solution in alcohol, for example, would leave you with highly inflammable overalls if some splashed on you and dried. Dissolved gases are released when pressure is taken off the solution – the soda water effect. The gas in acetylene cylinders is dissolved in acetone. The release of nitrogen dissolved in the blood gives divers the 'bends'.

Chemical terms:

Compounds:

These are substances that have been chemically bound together. The most familiar is rust, caused by iron and oxygen combining. The metal has oxidised; the rust is an oxide. Compounds can not only look completely different from their parent chemicals but also have different toxic effects – as with lead and its organic compounds. Lead is a soft grey metal; tetra ethyl lead, the petrol additive is an oily liquid.

Organic compounds are those which contain carbon atoms. Carbon atoms link easily with other atoms and more than half a million compounds are known. Organic chemistry started with the study of chemicals made directly from living things – organisms – and now gets most of its materials from coal and oil (which were once rotting organisms). Most of the new health problems are caused by organic compounds.

Inorganic chemicals are all those not containing carbon.

Hydrocarbons are compounds containing only hydrogen and carbon. Chemists can arrange them in many ways. One of the most important arrangements gives benzene and a series of related compounds. A different arrangement produces the series methane, ethane, propane, butane, hexane, heptane, octane. This series gets all sorts of things hooked onto it; alcohols give methyl alcohol (methanol), ethyl alcohol (ethanol – the one in drinks), and so on. Acetates give methyl acetate, ethyl acetate, and so on.

Aromatic compounds are all related to benzene. They include toluene, xylene and the trimethyl benzenes.

Halogens are the inorganic chemical group containing fluorine, chlorine, bromine and iodine.

Amines are compounds of ammonia.

In factories, organic chemicals are encountered most often as solvents. The main families, with some examples, are:

Aliphatic hydrocarbons: paraffins, white spirit

Aromatic hydrocarbons: benzene, toluene, xylene

Chlorinated hydrocarbons: trichloroethylene, perchloroethylene, 1.1.1. trichloroethane

Ketones: acetone, MEK, MIBK, cyclohexanone

Acetates: ethyl acetate, amyl acetate

Alcohols: methyl alcohol, iso-propyl alcohol

Glycol ethers: ethylene glycol monomethyl ether, ethylene glycol monobutyl ether (trade names cellosolve, oxitol, ethyl glycol, butyl glycol).

Farmworkers come across other chlorinated hydrocarbons in the form of insecticides like DDT, Heptachlor, and Lindane.

Some solvents carry particular risks for different parts of your body – see particularly benzene in next section – and all of them are narcotic. They can change your behaviour, making you sleepy, slow or 'drunk', and more prone to accidents, at quite low concentrations.

In the real work situation, health risks may take some unravelling. Many substances may be involved in different forms, as shown in the following examples.

1: Car battery

Casing: liquid/solid – pitch (dermatitis, skin cancer); solid/dust – blue asbestos, the most acid-resisting type, for reinforcing (asbestosis, lung cancer)

Plates: solids – lead and antimony; fumes – lead; dust – lead oxide (all highly poisonous)

Electrolyte: liquid – sulphuric acid (acid burns)

Charging: gas – stilbine from antimony (very poisonous); gas – hydrogen (explosive)

2: Welding

Welding can expose you to a rich cocktail of fumes, gases and physical hazards, as shown in the table below. Industrial hygiene surveys regularly discover dangerous concentrations of individual substances. More important is the suggestion from Dr J.Steel of the Industrial Health Unit at Newcastle

University that the combined effect of all the substances given off in arc welding, even if they are individually at 'safe' limits, may amount to a dose which is 40 times greater than a safe limit for daily exposure.

Welding and metal cutting hazards.
General dangers:
Threshold limit value – TLV – shown in bold after each entry
Ultra violet light: Damage to eyes ('arc eye' or 'welder's flash'). Skin cancer risk. UV is a special problem with argon gas shielding (argon arc).
Ozone: Present in all arc welding, most seriously in carbon dioxide (CO_2) and argon arc. Irritates nose and throat and damages lungs. Safe levels are regularly exceeded – if you can smell it, you are getting too much. **0.1ppm**
Carbon monoxide: Headaches, dizziness, slow reactions; can be fatal. Particular danger: CO_2 shielding. **50ppm**
Carbon dioxide: You suffocate if there's too much in air. Particular danger: CO_2 shielding. **5,000ppm**
Nitrogen dioxide: All arc welding, particularly at high amperage or with nitrogen shield. Nose and throat irritation, lung damage. **5.0ppm**
Iron oxide: If you can see the dust other toxic substances may be too concentrated. Apparently harmless on its own but can cause pneumoconiosis if other fumes, particularly nickel and chromium, are part of long-term exposure. **10.0mg/cu.m**
Coated rods and fluxes: Many coatings contain fluorides, zinc, lead, cadmium (health effects described below).
Phosgene: Trichloroethylene and perchloroethylene on degreased parts and in the air can be changed to phosgene by the heat of welding. This very poisonous gas can cause lung disease and death. People up to 200ft away have been affected. Stop work if very nasty smell comes off. **0.1ppm**

Specific dangers:
Stainless steel:
Chromium oxide – Fumes may contain up to 6 per cent chromates. Can cause nose ulcers and lung cancer. **0.1mg/cu.m**

Nickel oxide – Skin irritation, possible lung cancer risk. **1.0mg/cu.m**

Fluorides – Skin irritation, nose bleeds, general weakness. **2.5mg/cu.m**

Galvanised steel:

Zinc oxide – Can cause metal fume fever (described in next section). **5.0mg/cu.m**

Aluminium:

Fluorides, UV light – See above.

Ozone – See above.

Cadmium (on plated parts and in silver solder):

Cadmium oxide – Chest pains, coughing, dry throat, nausea and vomiting; kidney and lung disease. May be fatal. **0.1mg/cu.m**

Brass and bronze:

Zinc – See above.

Lead – Poisoning, nervous system damage. **0.15mg/cu.m**

Painted metals:

Lead – See above.

Mercury – Nervous system damage. **0.1mg/cu.m**

Zinc – See above.

Beryllium alloys:

Beryllium – Found in alloys with aluminium, magnesium and copper. Easily damages lungs. Can be fatal. **0.002 mg/cu.m**

Hard facing:

Manganese – Nervous system poison, loss of co-ordination, 'manganism'. **0.5mg/cu.m**

Local exhaust ventilation at the workpiece is essential in all processes. (See Section 6.)

Other hazards:

Burns: All processes. Wear flameproof aprons and gloves

Fire: All processes but particularly oxy-acetylene and oxy-propane

Explosion: Acetylene cylinders (handle gently; keep grease off internal fittings. If cylinder starts to heat up, get it outside, keep well away and try to cool it down with firehoses).

Electric shock: All arc systems

Noise: Excessively high levels in plasma arc only
Note:
TLVs are explained later in this section.

Concealed risk:

Identification of risks is made even more difficult by
the ways in which industry deliberately conceals chemicals
behind trade names and codes – or simply does not declare
ingredients.

Trade names are used to hide formulas from competi-
tors – and from customers who might be shocked to find out
how little had been spent on raw materials. Even the chemists in the customer's own laboratory may not know what a
branded chemical contains. We know of one product – a
polyurethane lacquer used on concrete formwork – whose
formula was not known to the firm that imported it from the
US. When forced to investigate, the importers found that the
lacquer would be a serious health risk if sprayed. There was
no warning of this on the can.

Codes are often used because management thinks the
shop floor will get confused if it has to learn the proper
names for things – or will get alarmed if it knows. Codes can
be even more confusing than straight labelling, especially
when the code extends to handling methods and first aid.
Code books get lost, which can be disastrous in an emergency. Ultimately the weakness of this system is that managements drawing up a hazard code will tend to underplay
the risks involved and you cannot easily check the judgement they have made.

Example – paint shops:

The solvent used as a thinner in paint shops in most
car plants is xylene, which is narcotic and also suspected
of causing cancer. Paint sprayers who occasionally feel a
bit dizzy or sick are probably suffering from the effects
of breathing xylene vapour. As long as the car manufacturers do not want this risk spelled out the paint firms
will not put a warning on the containers; they do not
want to be blamed for a walkout. In a different work
situation this failure to warn could be fatal: in the Swan
Hunter yard on Tyneside, three workers painting a
double-bottom tank in a ship's engine room were pois-

oned by xylene vapour. One died and his mates were unconscious for 15 and 18 hours.

All workers should know what they are handling. One of the first demands in any safety campaign should be for proper labelling which declares contents, health risks, safety precautions, and emergency action (first aid and fire fighting).

Finding out the exact identity of all substances used at work may be a long job, but trade names and codes can be 'cracked'. Methods and sources of information are suggested in Section 8, Action.

Concentrations:

When you have found out what vapours, fumes, gases or dusts may be in the air, you need to know how much of them you are getting and whether it is dangerous.

The concentration of a substance in the air is usually said to be so many parts per million (ppm). In this case both the pollutant and the air are measured by volume.

If you collected a million cubic centimetres of air from the workplace and analysed this sample you might find that it contained five cubic centimetres of, say xylene vapour. The concentration would be five parts per million (5ppm).

One million cubic centimetres is the same thing as one cubic metre. This is the amount of air you breathe each hour during fairly active, but not heavy, work. So, at the concentration of 5ppm you would be breathing in five cubic centimetres of xylene vapour every hour. That's about a teaspoonful of vapour – if you can imagine such a thing. Work in that atmosphere for 10 hours and you will inhale about 50cc – a couple of egg cups full.

Even though some of the vapour will be breathed out again, 50cc sounds like a lot of chemical to get into your body each day. Yet, in the case of xylene, the pollutant in this example, this would be considered a small 'dose'.

Whether a certain concentration of any substance is dangerous or not depends on several factors: how poisonous it is, how susceptible you are to the poison and whether you are getting that amount all day or only occasionally.

Almost any substance can be harmful if you get enough of it. Even water vapour, which is always in the air and is completely non-toxic, can be very dangerous for the person with chronic bronchitis who goes out in thick fog.

This is an extreme example of individual susceptibility. The xylene poisonings mentioned earlier may be more relevant: o one man died, o one was unconscious for 18 hours and one for 15. o Both survivors had transient liver damage but only one of them had kidney damage.

The distribution of your 'dose' through the working day is important. With carbon monoxide, for example, breathing a steady 30ppm for eight hours might give you a headache, or you might not notice it. Inhale the whole dose in a few minutes and it will probably kill you.

Pollutants collected from a sample of air may also be weighed. The concentration is usually given in milligrams per cubic metre of air (mg/cu.m). This is the way that concentrations of dust are most commonly measured. When really small quantities are involved the weight may be given in microgrammes (μg). Dust particles may also be counted, as in the case of asbestos fibres (see next section Lungs/asbestosis).

If one cubic metre of air from the workplace is found to contain 5mg of breathable dust, this is the amount you will breathe in during an hour's work, though some will be breathed out again.

'Safe limits'—TLVs:

Because it is expensive to keep the air pure, much effort is expended in devising 'safe' levels of contamination which, it is hoped, will not harm workers.

The most commonly used system is the 'threshold limit value', or TLV. The American Conference of Government Industrial Hygienists, which sets the limits, says a TLV is 'the level to which it is believed that nearly all workers may be repeatedly exposed day after day without adverse effect'. Exposure time is assumed to be seven or eight hours a day and 40 hours a week. Within each day the TLV for most substances can be treated as an average, according to

ACGIH; any exposure above the TLV should be balanced by periods below it.

Threshold values range from 0.001ppm (nickel carbonyl) to 5,000ppm (carbon dioxide). The levels for three common industrial solvents are: toluene, 200; trichloroethylene, 100; xylene, 100ppm.

Some chemicals, eg TDI (threshold value 0.02ppm) are so dangerous or fast acting at higher concentrations that the TLV cannot be exceeded at all without serious risk. ACGIH then gives the TLV a 'ceiling' designation which is really the same thing as the other kind of 'safe limit' you may come across – the maximum allowable concentration or MAC. The two must never be confused: exposures above a MAC limit could be disastrous.

There are many reasons why the TLV concept should be viewed with suspicion.

1. It accepts industry's economic assumption that it's all right to expose workers to contamination. Some of the limits are based on nothing better than 'reasonable freedom from irritation, narcosis, nuisance or other forms of stress'.

2. The levels are mostly based on inadequate information from animal experiments, observation of obvious symptoms in workers and some guessing inspired by experience of similar substances. ACGIH does not conduct research to detect long-term risks from small exposures. Even if it did, the chemicals would still be marketed while research was going on.

3. Even ACGIH does not claim that all workers will be safe: 'A small percentage of workers may experience discomfort from some substances at concentrations at or below the threshold limit, a smaller percentage may be affected more seriously by aggravation of a pre-existing condition or by development of an occupational illness'. The only way to protect this percentage would be to screen every worker for particular sensitivity or existing disease. (The working class is already the least healthy class in Britain.)

4. Even if the levels were safe for every worker, the system would only work if employers sampled the air regularly during each shift *and* supervised the exposure of each worker to ensure that no one exceeded the average for a day or a week. The firms who sell sampling equipment will tell you that most employers take no measurements at all.

5. Many factors can make a nonsense of TLVs. The air often contains mixtures of chemicals; sampling for all of them and 'calculating' the combined effect is a cumbersome and speculative procedure.

If other stresses are present, like heat, humidity, high pressures, ultra violet light or ionising radiation, the safety margins theoretically built into the TLV can disappear.

If you work a lot of overtime this will take your exposure above the dose on which the 40-hour exposure is based. (Ten hours overtime a week increases your dose by 25 per cent.)

6. TLVs have no legal force in this country although the Factory Inspectorate may use them as a guide when deciding whether to enforce the Factories Act requirement on protecting workers from 'injurious or offensive' impurities in the air.

7. Less than 500 substances have been given TLVs; thousands of dangerous substances have not.

It is clear that most workers are getting no protection from the TLV system. The whole idea is an uneasy compromise between what the more conscientious hygienists would like and what industry wants to be able to get away with. At no stage are workers asked what limits they would find acceptable – even from the point of view of discomfort, let alone risk.

Threshold limit values have been included in the Directory of Toxic Substances in the back of this book because they may provide a starting point in a clean air campaign, not because anyone involved with this book thinks they are safe limits. Dr Bob Hider and Dick Ranson of the Department of Chemistry at Essex University who prepared the Directory believe that 'TLVs are an excuse for industry to make people work in an atmosphere at certain levels of chemicals for eight hours a day, five days a week, year in year out, and it is for this reason that we really do not like the concept of TLV.'

The fact is you cannot be sure your health is safe until you know that the air you breathe is pure. The aim must be for 0ppm of any impurity. Employers can achieve this; they already do so when substances are too valuable to lose, or when contamination would ruin the product. Assembly shops in some ball bearing plants are sealed and filtered to the standards of an operating theatre. (Sampling methods are described in Section 6, Prevention.)

> o 'In order to obtain a workable system, the level now proposed (for asbestos) is such that possibly one per cent of those exposed to it will show the first clinical signs of the disease (asbestosis).'
> Craig Sinclair, **The Management of Hazard in Industrial Innovation,** Industrial Education and Research Foundation.

Environment:

Cleaning up your workplace may mean forcing the employer to install new extraction equipment. It is important to know what happens to the stuff that is extracted: if it just spews out over the neighbourhood it can undermine the health of families, particularly children, who are especially vulnerable to many poisons. Because the houses near factories are usually workers' houses, they get a double dose.

Concern for the environment can no longer be dismissed as a middle class luxury. It has often seemed that way in the past because the pressure groups are concerned to preserve what they've got from outside threats. For many workers and their families their whole environment is a threat; for them, environment means having the worst of everything: the worst workplaces, the worst housing, the most polluted neighbourhoods, the worst medical care, the worst schools. Not surprisingly, all this adds up to the worst health of all for the one class which depends absolutely on physical health for survival.

The fight against dangerous working conditions is just one part of the struggle for working class health and that struggle cannot be won while rotten environments are allowed to subvert health.

o The evacuation of working class families from their homes near the Enthoven lead smelter in Southwark, London, because their kids had dangerously high levels of lead in their blood probably doesn't reveal any new level of pollution, but a new level of awareness. o It is getting more difficult to spew filth into the air, as United Carbon Black found to its cost when local housewives blockaded its factory in the Port Tenant area of Swansea, in January 1973. Emission of muck into the air is supposedly controlled by the Alkali Inspectorate. There is no alkali inspector in Swansea – population 175,000.

As long as campaigns for a decent working environment and a decent living environment are regarded as separate, they will fail in the same way as much middle class protest. The employer's age-old threat of closing a dirty plant, as used at Swansea, can divide workers and protestors and so defeat them.

United working class action in the whole community – with links to other neighbourhoods to ensure that the filth cannot be taken elsewhere – can defeat the polluters.

One final point. **The staggering rate at which industry is now plundering and consuming the world's natural resources in the cause of growth and profits and at the expense of working and living conditions, cannot go on much longer.** o In as little as 20 years at the current rate of increase oil and other raw materials will be running out and workers will again be exposed to the cancer risk of extracting shale oil. Growth will be slowed, stopped or reversed. Union leaders who throw in their lot with the industrialists and politicians who promise prosperity through growth and who agree to sell jobs and working conditions in productivity wage bargains are just aiding the plunderers.

If wages are pegged to growth what happens when shortages force industry to contract? Big business is too busy to ask such questions. **Workers cannot afford not to.**

o In January 1973, the American Oil, Chemical and Atomic Workers Union staged the first national strike on a health and safety issue – against Shell Oil Company's refusal to meet demands for better health protection. A coalition of 11 environmental groups backed them. Because the Shell refineries could maintain 90 per cent production without the 5,000 OCAW workers, the damage done to Shell's public image and, through a threatened boycott of products, its profitability, was a useful extra pressure. o The strike ended in the first week of June when the company conceded most of the health and safety demands.

Conversions

1 metre (m)	= 39.7 inches
"	= 100 centimetres (cm)
"	= 1,000 millimetres (mm)
"	= 1,000,000 microns (μ)
1 cubic metre (cu.m)	= 1,000,000 cubic centimetres (cc)
1 cc	= approx 1 gram (gm) of water
1 gm	= 1,000 milligrams (mg)
"	= 1,000,000 micrograms (μg)

5

Disease

The last section dealt with ways in which dangerous chemicals, dusts, fumes and gases get into the workplace. This section describes what happens when they get into your body.

o **Explanation**
o **Introduction**
o **Cancer:**
Lung; skin; bladder; nasal.
o **The skin:**
Dermatitis; ulceration.
o **The Lungs:**
Pneumoconiosis; silicosis; asbestosis; byssinosis; farmer's lung; beryllium and cobalt; bronchitis; asthma; emphysema; gases.
o **Poisoning:**
Poisons, general; effects on your body.
o **Poisons:**
Lead; mercury; cadmium; benzene; phosphorus; organo-phosphorus compounds; arsenic.
o **Diseases caused by germs:**
Brucellosis; Weil's disease; anthrax.

Terms explained:

Two expressions used to describe diseases may cause confusion because the way they are used in everyday speech is not always the same as the medical meaning – **acute and chronic.**

An **acute disease or poisoning** is one that quickly reaches its most severe state – usually in a day or two.

Chronic illness or poisoning develops slowly – usually as a result of steady exposure to an irritant or poison, over a period of months or years. Some substances produce only chronic conditions – as with many of the dusts that affect your lungs. Many can give you acute poisoning if you get a large exposure and chronic (perhaps completely different) effects if you take in a little a day for a long time.

Diseases are also called **notifiable** or **prescribed** diseases.

A **notifiable disease** is one that your employer has to report to the appropriate inspectorate. The purpose of this is to help the authorities identify hazardous firms and processes, so you should try to ensure that all cases are notified.

Prescribed diseases are ones recognised by the Department of Health and Social Security as being **occupational** and therefore eligible for injury or disablement benefit. The occupation must also qualify as prescribed. There were 45 on the list at the beginning of 1973.

Using this section:

This section is to warn you of hazards so that you can check on precautions being taken and recognise any ill-effects at an early stage.

If you suspect that something is making you unwell: look up the substances you are working with (if they are not given here they may be in the 'Directory of Toxic Substances' at the back of the book) and see if they could account for your symptoms. If you think they do, go to a doctor without delay. Don't be embarrassed to tell him what you suspect, because he may not know the materials you work with.

o Do not use the book to make a diagnosis that nothing is wrong just because your symptoms are not mentioned or are slightly different.

If you don't feel well, for whatever reason, don't struggle on with your work. You are more likely to have an accident. Go home and get some rest. If you are at all worried about your health, for whatever reason, see a doctor. Tell him exactly what you do at work.

This section will be of most value if it is used as part

of a co-ordinated shopfloor attack on hazards in which a picture is built up of all the risk areas in the workplace and their safety record.

Introduction:

One of the main problems with dangerous substances used in industry is the very frequent changes that are made in methods of production.

There are thousands of hazardous chemicals. At first most of them are handled only by a few research workers, but then it may be decided to produce many tons of something because a new use has been found for it.

Instead of a few highly-trained technicians, thousands of workers come into contact with it; lorry drivers, storemen, part-time housewives, safety-conscious trade unionists, and tearaway lads.

Many of them don't know whether it is dangerous and often they don't even know its name. Dangerous chemicals time after time elude the best safety precautions, let alone the worst, and crop up in the most unexpected places, often causing illnesses that are quite unfamiliar to doctors.

We can describe the hard core of industrial diseases, many of which have been endangering workers for decades and, some, for centuries, but a complete textbook can never be written. The stuff you are working with today may be tomorrow's new disease.

Entry routes:

Harmful chemicals get into your body in three ways:

1. **Your lungs.** This is by far the most important route because it lets in not only substances that directly harm your lungs, such as chlorine gas and silica, but also poisons that attack other organs like your brain or your liver.

2. **Your skin.** This is the next most important route. Organic chemicals like nitrobenzene, aniline, phenol, tetraethyl lead, or nicotine easily penetrate your skin and can go on to harm other organs.

3. **Your stomach.** This method of absorption is much less important in industrial diseases. But you can absorb

E

poison into your system if you eat or smoke with dirty hands.

Effects:

There are four ways in which chemical substances can harm you:

1. Part of your body can be directly poisoned, either quickly when your skin is burned by acid, or gradually when small amounts of something like mercury slowly affect your brain and kidneys.

2. The chemical may be quite harmless when you first come into contact with it but the first exposure 'sensitises' you so that you become allergic to it. When you meet it again a few weeks later you have an allergic reaction, which may take the form of a skin rash, dermatitis or an attack of asthma. You may even have what amounts to a very serious fainting attack.

3. Chemicals can cause abortions and, worse, congenital defects and malformations in your child. Thalidomide had this effect and some chemicals used in industry probably carry the same risk. The developing embryo in your womb is probably more sensitive to very small amounts of poison than any part of your body. Because the damage is done in the very early stages of pregnancy, often before you realise you are pregnant, all women and not just the obviously pregnant should be stringently protected.

4. Many industrial substances cause cancer.

Cancer:

Introduction:

Other words for cancer are tumour, growth, carcinoma and neoplasm. The basic cause of cancers is not known but they very often result from long exposure to a small amount of a 'carcinogen', a substance that causes cancer. The best known are tar, shale oil and cigarette smoke. If you paint a spot on the skin of a rabbit with an extract of tar it will get cancer of the skin after some months. Extracts of tobacco smoke have the same effect.

When a cancer develops, in your skin for example, it

starts with a single cell – a piece of skin so small you can't see it – which begins to behave in a way that disregards the normal functioning of skin. It grows until it produces a mass of tissue – the cancer – which serves no useful purpose and eventually grows into the rest of your body and kills you. (Tissue is a word doctors use to describe the substance of your body – bone, muscle, everything). Tiny pieces break off from the growth and are carried in your blood to other parts of your body where they grow into more cancers, known as metastases.

Symptoms:
The symptoms of cancer depend on where it is, but you nearly always lose your appetite and a lot of weight – often very dramatically. (There are plenty of other reasons for losing weight). A cancer can kill you in a few weeks or it may take years. It can usually be cured if detected early enough.

Risk:
Many occupations expose you to carcinogenic chemicals. In some cases the carcinogen is so potent that its effects are obvious: benzidine, for example, is so efficient at causing cancer of the bladder that its use is prohibited in this country.

In other cases you are exposed to such small amounts of weak carcinogens that you have only a slightly higher risk of getting cancer. These risks are often difficult to detect.

o A statistical survey of machine room print workers showed that their chances of dying of lung cancer were 30 per cent higher than average. Lung cancer is a common disease, especially if you smoke cigarettes, but usually it doesn't develop until years after exposure to the carcinogen. For these reasons even 30 per cent more people dying from it would go unnoticed by the workers in a machine room: most of the victims would have retired or moved to other jobs before the illness developed.

We cannot wait years while scientists play with statistics and computers to establish the exact risk. The fine mist of mineral oil given off by the presses is suspected as the cause of lung cancer. But it could be ink particles or solvent vapours – or a combination of all three.

The technical and statistical debate misses the point: workers are expected to go on breathing an unpleasant atmosphere while the scientists find out how harmful it is. Insist on your right to breathe clean air and you will go a long way towards keeping your name out of the next statistical survey.

Oil mist is more of a problem in engineering. It is significant that the 'threshold limit value' allows 5 milligrams per cubic metre of air but conditions can be unpleasant with half this concentration.

The example is typical of almost all carcinogens. You have to be exposed for a long time and then there is a long latent period when nothing happens.

By the time you get the cancer you may have retired, you may have forgotten the six weeks, twenty years ago, when you worked in the tyre factory or the dye works.

Cancer of the lung:

Cancers of the lung (bronchial carcinomas) almost always develop just below the bottom end of your windpipe. Everybody in Britain has a good chance of dying from one. In most cases the actual cause is unknown, though if you smoke cigarettes you are much more likely to get one. Cigarette smoke contains tars which are carcinogens; so does the polluted air of our towns.

Occupations:

Several jobs increase your chances of getting lung cancer. Work in a machine room has already been mentioned. Others include the preparation or handling of chromates, nickel salts, arsenic compounds, radioactive dusts and, probably, carcinogenic organic chemicals. Asbestos dust causes this cancer and also the rarer cancer known as mesothelioma, described later.

Symptoms:

The actual symptoms are usually very slight at first. It is often found on a chest X-ray taken as part of a general check-up. A slight cough, with or without phlegm, or a slight hoarseness of your voice may be the only warnings and you are unlikely to take much notice. The first real warning comes when you start losing weight, by which time it is normally too late to do anything.

Perhaps one in a hundred can be cured by a major operation involving removal of one lung or part of it. Radiotherapy may prolong your life by as much as a year.

Cancer of the lung is a prescribed disease only for workers producing nickel by the Mond process.

Cancer of the skin:

Skin cancer is caused by long periods of contact with a variety of substances, including mineral oils, paraffins, tars and arsenic. Several kinds of radiation, including X-rays and ultra violet light, can also cause it (see Section 3).

The cancer will usually develop on a part of your body in direct contact with the substance, like your hands, arms, face or neck. Other parts can be affected if the substance penetrates your clothing; the skin of your scrotum, the bag that contains your testicles, is particularly vulnerable.

The cancer starts as a wart or as an ulcer that does not heal. Ulcers may have raised 'rolled' edges.

In the years between the two wars, scrotal cancer was so common in the cotton industry that it got the name of 'mule spinner's cancer'. Workers in charge of mule spinning machines got a fine spray of lubricating oil at crutch height so that their overalls and underwear became saturated. After years of exposure cancer developed in the skin of the scrotum. As many as a thousand may have died.

Compulsory substitution of more expensive lubricant for cheap shale oil, plus stricter health regulations, have greatly reduced the risk for cotton workers but there is still a real danger in other jobs.

The main risk seems to be from unrefined oils. In the past these were used extensively as cutting fluids in engineering machine shops. Oil companies were able to unload the rag-tag of their production in this market.

○ A successful legal action in 1968 by the widow of a GKN worker who died of scrotal cancer has led the main oil companies and larger employers to switch to safer *solvent-refined* cutting oils. *But there is no statutory requirement to use solvent-refined oils.* Some very carcinogenic fluids may still be marketed by 'less reputable' companies, or for special cutting tasks.

It is important to find out what kind of oil is being used in machine tools and to insist that it is the safer type. Even then, further precautions are advisable because the cancer risk in refined oils is not known. It is assumed to be small because years of use in the motor industry (where unrefined oils would not protect the delicate innards of engines and gearboxes) have produced few cases of skin cancer. On the other hand few motor mechanics get the continuous spray of oil on the front of their bodies that is experienced by operators of many automatic machines.

Safe or not, there is no reason why workers should submit to being sprayed with oil. Machines designed to protect the operator from this insult will not be produced until workers demand them.

Meanwhile many new cases of scrotal cancer can be expected among engineering workers as a result of past exposure to cheap cutting oils.

Precautions:

Try to keep oil (even 'safe oil') and carcinogens off your skin, clothing and overalls as much as possible. Wash regularly at work, making a particular point to wash before going to the toilet so that you don't get oil or other carcinogen onto your scrotum. Wash all over after work, particularly the scrotum. Change overalls regularly and don't put oily rags in your pocket. These requirements may show up inadequacies in the firm's arrangements for washing, showering and renewing overalls. (See Section 6.)

Check regularly for warts on your skin or scrotum and get treatment straight away. This is even more urgent if they start to bleed or grow. Skin cancers can usually be cured if treated early enough, so it is important to get into the habit of checking for warts, or ulcers that don't heal, and to keep on checking long after you retire or leave the risk area.

Prescribed and notifiable:

Skin cancer is a prescribed disease if you get it from

working with arsenic, tar, pitch, bitumen, mineral oil (including paraffin), soot or any compound product (including quinone or hydroquinone), or from radiation.

It is also a notifiable disease. In 1971, 70 cases were reported, three fatal. Since most victims die after they leave work this is a pretty meaningless figure.

Cancer of the bladder:

This very dangerous and unpleasant cancer is caused by a variety of organic chemicals, many of them used in the rubber and dyestuffs industries. Most of the known ones are listed below. The disease is also known as papilloma of the bladder.

The most notorious chemical causing bladder cancer is beta-naphthylamine, manufacture and use of which has been prohibited in this country since 1967. The chemical occurred as an impurity in an ICI product called Nonox S which was used by tyre and cable manufacturers throughout the 1930s and 1940s to stop rubber perishing. Unfortunately it had exactly the opposite effect on human bladders, as hundreds of workers are now finding out.

o Christopher Wright is one of the victims. He started work for Dunlop at Speke, near Liverpool in 1946 and was exposed to fumes from hot rubber containing Nonox S. Bladder cancer was diagnosed in 1966.
His bladder has been removed and he has to urinate through his anus.
In 1972 the High Court awarded him damages of £15,000 against ICI and a further £1,000 against Dunlop. The judge held that ICI should have known by January 1940 that the impurity in Nonox S was a cancer hazard.
Dunlop was found to have increased the risk by not advising all workers employed before 1949 to go for medical tests.
The Appeal Court judges found that ICI actually did know of the danger by 1943 and possibly as early as 1940.
Nonox S was not withdrawn until 1949.

The rubber industry succeeded in preventing publication of the facts until 1954 and, according to Dr Robert Case, the man who led the investigation that indicted the chemical, 'the Factory Inspectorate went along with this suppression of knowledge'. [British Society for Social Responsibility in Science Conference on **The Work Environment**, January 1972.] The Rubber Manufacturers Association insisted that Dr Case should leave out of his report a recommendation that investigations should continue in case there were other killers to track down. [Socialist Medical Association pamphlet **An Occupational Health Service Now.**] It is believed that current investigations will soon show that workers who entered the rubber industry after 1950 do not face any increased risk of bladder cancer.

The manufacture and use of beta-naphthylamine was not banned until 1967. Alpha-naphthylamine, the substance that contained the beta compound as an impurity, may be manufactured under strict control.

o Workers are now paying a dreadful price for the negligence of ICI and the rubber industry. One hundred and eighty three workers in the rubber and cable industries are known to have died of bladder cancer between 1945 and 1964. By the beginning of 1973 there were thought to be another 500 workers or widows with a claim against ICI.

Even this figure does not touch the full size of the horror. It is possible that as many as 80,000 workers were exposed to Nonox S during its profitable 20 years in industry. The worst of the epidemic is now over but it can take up to 40 years for the tumours to develop. The final toll will not be known until the 1980s.

Beta-naphthylamine and the other carcinogens in this family of chemicals (the aromatic amines) are absorbed through your lungs and skin and removed by your kidneys and bladder. This has the effect of concentrating them in these areas, with consequent risk of cancer, particularly in the bladder.

Symptoms:

Bladder cancers usually start as warts in the lining. The first symptoms are likely to be bleeding into your urine, or an attack of cystitis or a sudden inability to pass urine. Cystitis causes pain in your bladder and it hurts when you urinate.

Treatment:

In the early stages it may be possible to cure these

cancers with a relatively minor operation although a constant watch has to be kept for fresh growths. If you work with or have worked with any of the chemicals listed below it is essential to have tests done on your urine at least every six months so that the disease can be caught early. If you know anyone who might have worked in plants where Nonox S was used up to 1949, make sure they are having medical checks. Thousands of workers are still unaware of the risk they have been exposed to.

Known carcinogens:

The following are known to cause bladder cancer and are controlled or prohibited by the Carcinogenic Substances Regulations 1967:

Prohibited: beta-naphthylamine, benzidine, 4-amino-diphenyl, 4-nitrodiphenyl and their salts.

Controlled: alpha-naphthylamine (providing it contains no more than one per cent of the beta compound), ortho-tolidine, dianisidine, dichlorbenzidine and their salts, also auramine and magenta.

2-acetyl-amino-fluorine is also suspected as a bladder carcinogen.

Industries that have been or are at risk include, chemicals, rubber, cable making, textile dyeing and printing, gasworks, security printing, manufacture or use of a rat poison called ANTU.

Prescribed, not notifiable:

Bladder cancer is a prescribed disease if you contract it from the manufacture or use of the listed chemicals – with the exception of auramine and magenta which are prescribed only if you work in a place where they are produced.

If your employment is in the prescribed group you should be given Cautionary Card F2257 when you leave.

Incredibly, cases of papilloma of the bladder do not have to be reported to the Factory Inspectorate.

Wood dust:

Workers in the furniture trade often become ill after working with certain woods, usually imported from distant parts of the world, especially box wood substitutes. The dusts and oils given off by the woods can affect you in four ways:

1. The dust acts as a direct irritant – your nose and eyes smart and run. Irritation of your bronchi makes you cough and get short of breath.

2. The oil is absorbed by your lungs and circulated to your brain. Here it causes nausea and giddiness and disturbances of vision – you may see double, have temporary blindness or misty vision, or see strange colours. The effects last for a few hours.

3. The dust can cause dermatitis.

4. It can cause cancer of the nasal passages. The symptoms of this cancer are pain in your face, blocked nostrils and bleeding from your nostrils or down the back of your throat.

The cancer can be treated with radiotherapy or surgery. As usual with occupational cancers, it is a disease of later life, occurring as a result of long exposure to the dust. More than 40 woods have been implicated as irritants. Only beech is thought to be carcinogenic; incidence of the disease is declining as less beech is used in furniture.

If you get any of the symptoms listed under 1 and 2, press your employer to substitute a different wood or install better ventilation.

Prescribed, not notifiable:

Illness caused by working with gonomia kamassi (African boxwood) and nasal cancer caused by working in timber furniture factories are prescribed diseases. (Nasal cancer is also prescribed for workers making nickel by the Mond process.)

None of these conditions is notifiable.

The skin:

Skin is a remarkable material – elastic, waterproof and self-repairing – but it was not designed for the treatment it gets in industry. The worst hazard is skin cancer, described earlier, but less dangerous skin conditions cause untold misery on a far wider scale.

Dermatitis:

Dermatitis is an inflammation of the skin. It is the commonest skin disease and also the commonest industrial disease. It causes about 20,000 spells of absence from work each year, with men taking an average of about a month to get back and women about six weeks.

The disease can be caused by tens of thousands of chemicals and apparently harmless substances, including mineral oils, resins, pitch, cement, sugar and penicillin. It is often called eczema.

It usually occurs on the part of your body exposed to the chemical, though it sometimes spreads to other areas. The part most exposed is affected first, so it usually starts on your hands unless they are protected by gloves. With some dusts and fumes, the first signs may appear around the eyes, neck and face.

There are four kinds of risk:

1. Primary irritants – chemicals that are harmful in their own right. Most dermatitis is caused by this type of substance.

2. Substances that remove the oil from your skin – solvents, thinners, etc.

3. You become allergic to a particular substance and get an attack whenever you handle it. It may not affect anyone else at work. Sometimes the reaction is sudden and very violent: your whole body is affected and you may be sick.

4. Heat and radiation.

Symptoms:

Your skin becomes swollen, red and tender. It oozes or weeps and develops scab-like crusts. The effects may be confined to your hair follicles when it is very slight – the goose pimple spots on your skin go red and itch.

If the affected skin is invaded by bacteria they may produce spots, boils or blackheads, or increased tenderness.

Dermatitis does not involve any part of your body other than the skin and there is no danger at all of anyone else catching it from you. But it can be very embarrassing, especially if your face is involved and the skin is infected. Your skin may itch so badly that you can't get to sleep.

Prevention:

The longer or oftener you are exposed to the chemical, the more severe and long-lasting the dermatitis. It is often easy to find the substance responsible, but it can be extremely difficult. If the brand of some chemical you work with is changed you may be exposed to a different impurity, or something that someone else is using may find its way onto your bench. You or your mates may be able to find the cause much more easily than your doctor can; it is a good idea to make a note of who gets dermatitis and what they have been handling.

As soon as you stop handling the substance responsible, the dermatitis starts to get better; it leaves no permanent ill-effects – though you will remain sensitized to something that has caused an allergic reaction. Soothing creams may help but they are no substitute for avoiding the cause of the trouble.

When you return to work try to avoid contact with the oil or chemical that caused the attack. If you have to go on using it you should be protected by gloves or a barrier cream – though in many situations barrier creams are pretty useless. Tongs may be useful in some jobs. None of this advice is much good if you work a lathe or other machine where gloves cause accidents ; barrier creams *may* help but the best hope is to wash really carefully and often. Don't use strong solvents, paraffin or abrasives to get the skin clean, they will increase your chances of dermatitis by breaking down the skin's defences. If you use 'waterless' jelly-type hand cleaners, rinse them off well – apparently clean hands can otherwise be left with an invisible film of jelly and irritant.

When the work involves abrasive materials as well as irritating substances – for example the swarf that comes with cutting oil in turning, or the glass fibre that goes with resins in moulding work – the smallest scratches should be cleaned and covered with a plaster.

Cutting oil in machine tools must be mixed in the right proportions and changed regularly – not just topped up. In shops on piecework or tight measured day work a high urine content is not unknown. Doctoring the oil with antiseptic is not a good idea since it may cause irritation in its own right.

The skin's resistance to dermatitis is also lowered by jobs that force you to keep your hands in water, particularly if it contains detergents, or if they are always wet with sweat. Some people seem able to resist almost any irritant; others, particularly those prone to skin disease anyway, have a much greater risk of dermatitis. Some are even allergic to rubber gloves, hand cleansers, barrier creams, or supposedly soothing creams.

Many work systems and agreements will make much of the advice given here look unrealistic. The shopfloor offensive on hazards must see to it that the highest standards of care are built into the job – see Section 6.

Compensation:

Dermatitis is a *prescribed disease* so you should be able to get injury benefit while you are off work. The employer can notify the Factory Inspectorate if he wants to but he doesn't have to. It is difficult to see how risk areas in industry can be pinpointed under this system.

Even though dermatitis can be financially disastrous, for example if you have to take a less skilled job in order to avoid a particular irritant, you will be lucky to get compensation from your employer. 'Legal first aid' may improve your chances – see Section 11, Winning damages.

The main causes of dermatitis are:

o All forms of mineral oil, including diesel, lubricating and fuel oils.

o Chemicals, notably alkalis, chromates, bichromates and synthetic resins.

o Solvents, thinners and degreasers, such as 'white spirit', paraffin, trichloroethylene, turpentine and petroleum products.

o Tars, pitch and other coal tar products including chemicals in the phenol and cresol family.

o Soot.

o Radiation, including X-rays and radiant heat.

o Friction, particularly when dust or grit gets between clothing and skin.

Chrome ulcers:

Chromates and bichromates used in chromium plating, dyeing and tanning can give you 'chrome ulcers' or 'holes' as well as dermatitis. The liquid or dust from the process gets into cracks or cuts in your skin and forms deep holes which will take weeks to heal. You can also get irritation or ulceration in your nose.

Protective clothing should be worn to keep the chemicals off your skin. Insist that it is comfortable, clean and properly maintained; leaky gloves are not just useless, they increase the risk. Wash liquid or dust off the skin immediately. The slightest break in the skin should be washed carefully and covered with a waterproof dressing.

You can get 'holes' from working with alkalis, acids and formaldehyde. The same precautions apply.

Chrome ulceration is grouped with dermatitis as a prescribed disease. It is also notifiable: 89 cases were reported to the Factory Inspectorate in 1971.

The lungs:

Introduction:

The job of your lungs is to get oxygen into your blood and carbon dioxide out. They are constructed on the same pattern as a tree, with hollow trunk, branches, twigs and leaves. The trunk is the windpipe, the branches and twigs are progressively finer air tubes, or bronchi. These tubes penetrate all parts of your lungs, deep inside your chest. The leaves are the alveoli. These are minute air sacs which together form a very large area in close contact with the blood that flows all around them. Here the oxygen enters the blood and carbon dioxide leaves.

The air in your alveoli is kept fresh by breathing and oxygen from the air is carried to all parts of your body, dissolved in your blood. (It is actually combined with haemoglobin, the substance that makes your blood red.)

Only the very finest – invisible – dust particles can penetrate to your alveoli. The rest are filtered out by your nose, or stick to the fine film of mucus on the walls of your bronchi. The mucus carries them up to your mouth. Dust penetrating to the alveoli is collected by a system of very fine tubes called the lymphatics which carry it towards the central area of your lung, where the bronchi join the windpipe. It stays there for the rest of your life.

After a few years the lungs of all city dwellers are stained black by the fine particles of soot in the air. This is the result of atmospheric pollution – see below under bronchitis – but the soot itself seems to do no harm.

Other dusts are not so harmless. When silica or asbestos dust is deposited in your lymphatics, your lung reacts with small areas of inflammation. As this continues, fibrous tissue appears in your lungs, destroying their natural elasticity. The alveoli are also destroyed, so your blood cannot absorb so much oxygen – see below under emphysema.

Silica and asbestos are in your lungs permanently, which means that even a small amount will continue to irritate them for the rest of your life.

Pneumoconiosis:

Pneumoconiosis is the name given to a group of lung diseases caused by dust – **silicosis** (silica); **coal miner's pneumoconiosis** (coal dust); **asbestosis** (asbestos fibres); **byssinosis** (cotton); **bagassosis** (sugar cane); **farmer's lung** (mould spores).

Miners have been dying from it for at least 2,000 years, and probably since the Stone Age. The phrase 'blood on the coals' has a grim enough meaning for British miners but, apart from the terrible toll from accidents, about one in 10 – 30,000 men – suffers from some degree of **coal miner's pneumoconiosis**. Some 40,000 miners and ex-miners receive disablement pensions because of the disease. More than 700 new cases are diagnosed by the Pneumoconiosis Medical Panels each year. And each year doctors write 'fibrosis of the lung' on the death certificates of more than 1,000 miners.

Medical knowledge has come a long way since 1934 when a Medical Research Council report concluded that there was no evidence that inhalation of coal dust caused fibrosis. The disease is now recognised and the means of prevention are well understood. Dust suppression techniques succeeded in reducing the incidence of the disease but mechanisation is now undoing the good work. New machinery introduced since the early 1960s increases dust as well as productivity. Dust control techniques have not kept up and the result is a rising incidence of pneumoconiosis. The incidence per thousand workers rose by 35 per cent between 1969 and 1970, though these new cases date from conditions several years ago.

Symptoms:

The first symptom is an unusual shortness of breath when you exert yourself. It gradually develops over a period that may vary from six months to ten years into severe shortness of breath with the slightest exertion. Even walking slowly can be difficult and exhausting. Your cough brings up spit which may be flecked with blood; you lose weight. Lips, fingernails and the rims of your eyes become permanently blue, as though with cold.

Finally your heart is affected, as it is by any chronic lung disease. The effects of your heart failing are even greater loss of appetite, loss of weight, shortness of breath and weakness. Your ankles and liver may swell. At this stage in the disease, drugs may help a little but you cannot expect to live more than a few years. The full course of the disease may take as little as a year to kill you but 10 is more usual.

If exposure to the coal dust is stopped at an early stage the disease may not progress, although it may still shorten your life. Mild pneumoconiosis increases your chances of getting tuberculosis. Although TB can now be treated with drugs it will make your disability worse. The damage it does to your lungs can never be repaired.

Silicosis:

This is the oldest of the dust diseases; the first victims probably contracted it from silica dust while fashioning tools and weapons from flint. Inexcusably it continues to take a heavy toll of ruined and shortened lives.

Silica is the world's most abundant mineral and anyone working silica-containing rocks will be exposed to the hazard, whether they are after coal, uranium, gold – or the rock itself.

Apart from miners, many other groups are at risk, including quarrymen, tunnel workers and masons working sandstone, granite, slate or flint.

In foundries, the silica dust from sand blasters and sandstone grinding wheels proved so lethal that employers were forced to use harmless substitutes such as corundum. The risk remains in foundries because silica sand is still used in moulding. Even with grit blasting, large amounts of dangerous dust are released from castings during fettling. Mechanisation of sand handling by conveyors, for example, can increase concentrations in the air. New resin materials being added to moulding sands may bring different health risks.

Sand instead of grit blasting may still be used in the construction industry for cleaning buildings.

In steelworks much dust is generated during knocking out of refractory bottom plates and ladle wrecking. A pressure-fed respirator should be worn for ladle wrecking.

o Forty eight new cases of silicosis were diagnosed among foundry workers in 1970. Seventy six foundry workers had fibrosis of the lung on their death certificates that year.

o Potteries are the next biggest risk area in industry, with 29 cases diagnosed and the same number of deaths with fibrosis recorded in 1970. Incidence of the disease is being reduced but ventilation standards are in general still bad.

In manufacturing, fine silica sand used in white scouring powders and fillers for whitewall tyres can also put workers at risk – classic examples of needless hazards since the whiteness of the powder or the tyre doesn't make it work any better. Other abrasives, like pumice, work just as well but are not white.

Exposure time:

The longer you are exposed to dust the more certain you are to be affected. One single exposure will not do you any harm – as far as can be told. Workers in scouring powder factories using old, leaky plant that covered the place in dust have died after only a year's exposure. Others can work in heavy concentrations of silica dust for twenty years before they develop the disease. For most people ten years is enough. How susceptible you are probably depends to some extent on the previous state of your lungs.

Treatment:

There is no real treatment for silicosis, except to stop breathing silica dust at the first symptoms and hope the disease will not get any worse. Since miners and other skilled workers cannot stop their exposure without losing their livelihood, employers must be made to provide proper dust control.

Asbestosis:

Asbestos dust produces a disease very similar to silicosis in its effects on your lungs and your health – asbestosis.

o It is taking an increasing toll of workers: 64 are known to have died in 1965, 107 in 1970, 113 in 1971. The number of new cases diagnosed by Pneumoconiosis Medical Panels rose from 82 in 1965 to 153 in 1970 – more in one year than were diagnosed in the eight years up to 1938.

o In one company alone, a survey of 100 asbestos workers recently found 65 with X-ray abnormalities.

The disease can be mild if you have had only a slight exposure but it can kill you in as little as two years, affecting your heart as in silicosis.

There is a definite and real danger in all jobs where asbestos is handled extensively – see table on p 99.

There are two main forms of asbestos. **'Blue' asbestos (crocidolite) is so dangerous that it should be banned.** Small tonnages are still being brought into Britain which means that, somewhere, workers are handling this lethal substance. Thousands of tons have been built into old structures, ships and gas works, just lying in wait for the demolition worker. You can recognise it by its rich lavender blue colour but this may not show up when mixed with other types and it fades when exposed to extreme heat.

White asbestos (chrysotile) is also dangerous. Asbestosis is usually produced by a fairly lengthy exposure to the dust and individuals vary in their susceptibility. Six weeks may be enough if you work in heavy concentrations of dust.

Although such conditions have been illegal in factories

since 1931, some asbestos firms are known to have exposed their workers to dense dust until very recently and it would be naive to think that it could not happen today, somewhere among the thousands of firms handling the material.

Cancer risks:

About half the people who get asbestosis also get lung cancer. Because the lung cancer seems to require a smaller exposure it is possible to get it without having asbestosis first.

If you smoke and work with asbestos your chances of getting lung cancer are increased many times over.

Another sort of cancer known as **mesothelioma** is closely linked with very small quantities of asbestos. Mesotheliomas are growths in the lining of your lungs or belly. Almost all mesotheliomas are caused by asbestos and the blue type is said to be ten times more likely to cause them than the white variety. Some experts have claimed that five minutes inhalation of blue asbestos dust can produce cancers up to 20 years afterwards (report in *Guardian*, 23 February 1973).

You can develop mesothelioma without having any fibrosis in your lungs.

No one knows how many workers are killed by mesotheliomas – partly because it takes so long for them to develop, and partly because they are not always identified. A survey of male asbestos workers by the TUC Centenary Institute of Occupational Health suggests that, 30 years after first exposure, about one in 200 will be found to have died of mesotheliomas. ○ Among women who worked in the same factory between 1936 and 1942, deaths from lung and other cancers were four times as common as they would have been if the women had not worked with asbestos. They also had an excess of cancer of the ovaries.

With the discovery of unusually large numbers of mesotheliomas around asbestos factories and among the families of asbestos workers, and the link now being made with cancers of the stomach and alimentary tract, asbestos is emerging as the all-purpose killer, versatile in the ways of death.

All workers, not just those in asbestos processes, should be on their guard against the material, particularly during building alterations in factories and when new substances are introduced which could contain it.

o In 1972 workers at British Leyland's Cowley plant were exposed to blue asbestos when pipes were being de-lagged. When British Leyland and Carrier Engineering were prosecuted under the new Asbestos Regulations 1969, the Factory Inspector who discovered the offence said he would have preferred an unleashed tiger to have been in the plant to the blue asbestos that was on a walkway and floor.

The new regulations do not lay down a maximum limit for asbestos concentrations in the air but the Inspectorate works to a 'hygiene standard' of two fibres per cubic centimetre of air, averaged over four hours. The standard for blue asbestos is a tenth of this concentration, measured over 10 minutes.

Where the dust is found to be less than these levels the inspectors will not enforce the regulations requiring exhaust ventilation, respirators and protective clothing.

This implies that there is a safe limit for asbestos.

o At a conference on health risks in construction in 1971 Mr Bryan Harvey, Chief Inspector of Factories, was asked if it was possible to say that any concentration was safe. 'I certainly cannot get any of our medical advisers to make that statement: I wish I could,' he said.

Industry cannot afford to treat this useful raw material with the respect it deserves. The Department of Employment booklet, *Asbestos: Health Precautions in Industry*, seems to accept this: 'The economics of asbestos production and the processes that are commonly associated with it do not readily lend themselves to total enclosure.'

Workers cannot afford *not* to treat asbestos with the utmost respect.

It is important to see that the regulations are strictly enforced and to apply higher standards whenever possible – particularly on respirators. See next Section, Prevention.

Prescribed, not notifiable

Asbestosis and mesotheliomas caused by asbestos are prescribed diseases. Lung cancer is not because it is assumed that you will be receiving a disability pension for asbestosis by the time you develop the cancer. The assumption is false. (Disablement benefits and common law compensation for dust diseases in general are dealt with later.)

Other dangerous dusts:

Other mineral dusts can cause pneumoconiosis. They include talc, fireclay, asbestine, mica, china clay, graphite, synthetic silica. Mixed metal dusts given off by welding also cause a form of the disease – see p 111.

Byssinosis:

Byssinosis is a disabling lung disease caused by inhaling cotton, flax or hemp dust for several years and it is common among workers in cotton rooms and in blowing, carding, winding and spinning processes. One in five cotton operatives probably has the disease in some stage of development.

Symptoms are shortness of breath, cough and sputum, irritation of your eyes and nose, plus a fever. The disease is known as 'Monday fever' because you get attacks when you return to work after the weekend. During the week you appear to get used to the dust and you get better.

If you stop breathing the dust your lungs appear to recover completely, but if exposure continues the disease progresses: wheezing and shortness of breath last all week and don't stop when you get away from the dust. The final result is disablement, and an early death from emphysema (see below, p 145).

Dust control and ventilation in the cotton industry are still inadequate. New manufacturing processes have extended the hazard to operations beyond the stages of manufacture which used to carry the main risk. Higher processing speeds and inferior cottons have increased dust levels.

The Factory Inspectorate has adopted a threshold limit value of half a milligram per cubic metre of air – measured after cotton 'fly' has been filtered out.

Many mills, especially those spinning coarse cotton, will have problems meeting this level. Workers should insist that managements adopt a programme for meeting this limit, take regular air samples and disclose the results.

Prescribed, not notifiable

Byssinosis is a prescribed disease and 110 new cases were diagnosed as eligible for disability pension in 1970. Fibrosis of the lung was recorded on the death certificates of 37 cotton workers in 1970. The disease is not notifiable to the Factory Inspectorate.

Farmer's Lung:

Farmer's Lung is caused by breathing the dust of mouldy hay. It occurs when you become allergic to the mould spores and the result is severe coughing and shortness of breath with fever. You quickly recover from one attack, but after repeated attacks over a number of years your lungs are likely to become scarred as in all the other pneumoconioses.

After a long fight by the National Union of Agricultural and Allied Workers, the disease was recognised as 'industrial' in 1965. Many farmworkers are affected. In Ayrshire, where the warm, wet climate favours growth of the spores, about eight per cent of farmers and farmworkers suffer from it. (Farmer's Lung should not be confused with silo filler's disease. Fresh silage contains nitric oxide which forms nitrogen dioxide when air gets into the silo. This gas is described later under poisonous gases.)

Bagassosis:

Other mouldy vegetable products can cause Farmer's Lung and it may be a risk in handling bagasse, the sugar cane fibre used in making boards.

Malt workers suffer chest disorders from inhaling a kind of fungus produced during the germination of barley.

Chronic bronchitis, asthma, emphysema:

Chronic bronchitis is a disease of the air tubes of the lung – inflammation of the bronchi. One in three people over the age of 60 suffers from it and each year more than 30,000 die from it.

The first symptoms usually appear in winter with coughing, perhaps only in the morning at first, which brings up sputum. It goes on more or less all the year round, usually getting a lot worse in winter, when the sputum increases in quantity and turns yellow.

In the early stages you are not short of breath and the disease develops very slowly. The final stages are very similar to the final stages of pneumoconiosis, but they may develop so slowly that you die of something else. Often chronic bronchitis causes you to wheeze a lot as you breathe, and it then resembles asthma. It is not so much that you are short of breath but that you are unable to breathe easily. This is because the muscles that surround your bronchi contract and make the finest tubes very narrow, so that the air does not flow freely in and out.

Asthma:

In an attack of asthma, the bronchi can become narrow and then widen again in as short a time as half an hour, usually in response to something you are allergic to. The result is extreme shortness of breath. Substances which have this effect include TDI (toluene di isocyanate), used to make polyurethane foam; thiurals and thiuram disulphide used as accelerators in synthetic rubber, in the peptidation of rubber and as fungicides; maleic anhydride and piperazine; and enzymes used in making 'biological' detergents. These substances also make your nose and eyes run, as in hay fever.

Not prescribed, not notifiable

Emphysema:

Emphysema may be the end result of pneumoconiosis, asbestosis or chronic bronchitis. It can also affect you in later life after you have had only the mildest chronic bronchitis; it then appears to be a disease in its own right. Basically emphysema is the destruction of the alveoli – the lungs lose some of their ability to exchange oxygen for carbon dioxide. As a result the air passages become distended. The main symptoms are extremely severe and progressive shortage of breath and loss of weight. Your chest becomes a strange barrel-like shape – as if you have taken a deep breath and can't let it out. It also feels like that. (See the description of the last stages of pneumoconiosis, above.)

Not prescribed, not notifiable

Causes:

The main cause of chronic bronchitis is air pollution, especially by sulphur dioxide. This is the gas that erodes stonework in large towns like Leeds and London – you can imagine what it does to your lungs. Most of the sulphur dioxide in the air used to come from ordinary coal fires and the introduction of smokeless fuels has done a lot to reduce it. Car exhausts and oil-fired heating may be about to reverse the downward trend in sulphur dioxide concentrations in the centre of London and the Northern cities.

Six million tons of sulphur dioxide and about a million tons of smoke spew into our atmosphere each year.

Chronic bronchitis is not recognised as an industrial disease so you cannot get injury or disablement benefit when you are off work in the winter or forced to retire early. Miners in Australia can. In Britain it is believed that the link between coal dust and chronic bronchitis is not definitely proved and it has not been linked with other occupations in a way that satisfies the authorities. On the other hand it is a much commoner disease among workers than middle-class people who live and work in clean atmospheres. (See table below.)

It is quite possible to have chronic bronchitis, pneumoconiosis, or any other lung disease at the same time.

Disablement pensions:

All victims of prescribed dust diseases are entitled to a disablement pension under the Injuries Act – once their condition has been diagnosed by a Pneumoconiosis Medical Board. Having made the diagnosis the Board estimate your degree of disability in terms of percentage and your pension is graded accordingly. Percentages below 10 per cent all qualify for the 10 per cent rate of benefit – just over £1 a week.

But before you can get to the board a medical panel has to be satisfied that a full-size X-ray of your chest is abnormal enough to be true pneumoconiosis. X-rays are a notoriously unreliable guide to disability: workers with definite disability are rejected at this stage because their radiographs look almost normal. Others, with X-ray abnor-

Occupational factors:

There is a marked variation in the incidence of bronchitis in different occupations. The inception rates (attacks per 100 men) in a National Insurance Survey were:

All occupations together (average)	3.69
Miners and quarrymen	7.24
Labourers	5.59
Drivers	4.96
Foundry workers	4.71
Transport	4.11
Construction	4.10
Engineering	3.8
Service: office	3.79
Service: Food and drink	3.46
Woodworkers	3.27
Farmers	2.25
Sales	2.11
Professional	1.89

These broad categories conceal differences; for instance, in the last category, draughtsmen have twice the rate of teachers

malities, go forward to the Board and are diagnosed as having 'Category 2 simple pneumoconiosis'. Even though at this stage of the disease they may have no disability, they are rated as 10 per cent disabled.

Those who watch over the Industrial Injuries Fund were not happy with this situation – partly because of the injustices caused by 'rejection by X-ray' and partly because they did not like paying out the tiny '10 per cent' pension to those who were not yet disabled.

A committee of the Industrial Injuries Advisory Council spent five years looking into the definition of pneumoconiosis and, at the time of writing, its report is imminent.

Reliable advance information suggests that it has recommended a diagnosis system much more closely linked to disability. All claimants will be given a *lung function test*. This gives a much better indication of disablement than the shadows on an X-ray plate. There will be two main effects:

1. Unfair rejections will become less common.

2. Those with Category 2 simple pneumoconiosis but no impairment of lung function will not get a pension. The committee made other recommendations which may help to undo some of the injustices of the old diagnosis methods:

1. Although bronchitis is still not recognised as an industrial disease, workers with Category 1 or 2 pneumoconiosis and reduced lung function thought to be caused by bronchitis should get a pension.

2. Young men, say 25 or 30, who quickly develop Category 2 shadowing, even without reduced lung function, will be recognised as being at risk from further exposure and recommended to leave their dusty trade. This situation will be recognised as disablement and therefore pensionable.

Whether these recommendations lead to a more just system will depend, as before, on the way the panels and boards interpret them. It is doubtful if the proposals for taking bronchitis into consideration have been written strongly enough to overcome traditional reluctance to pay out for this condition. Continuing reliance on the old X-ray categories as the easiest way to distinguish between disablement caused by prescribed dust diseases and that caused by non-prescribed conditions could still cause injustice.

The only way out of the nightmare caused by this penny-pinching bureaucracy is to build a *real* welfare state (see last few paragraphs of this section).

The constant fight for fair compensation which absorbs so much time and energy in the trade union movement is important; but nothing suits the employers better than having the workers' attention diverted away from the *cause* of such diseases.

A concerted attack on dust, backed with demands for the highest possible standards of medical supervision in dusty trades, can prevent disablement. Compensation can only ease its financial burden.

Common law compensation:

Meanwhile the chances of obtaining compensation by taking your employer to court are improving slightly.

Asbestosis:

In July 1970, seven men with asbestosis were awarded a total of £86,469 against the Central Asbestos Company whose numerous and persistent breaches of the 1931 Asbestos Regulations at its East London factory caused the disease. Many other workers and widows are claiming damages against asbestos companies.

Coalworker's pneumoconiosis:

Early in 1974 a crucial test case will determine whether thousands of coal miners can win damages for pneumoconiosis. With massive backing from the National Union of Mineworkers, four Durham miners are suing the National Coal Board on the grounds that its negligence – or that of the old coal owners – gave them pneumoconiosis.

Bronchitis:

Formerly the courts echoed the official opinion that chronic bronchitis was not an occupational condition. There was not much point in suing your employer for lost earnings or early retirement.

Not any more.

o In March 1973 a retired moulder and sandmiller was awarded damages in the High Court because, it was held, dust at work not only gave him pneumoconiosis but worsened the main cause of his serious disability – chronic bronchitis and emphysema. Charles Wallhead was awarded £5,000 damages against his former employers, Ruston and Hornsby of Lincoln. Since early 1972 his wife had had to wash and shave him and he now had to sleep in a sitting position, on the ground floor, said the judge.

Recognition by the courts that chronic bronchitis can be caused by working conditions, and that an employer is liable if he fails to guard against this risk, opens the legal doors to thousands of similar cases – but does not guarantee success. See Section 11, Compensation.

Beryllium:

Beryllium is a very light metal used in the manufacture of special metal alloys, and beryllia ceramics. The materials are used in various specialist applications, including valve and semi-conductor components. Use in fluorescent tubes has been stopped.

Workers preparing the metal from its ores have been affected but the main hazard comes from handling the highly toxic beryllium oxide and certain beryllium salts. Poisoning may be either acute or chronic.

With acute poisoning you progressively develop shortness of breath over a few days. You feel very ill and have a cough that brings up blood-stained sputum. The dust or fumes directly damage the alveoli of your lungs, giving you a sort of 'instant pneumonia'. There is no treatment and you may well die. If you recover you may go on to develop the chronic form.

Chronic berylliosis causes lung damage similar to emphysema, coming on at least six weeks after exposure and developing over months or years. Several years can elapse between exposure and the start of the disease.

o In one of the three cases of chronic berylliosis notified to the Factory Inspectorate in 1971, the disease was diagnosed in 1969 – 13 years after the worker's last exposure. Of the other two cases, one came from the same factory and the third worked in a foundry where he had been exposed to both beryllium and cadmium fume.

The average concentration of dust in the air during a working day should not exceed two micrograms per cubic metre and, as some people may be susceptible to less than that, ventilation must be very efficient. Concentrations must be checked regularly.

Beryllium poisoning is both prescribed and notifiable.

Cobalt:

Cobalt is not so dangerous as beryllium but it also affects your lungs. The condition is known as 'hard metal disease' and its effects may be similar to pneumoconiosis.

The main risk comes from grinding of tungsten carbide tools in which cobalt is used as the 'cement'. Good exhaust ventilation should be installed to extract the dust from grinding. **The disease is not prescribed or notifiable.**

Poisonous gases:
There are two main groups:
1. Irritant gases. Gases like nitrogen dioxide, am-

monia, sulphur dioxide, hydrogen chloride, and chlorine
have a very strong and unpleasant smell and are actually
painful to breathe in. You will instinctively try to stop
breathing and get away, but if you are forced to inhale them
you get a sort of 'instant pneumonia'. With nitrogen dioxide this does not start until six or seven hours later. Some
of these gases are used very extensively in the heavy chemical industry and all of them are met with in innumerable
other places. Ammonia is used in making fertilisers; hydrogen chloride is given off from hydrochloric acid, used to
'pickle' metal before it is plated. For other risk areas, see
Directory of Toxic Substances at the back of the book.

2. Gases that are easy to inhale. Carbon monoxide,
hydrogen sulphide, hydrogen cyanide, arsine, phosphine,
nickel carbonyl, are actually much more lethal than the first
group although they may have no smell (carbon monoxide),
an unpleasant sickly smell (hydrogen sulphide) or a rather
pleasant smell of almonds (hydrogen cyanide) even at concentrations low enough to be safe. In contrast to the first
group, these gases are not difficult to inhale and you can be
dead in a matter of minutes – particularly from hydrogen
cyanide.

Nickel carbonyl is used in the extraction of nickel;
arsine is found in the holds of ships when sea water gets
into a cargo of iron ore containing arsenic; hydrogen cyanide is used in fumigation, in the chemical industry and in
electro-plating.

(Non-poisonous gases, like nitrogen, argon or methane, can also kill you: if they are allowed to displace the
oxygen from the air you can be asphyxiated. Pockets of carbon dioxide in a mine are known as 'choke damp' or 'black
damp', methane is known as 'fire damp'. Oxygen can be
absorbed from the air by the rusting process inside sealed
iron and steel vessels, so do not assume that such places will
be safe to enter just because they have not contained anything poisonous.)

Poisoning:

Introduction:

This part deals with substances that circulate in your blood stream and attack organs other than your lungs or skin – even if they got in by those routes.

Your body has a limited number of ways in which it can go wrong. Different poisons can affect the same organs to some extent, so that their effects have a lot in common. Lead and benzene for example both affect your bone marrow and make you anaemic.

The liver:

Almost every disease of your liver will make you jaundiced. When this happens the whites of your eyes, and then your skin, goes yellow. At the same time you will probably lose your appetite and feel ill. In extreme cases, your ankles and belly swell up, you may become unconscious and die. Poisons which can do this to you include TNT, chloroform, carbon tetrachloride and tetrachloroethane.

Toxic jaundice is notifiable. Poisoning by tetrachloroethane is prescribed.

Chemicals in this group can damage your liver severely enough to kill you inside a week. (Weil's disease, a hazard to sewermen and farmworkers – see page 170 – has a similar effect.)

The kidneys:

When your kidneys are poisoned – by mercury for example – the most common effect is perhaps 'acute renal failure', which means that you pass very little urine, or none at all. What you do manage to pass may be bloodstained. Your face and ankles swell, you lose your appetite and feel ill.

These symptoms can also be brought on by shock following a serious accident, particularly when you have lost a lot of blood.

Chronic kidney disease begins very slowly. You gradually lose the ability to concentrate your urine: the first sign may be having to get up more often at night to pass urine.

After a few years chronic kidney disease can give you high blood pressure – hypertension.

Blood:

The red colour of your blood is due to the pigment haemoglobin which is contained in the red blood cells. These are made in the bone marrow and if production is interfered with you become anaemic. Anaemia can result from not having enough iron or vitamin in your diet, but in industry it can be caused by poisons like benzene. Toxic anaemia is notifiable.

When your blood gets short of haemoglobin it is not so good at distributing oxygen around your body. You may not notice the effects of a slight shortage, but severe anaemia makes you tired and breathless. When the poison stops entering your body or when you take iron or vitamin tablets the marrow usually recovers.

Some poisons can damage your marrow permanently and the result is known as 'aplastic' anaemia. Your haemoglobin has to be artificially replenished with blood transfusions for the rest of your life, which may be short. Aniline and nitrobenzene have a direct effect on your haemoglobin. They link up with it chemically so that it cannot carry oxygen. Your eyes, fingertips, ears and lips turn blue. You feel unwell, with headache, weakness, dizziness and breathlessness. When exposure is stopped, the haemoglobin recovers. No permanent damage seems to be done though some experts think repeated attacks can lead to anaemia.

Other cells in your blood are the white cells and platelets. Lack of white cells lowers your resistance to bacterial infection:

The results vary from a severe crop of boils to fatal septicaemia or pneumonia. Platelets make your blood clot properly so that you stop bleeding after you are cut. A shortage of them makes you bleed abnormally: you bruise very easily, get a rash of minute haemorrhages in your skin, bleed into your urine, or cough up blood. You can also get brain haemorrhages—sometimes fatal.

White cells and platelets are affected by the same poisons that make you anaemic. Benzene is the most important – see p166. More rarely the same chemicals can give you leukaemia. Leukaemia is a sort of cancer of the blood and usually appears many years after exposure to the chemical or to radiation. Acute leukaemia kills you in a few weeks or months but, if treated properly, some chronic forms of the disease will allow you to live for years.

Brain and nervous system:

Your brain and nervous system can be affected in a variety of ways by poisons. Any illness has some effect on your brain, even if it is only to make you anxious.

If you are poisoned, you may be so terrified that your racing pulse, trembling, sweating skin and heavy breathing are the most obvious things wrong with you. Fear also makes you excited, and if you make some incoherent remarks this may be mistaken for delirium. Doctors often use the word 'confused', by which they mean that your mind is wandering – you don't know where you are and whatever you say is nonsense to anyone else.

Other general effects of poison on your brain – which apply to any illness – include feeling faint and giddy, losing your appetite, and having difficulty in concentrating or sleeping.

Doctors can distinguish four sorts of effects of poisons on your brain and nervous system.

1. **Minimal effects** – slight loss of ability to make judgements, to concentrate, to do simple arithmetic. You may be forgetful. The danger lies in not realising that anything is wrong – as in driving when you are drunk.

An agricultural worker was marking out the areas of crops to be sprayed by an aeroplane when he got soaked with the organo-phosphorous insecticide. He noticed that he wasn't able to add up the acres of crops that had been sprayed but he did not suspect he had been poisoned. At the end of the day he drove a tractor straight into a ditch and was lucky not to be injured. The organo-phosphorous insecticides include Parathion, TEPP, HETP, OMPA, EPN, Systox, Mipafox, Malathion.

When your brain is more seriously affected you may have a headache, feel giddy, be unable to stand up, feel sick, have a singing in your ears or be unable to think.

2. Maximal effects of poisons on your brain – epileptic fits, coma and death. Some poisons first make you feel very drunk and unwell, then you go into progressively deeper coma until you stop breathing and die. Often you have fits before becoming unconscious: you fall to the ground, your limbs shake uncontrollably and you wet yourself. You might begin to wake up in the next half hour if you are not severely poisoned.

Many substances have this effect if you take in enough of them. The organo-phosphorus insecticides mentioned earlier can kill you in this way in an hour. Volatile organic chemicals are dangerous, especially the chlorinated hydrocarbons like carbon tetrachloride, chloroform, 'trike' (trichloroethylene), ethylene dichloride and tetrachloroethane. These substances are used to dissolve things like oils, rubbers, glues, paints and fats. They can also dissolve their way quite quickly through rubber boots or gloves, and can be absorbed by your skin as well as your lungs.

In the same family of chemicals is methyl bromide, used in fire extinguishers, refrigeration, chemical production, fumigation and as an insecticide. It is highly toxic, you can't smell it until there is already too much in the air and the effects usually don't hit you until several hours after breathing it or getting it on your skin. Substitute materials should be used, but if you have to work with it the process should be enclosed. Protective clothing won't keep the gas out.

Phenol splashed on your skin rapidly affects your nervous system: within minutes the signals sent out by the brain can get so weak that you stop breathing. Instant first aid is vital if you get splashed – see Directory of Toxic Substances.

3. Poisoning of specific, localised parts of your nervous system. You may for example lose the use of some of the nerves in your arms or legs. This condition is known as peripheral neuritis or polyneuritis and its effects will depend on which nerves are affected.

If the nerves of sensation are involved the affected part, usually a hand or foot, goes numb. You usually get

F

a tingling feeling before numbness really sets in.

If the nerves controlling your muscles are affected you may experience a form of localised paralysis. This is one of the symptoms of lead poisoning.

Carbon disulphide (poisoning is notifiable and prescribed) used in large amounts in the viscose rayon industry, can have both kinds of effect. (It is also suspected of causing heart disease.)

One of the most recently discovered effects of the chlorinated hydrocarbon insecticides may also belong in this group. It is known by the nickname of 'Derbyshire droop' after the farmworkers in that county who found they were unable to get an erection after spraying insecticides. All recovered when taken off spraying – but one took a year.

4. Damage to your eyes, which are part of your brain and nervous system. There are many different symptoms, including blindness, double vision and 'tunnel vision' – you see only what is exactly in front of your eyes.

Methyl alcohol (wood spirit) causes all these, plus stomach pains and unconsciousness, usually about 24 hours after being absorbed from your stomach. If you recover, your eyesight may well return to normal. With smaller exposures over several days, the symptoms appear more slowly. Irritation of eyes and skin is a warning that you are getting too much.

Methyl alcohol is used as a solvent and in the production of other chemicals, including formalin.

(You can also be blinded by many corrosive substances, if they splash into your eyes and destroy their transparency. The list is a long one, including acids, alkalis, molten metals, and liquid gases like sulphur dioxide and ammonia. The worst and most common corrosive is caustic soda – sodium hydroxide.)

Lead:

Lead is dangerous in all its forms – the metal, its oxides, salts and organic compounds. One of the oldest of industry's toxic hazards, it remains the single biggest cause of poisoning at work while arousing increasing concern as a community health risk.

Because your body gets rid of it very slowly, lead is a cumulative poison. Without going to work in industry, everyone picks up a tiny daily dose from the food they eat and the air they breathe. Most of the lead that you eat with your food passes straight through your gut but the little that is absorbed ends up in your blood where it joins the lead absorbed by your lungs.

It is possible to accumulate more than 40 micrograms of lead in every 100 millilitres of blood, just by living in a town or city. You only have to double this concentration to be on the threshold of serious poisoning (or be well over it if your personal threshold is low).

If you actually work with lead processes this can happen very easily. Most cases of poisoning are caused by inhalation of fumes or dust in the working atmosphere.

All the workers in a lead smelter for example will have slightly higher levels of blood lead than ordinary city dwellers. A minimal increase in blood lead doesn't appear to be dangerous but there is no certain level above which the effects of poisoning appear. Some workers are healthy with quite high levels of lead and others develop serious illness at levels only slightly above 'normal'.

Normally your body keeps the level of lead in your blood within reasonable limits by storing any excess in your bones, where it slowly accumulates during your life but – usually – does no harm. When you absorb lead too rapidly for this method of disposal to work, the level of lead in your blood rises and it begins to poison you. One of the first effects is to poison your bone marrow, which interferes with the production of red cells and makes you anaemic.

It also attacks your nervous system, causing localised weakness – usually in the muscles of your wrist. Many scientists believe that, long before this obvious sign emerges a lot of people will have undergone subtle behaviour changes caused by the effects of the poison on the brain itself.

While the scientific debate goes on, throwing increasing doubt on present 'safe' limits for lead exposure, workers should aim for the smallest possible concentrations in the air and in their blood. Individually, 45 micrograms/100 millilitres is high enough, but a better warning of bad conditions is the average level for a group of workers. If this goes above about 30 conditions probably need investigation.

If you work in lead processes you should be given a general medical examination at intervals varying between weekly and quarterly, according to the regulations for each process. A blood test may be given for haemoglobin (to see if you are becoming anaemic) or for lead in the blood. You will probably be taken off work with lead if haemoglobin falls below 12 grams per 100ml or if lead rises above 80 micrograms per 100ml. When the levels return to normal you can be returned to your usual work.

Lead workers are now fighting for two important rights:

1. That the results of blood tests should be disclosed in full and the figures explained to their satisfaction.

2. That they should continue on full pay when suspended from lead processes because of over-exposure.

Symptoms:

The first symptoms of poisoning are a feeling of tiredness, and vague muscular aches followed by constipation, colic, headache and paleness. The colic is a very bad stomach pain which usually comes on after a few days of constipation. The pain can last several days but an injection of calcium cures it in a few minutes. It may be difficult for a doctor to be certain you have not got appendicitis or a perforated stomach ulcer. Anaemia from lead poisoning is not usually serious, but it may make you tired and breathless. The other symptoms are usually much worse. Muscular weakness, or 'lead palsy' does not usually occur until you have worked in a lead process for some years. Typically it affects the muscles of your right wrist so that your hand droops when you try to hold it up. 'Wrist drop' can be disabling if not properly treated.

The muscles first attacked are actually those you use most. For most manual workers this means those of the right wrist but during Prohibition in the USA it affected the ankle muscles of cabaret dancers who had been drinking whisky made in a lead still.

The most serious form of poisoning is lead encephalopathy, which will probably kill you. Symptoms are delirium, paralysis or numbness of parts of the body, fits and coma.

Occasionally, the symptoms of lead poisoning come on unexpectedly. This can happen if you have 'flu or are forced to lie in bed for a few weeks for some other reason and the lead stored in your bones is released.

Children:

Children are particularly vulnerable to lead poisoning. Not only can they pick up more than adults in the same environment – from lead-paint on imported toys, pigments in gummed papers and street dust on their fingers – but they need a smaller amount to become ill. Poisoning can cause mental retardation and, after perhaps ten or twenty years, kidney disease. Lead poisoning can also cause kidney disease in adults and a link with liver disturbance is suspected.

Check what happens to the dust and fumes extracted from your workplace – they may be spewing out over the places where children play. Don't go home in your work clothes – see references to washing facilities and overalls in the next section.

Tetraethyl lead:

The effects of tetraethyl lead poisoning are quite different from those described above. It is an oily liquid which is easily absorbed from the skin and sometimes the lungs. It acts rapidly on your brain and has often killed workers in a matter of hours. The symptoms are the same as those for any severe poisoning of the brain – delirium, fits and coma.

The chemical is added to petrol as an anti-knock agent and this is why car exhausts provide one of the main sources of lead in the air. In industry the greatest hazards may be for those who don't realise they are handling it: motor mechanics have been poisoned after regularly washing their hands in petrol. US garage hands were found to have blood lead levels way above average. Storage tanks that have contained TEL will remain contaminated long after they have been completely emptied of liquid.

Other organic compounds of lead, such as lead stearate, used as a filler in plastics, are also dangerous.

Occupations:

Industry is consuming ever-increasing quantities of lead (see p98) and poisoning can occur in a wide variety of processes. They can be divided into four main groups:

1. Raw materials. Mining and the production of lead from its ores and as a by-product of zinc smelting. These processes can generate large amounts of lead fume and dust, as was demonstrated by the outbreak of lead poisoning at Rio Tinto Zinc's Avonmouth smelter in 1972 and by numerous cases of occupational and environmental pollution by the lead industry which have been exposed since then. Smelting contributes the biggest share of poisonings.

2. The hundreds of manufacturing processes where lead is used, particularly where there is exposure to molten metal – everything from car batteries to printers' type. The danger occurs when the metal is heated to considerably above its melting point and fume is generated. Such temperatures are unusual in ordinary plumbing but 'chemical plumbing' – lining vessels with lead – is a very hazardous job, producing large amounts of fume in a confined space. The list of activities is almost endless and always changing.

3. Pigments and paints – the manufacture and use of paints and surface treatments containing white and red lead. Although the use of these pigments has been greatly restricted since the days when they were freely used to paint children's toys, they are still a hazard. Many household leases still specify exterior decoration with a good quality lead paint. Pink primer for joinery still contains it as do special protective finishes for ships and engineering structures. Welding or flame-cutting of treated metal can give off dangerous fumes. Old paintwork can be dangerous if you burn it or scrape it off dry and old lead-painted joinery should not be chucked on the bonfire.

4. Production and use of organic compounds: Chemical industry, refining, plastics, garages.

Prevention:

Because you will get most of your lead intake from the air you breathe at work, the main responsibility for prevention lies with your employer. If concentrations in the air are too high, nothing you do will prevent you accumulating too much lead in your blood.

Filter-type respirators provide inadequate protection and you should not be expected to wear one for long periods – see next section.

The aim must be to make the air safe to breathe without protection. There are various definitions of 'safe'. The list of TLVs prepared in the US and republished here by the Factory Inspectorate gives 0.15 milligrams per cubic metre of air but this is 75 times as much as the level which the US Government Environmental Protection Agency recognises as a health hazard in city air, and more than 150 times the limit for Russian cities. Clearly the TLV is an absolute upper limit.

These figures are obviously important but they are not much use to workers unless management is regularly sampling the air and making the results available to them in precise terms. It is no use to be told that 'tests were satisfactory' unless you know the standards by which safety was measured. See 'air sampling' in next section.

Personal precautions:

If the air is clean, the rest is easy. All you have to do is see that lead material from the process does not get to your mouth. Wash well, scrubbing under your fingernails, before eating or smoking. Don't work on an empty stomach. Plenty of calcium, eg milk and cheese, helps the disposal of lead in your bones. Watch for a blue line around the gums, close to the teeth.

Action:

The most important thing to do when someone develops lead poisoning, or is taken off because of high blood lead, is to stop it happening again. Stop the process responsible until adequate safety measures are taken or methods are changed.

Notifiable, prescribed.

Lead poisoning must be notified to the Factory Inspectorate. It is important to see that cases are in fact reported.
o Cases reported by industry in 1970 totalled 74 and there was a sharp rise to 122 in 1971. Part of the rise was caused

by a Factory Inspectorate investigation into the health of lead workers which 'sometimes led to the notification of other cases'. (1971 annual report.) The recent figures should be compared with the total for 1956 – only 49.

Most lead processes are covered by special health regulations which lay down intervals for medical examinations and usually exclude women and workers under 18. A copy should be on the wall; it is important to see that the regulations are followed.

Lead poisoning is prescribed.

Mercury:

Mercury (quicksilver) is the only metal that is liquid at room temperature. Although it seems harmless enough when you handle it occasionally it is a very dangerous poison. It evaporates easily at room temperature and a hazardous concentration of odourless vapour can quickly build up in the air. This can happen when large amounts are exposed without proper ventilation or when spillages are allowed to collect in benches and floors. Some of the compounds of mercury are even more dangerous.

Poisoning:

Poisoning is usually caused by inhalation but skin contact is also a risk. It can affect your body in three ways.

1. Diarrhoea, vomiting and gum disease. You have mouth ulcers and swollen bleeding gums that can lead to all your teeth dropping out.

2. Kidney disease – you lose your appetite and feel tired and unwell. Your ankles swell.

3. It affects your brain. The first sign is usually a fine tremor which makes your hands shake so that you can't lift a cup of tea without spilling some. It spreads to your legs so that you can't walk. At the same time you may become very shy, easily embarrassed and irritable. This strange illness is known as 'erethism'. It was once so common among people who felted rabbit fur for hats by dipping it into tubs of mercuric nitrate, that the expression 'mad as a hatter' became part of the English language.

The hatters are now sad history but the growing use of mercury and its compounds (see p 98) not only puts more workers at risk but also threatens the health of whole communities.

> o In 1953 there was a serious outbreak of mercury poisoning among the peasants and fishermen of Minimata Bay in Japan; the effluent from a plastics factory polluted the bay so that the fish contained high levels of mercury. Fish formed a large part of the community's diet and poisoning struck on a massive scale.
>
> Victims suffered tremors, paralysis, numbed limbs, blindness, deafness and convulsions. Dozens died, hundreds were disabled, and an unknown number of children were born mentally defective.
>
> The polluters refused all compensation until 3,000 fishermen and peasants stormed the factory and were beaten off by police. The company paid out £100 per adult victim. Finally, in 1973, seventeen years later, a long campaign of legal action extracted £1½ million and an apology from the company.

Coastal mercury pollution is now so bad that fishing is forbidden in some areas and all Japanese have been warned to restrict their consumption of sea food. Fishing bans have also been placed on certain lakes in Canada and Sweden.

Uses:

1. As a metal, mercury is used in scientific instruments, thermometers, barometers, direct current galvanometers, mercury-arc rectifiers, and contact breakers. The chemical industry uses it on a large scale to produce chlorine and caustic soda.

2. Mercury compounds. These account for the biggest consumption of mercury and the worst pollution hazards. Compounds are found in surgical dressings and ointments, pigments, anti-fouling paints for ships. Mercuric sulphate is used as a catalyst in the production of acetaldehyde, an important organic chemical for the manufacture of PVC plastics and many other products.

The organic compounds – methyl, ethyl, tolyl and phenyl mercury – are used as fungicides, particularly in the preservation of seed corn. They are among the most dangerous chemicals known, especially the first two.

Legal:

Mercury poisoning is a notifiable disease. Three cases were reported by industry in 1970 and four in 1971. Not all cases are reported and there is still a very real risk of poisoning, as shown by this quote from the 1971 annual report of the Chief Inspector of Factories:

> o A number of factories using mercury in the manufacture of scientific instruments have been surveyed. In some instances environmental levels of over four times the TLV of mercury vapour were found and some firms did not seem aware of the serious health hazard that could be created by such high concentrations.

Prevention:

The TLV for mercury vapour and compounds is 0.05 milligrams per cubic metre of air (organic compounds 0.01-mg/cu.m). As with all poisons affecting the nervous system this is likely to be revised downwards in the next few years and the lowest possible concentration should be fought for.

The whole work system must be very carefully designed to minimise exposure of liquid mercury to the air; containers must be sealed when not in use, handling equipment must be designed to prevent spills and the whole work area constructed so that there is not a single place where spilt liquid can lodge except the water traps in benches. Mercury should be heated only in sealed systems.

The metal should be handled only with very good local exhaust ventilation – for example fume cupboards in barometer filling – and general ventilation of the workroom to the highest standards.

Poisoning by mercury or its compounds is a prescribed disease.

Poisoning – other metals:

Many other metals are poisonous or irritating. You should look up any that you work with in the Directory of Toxic Substances and check for additional references in the Index. One more metal is so dangerous that it must be dealt with in more detail – Cadmium.

Cadmium:

Two Scandinavian toxicologists have said that 'cadmium has probably more lethal possibilities than any of the metals.' Many in industry do not even know it is hazardous and this may be because until recently it has been used in relatively small quantities and harmful effects have gone un-detected or unpublicised. World production is now doubling every decade and there are probably a thousand plants making or using it in Britain today.

Commonly produced during zinc smelting, the metal is used in plating, solders, bearing alloys and alkali storage batteries. Its compounds, notably cadmium oxide and sul-phoselenide are used as pigments and are found in paints, wood finishes, varnishes, plastics and sprays for fruit trees.

The main risk is from inhalation of fumes or dust. In acute poisoning damage to the lungs can quickly prove fatal, as it did for a welder who cut through cadmium-plated bolts inside one of the boxes during construction of the Severn Bridge. If you recover from the acute effects you are likely to develop emphysema (see this section, p 145).

Long-term exposure to smaller concentrations can harm you in many ways: emphysema, chronic kidney disease, liver damage, weakening of the bones, anaemia and cancer of the prostate. It causes genetic defects in animals. Almost trivial by comparison, you may lose your sense of smell and your teeth may be stained yellow.

Treatment is often unsuccessful..

Because of the wide range of effects, individual susceptibility and lack of research, it is doubtful if anyone can set a safe limit for airborne concentrations. The TLV is 0.2 milligrams per cubic metre of air (0.1 for the oxide) but there is evidence that regular exposure to such levels is dangerous.

Notifiable, prescribed

Cadmium poisoning must be reported to the Factory Inspectorate. Industry notified five cases in 1970 and three in 1971, but these figures will not indicate the actual numbers with kidney disorders and other chronic symptoms.

It is a prescribed industrial disease.

Metal fume fever

This is an acute illness which feels very like the 'flu and lasts up to two days. It starts an hour or more after breathing metal fumes: you feel cold, tired and weak and have a headache. Your temperature rises and you feel thirsty and sick.

The fumes of brass are the commonest cause; the more zinc there is in the brass the worse they are. Zinc, copper, magnesium, aluminium, antimony, cadmium, manganese, nickel, selenium, silver and tin have caused the disease. It seems your lungs are not damaged by the fumes in an attack of the fever caused by a small 'dose'.

The disease tends to affect you when you return to work after a few days off; you probably become acclimatised to the fumes during the working week. (A similar fever can be produced by the fumes of PTFE (polytetrafluorethylene) if the polymer is allowed to get onto cigarettes. The temperature at which cigarettes burn is enough to produce poisonous vapours from the PTFE which you inhale directly.)

Benzene

Benzene is used as a solvent for glues, resins, rubbers, paints, fats and other substances. It is so dangerous that substitutes have been found for many applications; regulations are to be introduced which will restrict its use.

Part of the danger – and much of its attractiveness for industry – lies in its extreme volatility. Quick evaporation makes paints and glues dry out quickly, but it also enables the vapour to rapidly reach dangerous concentrations.

Inhaling a large dose of benzene will make you unconscious and soon kill you; smaller amounts make you feel ill, confused and disorientated. Prolonged exposure is likely to damage your bone marrow (see page 153).

Substitution by less harmful substances is the only real answer to this hazard. Toluene is one of the main alternatives, being less volatile and less poisonous, but commercial grade toluene may contain benzene as an impurity. It is also present in petrol. Increasing amounts of this poison are being added to petrol to boost octane ratings and compensate for lower levels of tetra ethyl lead required to meet anti-pollution laws.

Benzene is also referred to as benzol. It should not be confused with benzine, spelt with an *i*, and pronounced the same – which is far less hazardous.

Chronic poisoning by benzene is notifiable. Two cases were reported to the Factory Inspectorate in 1970 and none in 1971. This does not mean that the risk has disappeared.

Narcotic effects:

All organic solvents, including benzene, are narcotic. Like alcohol, they can change your behaviour, making you sleepy, slow, 'high' or drunk and, as with alcohol, more likely to have an accident.

The risk is greatly increased if you drink alcohol. Chlorinated hydrocarbons, like trichloroethylene, are a particular hazard. You can feel perfectly all right after working in 'trike' vapour but when you have a beer at lunchtime you can get a splitting headache and even collapse. The danger is worse if you have a few drinks and then go back to inhale some more chemical.

Narcotic fumes at work plus one brandy could be enough to get you prosecuted for drunken driving.

The risk of liver damage can also be increased by this additive effect.

This doesn't mean that workers have got to give up drinking. Employers have got to give up work systems that expose you to intoxicating chemicals. While they are being weaned of their addiction to cheap engineering you may have to be on your guard against these effects – *even if you haven't had a drink.*

Phosphorus:

Phosphorus itself is dangerous in its white or yellow forms. Red phosphorus is very much safer and should be used wherever possible. White phosphorus was once a hazard in match making but it has been outlawed in the British match industry for 60 years. It is still a health risk in the manufacture of phosphor bronze, flares, incendiary bombs and napalm.

Its main effect is to cause 'phossy jaw' – your lower jaw bone slowly and very painfully drops out. The first signs are a red spot on your gums and toothache. Eventually, holes appear in your gums or in the skin over your lower jaw and the dead bone of the jaw breaks up and falls out of the holes.

Meticulous care of your teeth can slow up the disease or stop it altogether. The dentist has to fill every cavity very carefully as soon as it appears.

Although phossy jaw is a **notifiable disease,** there are companies that avoid reporting cases by making sure that workers are treated by a dentist at the first sign of trouble. This is a big risk to take with the lower half of a worker's face; it means that there is unnecessary – and illegal – exposure to white phosphorus. (When some of the phosphorus products such as napalm are designed to burn whole communities alive we should not be too shocked at failure to observe small details of law and humanity.)

Workers must make sure that all cases are reported. Six were reported in 1970 and three in 1971.

Phosphine is a very dangerous gas – see Lungs/gases.

The organic compounds of phosphorus are powerful nervous system poisons which interfere with the chemistry of nerve cells to produce a variety of symptoms – see Poisoning/brain and nervous system.

These chemicals are widely used as insecticides and should be treated with the utmost respect. They can easily penetrate your skin as well as getting in through lungs and mouth. All skin should be covered with protective clothing which should be cleaned daily. There should be provision for changing clothes and having a shower before meals – a requirement which may be difficult to achieve on farms. (When all the health risks of modern chemical, mechanical farming are taken into consideration – plus the traditional hazards of infectious diseases – it is clear that such facilities should be available anyway. Contract spraying gangs working a long way from base could have mobile units like those used in the construction industry.)

Tri-ortho-cresyl phosphate (TOCP) can be a hazard in the chemical and oil industries. It is used as an additive in lubricating oils and hydraulic fluids. In Morocco in 1959 10,000 people were poisoned and 2,000 of them permanently disabled after US Army surplus hydraulic fluid was sold as cooking oil. It is one of the highly toxic substances found leaking from the industrial chemical tip at Maendy quarry in South Wales.

If you are often exposed to organo phosphorus compounds you should have regular blood tests to check the level of a substance called cholinesterase which is vital to the functioning of nerve cells. If the level is low you should be removed from exposure until it returns to normal.

The Department of Health and Social Security notifies the Ministry of Agriculture of any cases of organo phosphorus poisoning. Four cases reached the Ministry's statistics by this roundabout route in 1970.

Prescribed, notifiable

Poisoning by phosphorus, phosphine, and organic phosphorus compounds are listed as one prescribed disease. The effects of tri-cresyl phosphate and tri-phenyl phosphate are each listed separately. All are notifiable diseases.

Arsenic:

White arsenic (arsenic oxide) is the most important and dangerous compound of arsenic. It is a hazard in smelting, optical glass making, the manufacture and use of insecticides and weedkillers and in the fur trade.

Acute poisoning affects your stomach and intestines, causing vomiting, diarrhoea and severe pain. You can die from these effects but the poison also affects your brain, causing fits and coma. If you recover you are likely to get numbness of your hands and feet, with muscular weakness. There are also remarkable effects on your skin – a dry scaliness, possibly with the development of warts.

Chronic exposure is more likely to produce the brain and nervous system effects. Arsenic dust on the skin for a number of years can lead to spotty pigmentation of the skin, dermatitis, ulceration in sweaty areas and skin cancer. Face masks and other protective equipment should not be of rubber because this can encourage ulceration.

There is a high incidence of lung cancer in workers exposed for a long time and heart disease is also reported.

Arsenic poisoning is both prescribed and notifiable. No cases were reported in 1970 or 1971.

Diseases caused by germs:

Brucellosis:

Brucellosis is really a disease of sheep, cattle, pigs and goats but it is easily caught by people who work with animals. More than 60 per cent of vets are believed to suffer from it. You cannot pass it on to another human. The disease usually results from contact with infected animals – which may appear perfectly healthy – but you can also get it from the unpasteurised milk of a cow or goat that has the disease.

Brucellosis is usually like a very bad and prolonged bout of 'flu: you may have a fever every day for a week, with headache and lack of energy. Many farmworkers have had it without realising; only a blood test will show if you have.

Sometimes the disease takes a much more serious form and illness may last for years. You feel generally rather weak and then every few weeks you have a fever with sweating, headaches and joint pains. A course of antibiotics often cures it. Rarely it can kill you. Severe depression is a common side effect and one farm worker committed suicide because he could not bear the disease any longer.

Employers do not have to report the disease but it is recognised for injury or disablement benefit. Compulsory eradication has now started after much opposition on grounds of cost.

Weil's disease:

Weil's disease is caused by a bacteria that infects rats and is excreted in their urine. It is a hazard in any place infested with rats, particularly if there is stagnant water in which the bacteria can live for several weeks. It is a particular risk for sewer men, miners and farmworkers, but demolition workers, river board workers and many others should regard it as a potential danger.

Infection usually enters through a cut or scratch, and, up to two weeks later, you suddenly get a fever with headache, muscle ache, nausea and vomiting. Your eyes are often very painful and you may get a spotty and blotchy rash on your limbs and body and have a cough.

Only rarely are people seriously ill but you can become jaundiced, your kidneys fail and you may die. Early treatment with penicillin is essential in all cases.

Your doctor is unlikely to think of Weil's disease unless you tell him this is a hazard of your work. Sewermen usually have a special card they can show their doctor and this should be standard practice. o Essex River Board workers were issued with cards after one of them caught the disease in 1972.

> o A Kingston, Surrey, council worker who died in 1972 after cutting his hand while clearing a river bank was first treated for pneumonia five days after the cut. He then developed jaundice but it was not until he was admitted to hospital in a critical condition that Weil's disease was diagnosed. His chances of survival were then put at 30 per cent, and he was not lucky – he died.

Workers in the main risk area, sewers, do not come under any workplace safety law and cases are not reported to any inspectorate. o In agriculture four cases were reported in 1969 (2 fatal); seven in 1970 (1 fatal); five in 1971 (none fatal). In mines there was one case in 1970 but this was only the third in 10 years.

Weil's is one form of the disease known as leptospirosis. Another kind is caught by people who work with dogs. Both are **prescribed** occupational diseases.

Anthrax:

Anthrax is a disease of horses, goats and sheep and you can catch it from spores in animal products imported from countries where the disease is not controlled. You can also get it from the animal itself but that is not likely in this country.

Wool is the most common hazard, which is why the disease is also known as 'wool sorter's disease'. Others are hair, bristles, hides, skins and bones. There can be a risk wherever these are handled, including docks, transport, warehouses and factories making glues, fertilisers and textiles.

If you inhale the spores you get a very bad form of pneumonia but they usually get into your body through a cut or abrasion. The result is a painless red lump in your skin that ulcerates and then slowly heals. Penicillin cures it so easily that many cases are not reported as they should be by law. This hides a dangerous work situation from the authorities, who might otherwise be forced to step in and order better protection. The danger is that the disease sometimes spreads to the rest of your body, when it is usually fatal.

o Four cases were reported by industry in 1970, none fatal. o No cases were reported in 1971. The disease can still be a killer.

> o In 1972 a young woman died in an Oldham hospital after returning from a holiday in Tunisia. She contracted the disease after handling animal skins in a street market.

Prevention
Precautions can eliminate the risk in industry:

1. Hazardous imported animal products should be sterilised. Some, notably goat hair, *must* be sterilised under new regulations.

2. Workers should be immunised. For full protection you should have three doses at intervals of three weeks, a fourth dose after six months and then reinforcing doses each year. Some doctors may still be using an outdated programme that does not develop protection quickly enough.

3. There should be a warning placard on the wall of the workroom and you should be issued with a cautionary card. These are legal requirements but casual workers are often not given a card or warned of the risk.

Prescribed and notifiable.

Other infections:
Other infections can present special risks in different occupations. People who work with horses may get a disease called glanders; zoo workers could risk psittacosis, a disease of parrots; farmworkers run a higher than usual risk of tetanus (one died in 1971) and ringworm (eight cases reported in 1971). Doctors, nurses and other medical workers are at risk from many infectious diseases.

Of the above diseases and occupations only glanders

and tuberculosis (for medical workers) are prescribed: the widow of the farmworker who dies of tetanus can get Death Benefit only by proving that the disease resulted from a particular *accident*; the nurse who gets hepatitis cannot get Injury Benefit. (You might think she would qualify if she caught the prescribed disease of anthrax from one of her patients but her *occupation* is not prescribed. If work brought her into contact with an infected *animal* she would be eligible.

Manual labour:

Other diseases are produced not by chemicals or infection but by manual labour itself. They include beat hand, beat knee and beat elbow, the swellings that miners get from working on their hands, knees and elbows; cramps and inflamed tendons (tenosynovitis) caused by repetitive movements of fingers, hands and arms.

Miners' diseases:

Tenosynovitis can be a problem in many industries, especially when the work rate on repetitive movements is speeded up, but miners are probably more familiar with it than most. Other diseases of miners are nystagmus (rapid and involuntary oscillation of the eyeballs resulting from poor lighting), and ankylostomiasis (hookworm). Hookworm used to be a problem in tin mines; it is now unknown in coal mines. In the financial year 1970-71 the totals for miner's diseases other than pneumoconiosis were:

Beat knee	1,137
Beat elbow, beat hand, tenosynovitis	344
Nystagmus	4
Dermatitis	1,416

The beats, cramps, tenosynovitis, nystagmus, ankylostomiasis and dermatitis (dealt with earlier – see Skin/dermatitis) are all prescribed diseases.

Not prescribed:

There are many other occupational diseases which are

not recognised for benefits at the industrial rate. Damage by noise and vibration (see Section 3) may be prescribed in the near future but others, like bronchitis and rheumatism which occur widely in the general population, are a long way from recognition – even for occupations where the incidence is high, eg bronchitis among miners.

Mental stress caused by work pressures is increasing at an alarming rate (see Section 2) but is never likely to be separated out from domestic and other forms of stress. How could it be? An industrial cause does not make mental illness feel any different. Lung cancer is just as disastrous for a worker and his family if it is caused by nickel carbonyl (prescribed) or asbestos (not prescribed).

Human needs are the same, whatever the cause; the higher rate of benefit for prescribed conditions simply makes it slightly easier to meet them. Because of this, the unions expend much energy on campaigning for recognition of particular diseases (and this book takes up valuable space explaining the system and its demarcations). Much medical time and skill is tied up in devising the rules so that non-occupational conditions cannot slip through.

Health, security:

A welfare state that ungrudgingly met the needs of all people, whatever the cause of their misfortune, would free all this energy and skill for the real task of preventing illness.

Meanwhile, Industrial Injury Benefits are dealt with in detail in Section 12.

The methods that should be used to protect you from poisoning and disease are described in the next section. Suggestions for a co-ordinated attack on all hazards are given in Section 8, Action.

6.

Prevention

The two previous sections dealt with the ways in which harmful substances get into the work environment and the effects they can have on your health.

This section describes the ways in which management should prevent contamination of the workplace and protect you from the risk of disease.

The first principle is that all hazards should be controlled at source by proper design of the whole work system.

In the vast majority of industrial jobs you should be able to work safely and comfortably without any more protection than overalls, gloves, boots and safety spectacles. If a job requires you to wear uncomfortable equipment like respirators for long periods, there is usually something very wrong with the safety engineering. (The fact that there may also be something wrong with the personal protection, in that it is more uncomfortable than it need be, does not alter this principle.)

Work should be pleasant and that means modifying processes so that hazards don't get out rather than modifying you so that hazards don't get in.

Methods of control come under the following headings and usually in this sequence:

1. Substitution
2. Suppression
3. Extraction
4. Measurement

1. Substitution:

The best way to remove or reduce hazards is to stop using them or to use something else – for example ceramic-based materials, gypsum, concrete and glass fibres instead of asbestos; toluene instead of benzene; synthetic abrasives instead of sandstone; zinc oxide for white lead in paints. When this can't be done other methods will be needed.

2. Suppression:

This covers a variety of methods for preventing impurities getting into the air. Equipment can be completely sealed or enclosed as in many chemical processes, and in work with radioactive materials. Total enclosure is rare in manufacturing because equipment would be expensive or production very slow. The principle could be used much more widely – for example by pumping liquids out of drums using sealed connectors instead of pouring. Pneumatic or screw conveyors can be used instead of belts.

Dusts can be eliminated by mixing them into liquids and slurries but they will turn back into dust again if splashes are allowed to dry out on floors and benches. Damping down of dusts before handling will reduce the amount that gets into the air, but once it is there, water sprays will not control it – particles can move through a curtain of water.

Damping down of dangerous dust on the floor is neither suppression nor control. It is often no more than an excuse to leave it lying around a bit longer instead of cleaning it up. Spraying it with a hose can actually jet dust into the air.

When it gets to the stage described by workers in battery plants, of a sludge of lead oxide on the floor, this approach amounts to gross negligence.

3. Extraction:

Local exhaust ventilation is the most important method of control; contaminants are caught by the air moving into the extraction system the moment they escape from the process. Systems vary from almost total enclosure of the pollution source, with small openings at the front where you handle the materials, to booths where the front is completely open, and hoods which provide no enclosure but rely entirely on air flow to capture the pollution. In addition a variety of dust-producing portable tools like grinders, rock drills and welding gear can be fitted with integral or 'clip-on' extraction equipment.

All these systems can stop pollutants getting into the air you breathe. It is probably true that most installations fail to do this. Exhaust ventilation is more than a hood, a pipe and a fan; to work properly all three components must be designed to work together in relation to a particular source of dust or fumes.

This means that managements must pay expert ventilation engineers to design, install and test the system. That many believe this is unnecessary or too expensive is evident from the figures for lung disease and poisoning given in the previous section. Some installations actually make life more dangerous by drawing dust or vapour through your breathing zone and into the duct.

If dust collects in booths or on the floor, the system is not working properly. You can check the performance of spray booths by seeing if the pigment stain has spread beyond the enclosure. With pollutants that leave no trace, smoke from a cigarette will show whether air is moving inwards or outwards at the edges of the booth (not suitable where inflammable or explosive substances are used).

Once engineers have installed a proper system it must be inspected (at least weekly) and maintained by people who understand how it works. Ducts get clogged up or leak, fan motors lose power; many installations are allowed to deteriorate to the point where they achieve no more than a false sense of security.

All extraction plant must have a proper filter unit and regular maintenance is vital if pollution is not to be passed on to the outside world – or back into the workroom in the case of recirculating systems.

Good **exhaust** ventilation should prevent any escape of pollution to the air. If any does get out, good **general** ventilation of the room will dilute vapours or gases. But dusts will settle out and accumulate on surfaces, to be recirculated by air currents. Ordinary sweeping will make the dust situation worse and cleaning should be done with an industrial vacuum cleaner. These are fitted with high-efficiency filters and designed not to create a draught. Some can pick up wet as well as dry waste.

The Factories Act requires:

1. Adequate ventilation of workrooms must be secured by the circulation of fresh air.

2. All practicable measures must be taken to protect workers against inhalation of dust, fumes or other impurities likely to be injurious or offensive.

3. Local exhaust ventilation must be provided and maintained *where practicable*.

Local exhaust ventilation is always practicable in engineering terms though courts may accept arguments based on economic practicalities. Efficient exhaust draught is mandatory under special regulations for various hazardous trades including lead, asbestos and pottery processes.

4. Measurement:

No prevention system is complete without regular *air sampling* to see if it is actually working. **Most workers have never seen air sampling equipment. This is hardly surprising because there is usually no legal obligation on the employer to test the air.** The new Asbestos Regulations 1969 contain no statutory requirement to take samples, though the Factory Inspectorate has published a 'hygiene standard' which it uses in deciding whether conditions are dangerous. (See Section 5, Disease, p 142.)

The amended Chromium Plating Regulations which came into force in 1973 do actually require the employer to carry out regular atmospheric monitoring for chromic acid spray. Workers in the 1,200 companies which do chromium plating should see that this requirement is enforced.

The principles of air sampling are quite simple. You draw a known volume of air through an instrument and trap the impurities. By weighing, chemical reaction or other methods the amount of impurity can be determined and then, because the amount of air it came from is known, it can be expressed as a concentration (see Section 4, Chemicals, p 114).

In practice it requires considerable skill to get a true

picture of pollution in a particular plant under different operating conditions. A full survey should be done by a qualified industrial hygienist with the necessary laboratory back-up.

One of the best methods for testing individual exposure is the **personal sampler.** A battery powered pump worn on a belt round your waist draws air from a 'pick-up' near your face for an entire shift. The total amount of contaminant – dust or vapour – in the breathing zone during a shift can then be determined.

Only a handful of big firms employ their own industrial hygienists so consultants will usually have to be brought in to do periodic surveys and be kept on call to investigate any problems that may develop – for example when production methods are changed.

As with noise surveys (see Section 3, p 60) getting management to order a survey may require some pressure. When dangerous conditions are suspected one form of pressure is to notify the Factory Inspectorate. The Inspectorate may employ its own hygiene unit to investigate conditions or recommend the employer to bring in consultants. If this doesn't work traditional industrial action may be needed.

When a plant has been surveyed and proper engineering controls installed to ensure pure air, **continuous monitoring devices** can be placed in all areas where plant failure would release toxic materials. The equipment sounds a warning the moment concentrations reach a preset danger level. It is important to check such monitors are not set for phoney safe levels. They are available for a wide range of gases and vapours, which now includes TDI. Management may oppose them on grounds of cost.

In between full-scale hygiene surveys, management should make regular spot-checks for pollution – at least once a shift if serious hazards are present.

The most common type of instrument for spot checks on airborne chemicals works rather like a 'breathalyser'. A small **hand pump** is used to draw a measured volume of air through a glass tube containing chemicals which react with the one you are sampling for. The reaction in the **'detector** tube' produces a colour change and the length of this stain gives an immediate indication of the pollutant's concentration.

Nearly 100 gases can be detected in this way, though probably less than 20 tubes are accurate enough to provide more than a preliminary check. As with the breathalyser, a high reading is the signal for further investigation but, unlike the breathalyser, management cannot be allowed to 'drive on' when the reading is low. The real concentration could be as much as 30 per cent higher than indicated by the tube.

The real value of detector tubes is in finding out *whether* a poison is in the air, not how much. The inaccuracy of most tubes is a problem only when management is trying to get away with as much pollution as it can within the TLV system (see page 115). If the aim is zero concentration of poison in the air then detector tubes are a good way to find out if it is there.

There are two kinds of hand pump. One looks like a small pair of bellows and the other like a short fat bicycle pump. Both are simple to operate and they could be used by workers when management refuses to admit that a particular pollutant is in the air, insists that levels are 'safe', or will not agree to have samples taken.

The bellows-type pump, as used by Factory Inspectors, is slightly cheaper than the other type, and detector tubes are supplied in smaller lots, but a pump and one or two boxes of tubes won't leave you much change from £30. Unions do not at present have this equipment and it would have to be bought specially, either out of union funds or from a shopfloor whip round. Whether this is a worthwhile move will depend on the situation. It is worth considering.

Addresses of the two main suppliers are given on page 328. It is probably best to contact both and buy from the one who seems most willing to come and give technical advice.

You can buy an attachment to convert a hand pump so that it will collect **dust samples** on membrane filters but the samples have to be interpreted by a specialist industrial hygiene laboratory. If you sent the membrane filters, with full details of all suspected contaminants and the sampling equipment and methods used, the laboratory should be able to tell you what substances you collected and probably make some estimate of concentrations at the times when you took the samples. The whole process might take many days and the result might not be very accurate – but you could prove whether a dangerous dust was present in the air or not.

If you decided to try it, the TUC Centenary Institute in London (see p 329) would be able to interpret samples on membrane filters.

Personal protection:

Protective equipment is available that enables people to handle almost any substance or go into any atmosphere with safety. Providing it is only used for special operations and emergencies, that is a good thing. If risks are controlled at source, elaborate personal protection should be unnecessary in the ordinary course of the job. Exceptions to this rule are when the hazard cannot be controlled – for example cold weather on building sites and trawlers (see Section 3, Temperature) or when a second line of defence is needed against extreme risks like radiation.

Whatever clothing or equipment is needed to protect you from the particular risks of your job, management should provide it free. Many firms tell you that a lot of time is being lost through foot injuries and then go on to suggest that you should buy safety boots or shoes from management at subsidised prices, with free membership of the 'Golden Boot Club' or some other fabulous incentive scheme to save you from a crushed toe. If a firm's work systems endanger your feet it should pay the whole cost of protection.

Respirators:

Respiratory protection is uncomfortable and unpleasant. It makes conversation with workmates nearly impossible and, in some cases, actually dangerous because of increased leakage around the face seal. It should be accepted only for very short periods during a working day, and then only if you are absolutely satisfied about safety.

If the employer wants a process operated continuously by workers in respirators he will have to accept a rota system that gives short individual periods on the process, long periods on other work and, overall, a short working day.

Workers are often given totally unsuitable equipment and it is important to be able to recognise the different types, and their limitations.

Filter respirators (known by the fancy name of ovi-nasal respirator or, colloquially, 'pig's snout'). Rubber face mask which covers mouth and nose. Wearer has to draw air in through one or two filter cartridges fixed to the mask. Filters are designed to stop dust and **cannot stop gases and vapours.** None will trap 100 per cent of any dust – if they did you would not get much air through.

The filter must be able to trap the size of particles producing the risk and the percentage let through must not be enough to endanger health. (Gauze pads are no good for toxic dusts but it may be worth trying them where dust is a nuisance, on building sites for example). The efficiency of the filter is often made quite irrelevant by the amount of air that leaks in between the mask and your face, especially when you talk. Masks must be issued individually to workers and checked for fit against the face; if this seal is to work they must be worn so tightly that they are uncomfortable. Masks with a pneumatic seal may be more effective and less uncomfortable.

> o 'If you've got your mask on for an hour you are exhausted because it restricts your breathing.'
> Ken Fletcher, senior chargehand at H.J.Enthoven lead works, South Darley.
> o 'It was very uncomfortable to wear. If it was too tight you couldn't breathe and if it was too loose it slipped off with the sweat.' Bob Smith, former employee of Central Asbestos, London.

For all their discomfort, Ken Fletcher still got lead poisoning and Bob Smith is dying of asbestosis.

Positive pressure powered respirator: Air is driven through a filter to the facepiece by means of a battery-powered air blower carried on a belt round your waist. Breathing is easier and face-seal leakage is outwards. For reasons of comfort and safety this type of respirator should be regarded as the minimum standard for protection from toxic dusts or for strenuous work. Even this equipment lets through some dust and is not good enough to protect you against all dust conditions.

For any work with blue asbestos where the employer cannot demonstrate a complete absence of contamination, you should be equipped with air-line breathing apparatus. Because there is no known safe limit for white asbestos it may be wise to treat it in the same way.

Air-line breathing apparatus. Air is fed under pressure through a hose to a hood or facepiece, enabling you to work in atmospheres containing toxic dusts, vapours, gases or insufficient oxygen. A welder's mask can be supplied in the same way. Air is usually supplied by a compressor and it must be filtered to remove oil. In corrosive or irritating atmospheres the gear must protect eyes and skin as well. This type of equipment gives good, if extremely restricting and oppressive, protection but it is important to remember that in very poisonous atmospheres failure may mean death.

Self-contained breathing apparatus. There are various kinds having a built-in supply of oxygen, liquid air or compressed air. Normally used only in emergency they have a limited capacity, ranging from 25 minutes to two hours. Should be available and clearly marked in all places where there is a risk of sudden and disastrous contamination. Must be checked and maintained on a regular basis.

> o On August 2nd 1972 Ben Eynon, Fred Stitfall and Peter Davies died in a gasholder at the British Steel Corporation's East Moors works because the oxygen breathing equipment issued by the BSC was faulty. After hearing that the equipment worn by Peter Davies in his rescue attempt was the worst ever tested by the Mines Rescue Centre at Doncaster, Cardiff magistrates fined the BSC £250.

You should never be sent into a toxic atmosphere without a safety harness and life line and someone standing by to haul you out.

Canister respirator: This consists of full-face mask, flexible hose and a canister containing absorbent chemicals which remove gas or vapour from the air before you breathe it. The correct canister must be used for each contaminant or you will get no protection; colour coding of canisters shows what they are for. These respirators will not remove concentrations greater than one per cent by volume and the absorbent material is quickly exhausted – usually in 30 minutes, some in only 15 minutes. They should never be used in confined spaces and, of course, they can do nothing for you if there is a shortage of oxygen. Canisters will not trap dust particles unless a special filter has been added.

Cartridge respirator. Looks like a 'pig's snout' dust respirator but the cartridge is designed to absorb gases and vapours. Gives even less protection than the canister type and for shorter periods. Managements often issue this equipment for conditions with which it cannot cope. Be very wary of this equipment. If you do use it, make sure the cartridge is right for the type of contaminant, its concentration and your length of exposure.

Clearly respiratory protection cannot be dished out casually. Management must know exactly what the conditions are – substances, concentrations, particle sizes, and so on – before they can specify the right equipment and demonstrate to workers that it does in fact give the required protection. **So, once again, management must be made to face its duty to carry out air sampling.** Issuing respirators requires an equal knowledge of workers' health because they should not be worn by anyone with respiratory or heart conditions – another reason why issue must be on an individual basis.

All respirators should be inspected, cleaned and sterilised regularly.

Eye protection:

Every eye injury is a serious injury because the smallest scratch can lead to permanent damage to your sight. The Factory Inspectorate has estimated that there are 1,000 eye injuries a day in workplaces covered by the Factories Act. While this figure is an indictment of the work systems that produce such injuries, it also reflects the fact that most employers do virtually nothing to protect their workers' eyesight. The vast majority of injuries can be prevented by very simple safety spectacles with side shields. These can and should be as comfortable and optically-correct as ordinary prescription glasses, which are already worn by nearly 40 per cent of workers in manufacturing.

Many workers have been put off eye protection by half-baked safety campaigns where tatty equipment, bought at the cheapest possible price, is dished out by stores and the whole place plastered in posters to 'drive the message home'. Not surprisingly, the message that gets through to most people is that eye protection is uncomfortable, makes it difficult to see, distorts vision or gives you a headache.

Safety spectacles and, for special risks, goggles, should be introduced only after the hazards of every operation have been surveyed, real efforts have been made to control them and workers have been given a chance to choose acceptable equipment. Issue must then be on an individual basis, with great care being taken to ensure comfort and proper fit.

Because people who wear ordinary glasses will need prescription lenses in their safety spectacles and many others may need them without realising it, vision screening should be included in this programme. Screening reveals unsuspected eyesight faults that cause stress, headaches and accidents – three-fifths of the 'accident-prone' workers in a metal works had poor vision – **but there should be a firm agreement that no worker will be penalised for any disabilities that are discovered (among 1,400 workers screened in one firm, seven were found to be blind in one eye).**

The new Protection of Eyes Regulations which are due to come into force in 1973 only in workplaces covered by the Factories Act, require employers to provide eye protection for a wide range of hazardous processes that have never before been covered by regulations. They contain the important provision that eye protection must be issued individually to each worker who has to perform any of the tasks listed in the regulations. Throughout large sections of industry almost every worker will have to be equipped with, and will have to wear, the protection for the listed jobs. Employers will find this expensive and it is vital that you are not palmed off with the cheapest goods that will meet the requirements. People who wear spectacles all the time should be asked for their opinion on the acceptability of anything that is offered. Dispensers for cleaning and demisting pads should be installed in workrooms, though this is not part of the regulations.

Overalls:

Overalls are such an everyday item that you may not think of them as protective equipment. Often they are not and management indifference to this kind of protection can actually increase risks – as when women workers on drilling machines were given overalls with long sleeves which got caught in drill chucks.

Overalls need to be selected and maintained with as much care as any other safety equipment if workers – and their personal clothing – are to be protected from danger-ous contamination – or just plain dirt – from the job. **This is a management responsibility and there is no reason why workers should continue to subsidise industry by providing their own protection.**

For the millions of workers in daily contact with min-eral oil, overalls provide the first line of defence against skin cancer, particularly cancer of the scrotum. Absorbent cot-ton is not a particularly clever defence but if overalls are changed and cleaned at least once a week (more often for really oily work) they stop the oil getting through to your clothes and skin.

Every trace of oil must be removed when the overalls are cleaned. **Ordinary washing or laundering removes only half of the contaminant:** tests on a freshly-laundered pair of overalls found that they still contained three ounces of a viscous dark brown mineral oil which contained fine silica particles and minute metal turnings. Overalls must be **dry-cleaned** if the dermatitis and cancer risk is to be removed. This is so important that management must be made to pay for a contract overalls service where the supplier guarantees to dry clean. It is thought that only one third of industrial workers are covered by overall rental schemes paid for by the employer. Many of these services do not dry clean.

Workers on high speed machining equipment, like bar automatics, which throw out a spray of coolant oil, need extra protection. Impervious aprons are available but many operators find they interfere with their work. As a solution

to this problem British Leyland researchers helped develop
overalls made of polyurethane-coated nylon.

> o 'These were found to be excellent in terms of protect-
> ing the worker without too much physical discomfort
> but the price was unacceptable to the management.
> Three garments were required per man at £10 each and
> special cleaning facilities were also needed. So far, a
> satisfactory solution to the problem of providing the
> protection we believe necessary has not been found.'
> Mr G.L.Leem of British Leyland, Royal Society of Med-
> icine, Meeting on Protective Clothing and Equipment,
> 12 January 1970

What this means is that British Leyland management
did not think it worth paying £30 for clothing which would
not only protect the worker who runs the biggest risk of
scrotal cancer but also free him from the reek of sulphurised
fats in cutting oils. Some bar auto operators say the only
time their bodies don't smell of it is at the end of their annual holiday.

Another important reason for forcing management to
take responsibility for supply and cleaning of overalls is the
risk of taking toxic contaminants home with you. High
blood lead levels among children of lead workers are believed to be caused by dust from work clothes which would
seem to indicate that the regulations on protective clothing
and other safeguards are not being observed or are not
strict enough. It has also been suggested that wives of asbestos workers may have contracted mesothelioma from washing their husband's dusty overalls. Under the new Asbestos
Regulations employers must clean all protective clothing on
the premises or have it sent out for cleaning in sealed containers boldly labelled to show that they contain asbestos-
contaminated clothing.

The take-home risk applies to any toxic substance,
particularly dusts, and also to germs and spores like anthrax. It is important to see that any special regulations are
observed and to extend the principle to jobs not covered by
regulations.

Washing and changing:
You should be able to leave work as clean and as free
from contamination as when you arrived. Most employers

provide the bare minimum required by law in the way of washing, changing and locker facilities. In spite of the fact that many of the regulations were written more than 30 years ago, many places do not meet even the minimum standards and the average is a disgrace to convenience and hygiene.

When workers demand improvements they are treated as though good facilities are a luxury instead of an essential element in fighting dermatitis, skin cancer and poisoning. Management washrooms and WCs are usually provided to a much higher specification in spite of the fact that they face none of these risks.

The first step is to ensure that the regulations for any workplace are being met. Further improvements will come not from the law but from workers' demands for completely new standards. These might include provision of showers in all dirty, dusty and oily trades; enough WCs and washbasins to eliminate queues at breaks and knocking off times; and washing and changing periods at the beginning and end of the shift, in paid time.

   o When workers at the H.J.Enthoven lead factory at South Darley, Derbyshire, realised the risk of carrying lead home to their children they gave management two weeks to improve arrangements for changing and washing, with the threat of a strike if they did not comply.
   o The National Coal Board's failure to provide a shower-bath at its Prestongrange brickworks cost it £5,000 in compensation after a long legal action by Mr James McGhee of Prestonpans, who contracted dermatitis after working in the brick kiln. In the House of Lords it was said that 'The fact that the man had to cycle home caked with grime and sweat added materially to the risk that this disease might develop.'

First aid:

First aid is an essential part of disease prevention: the smallest cut, scratch or bruise should receive attention from someone who knows what he or she is doing.

Statutory safety standards lay down various requirements for first aid boxes and personnel according to the number of people employed and the type of work being done.

These standards are seldom good enough for the kind

of care that is needed – for example the Factories Act requires no more than one first aid box for 150 people and the person in charge of the box does not have to be trained in first aid unless there are more than 50 workers.

It would be more realistic to have a box and a worker trained in first aid (in the firm's time) in every workroom. In a place of any size there should be a first aid room permanently staffed by an industrial nurse. The nurse can not only give skilled first aid but also keep the comprehensive accident records needed to identify areas with dangerous work systems (see Section 7, Accidents).

Where toxic or corrosive chemicals are used it is important that any special first aid treatments that may be needed, eg amyl nitrite capsules, are available. (Treatments are given in the Directory of Toxic Substances.) Eye wash bottles and emergency showers should be available close to all hazard areas – and in working order. ○ A man died after being splashed with phenol because, when the helpers got him to the emergency shower, they found the water supply was turned off.

Under the Chemical Regulations, a cautionary notice giving instructions on first-aid treatment for gassing and burns must be displayed in all places where strong acids or dangerous corrosive liquids are used.

A placard giving instructions for treatment of electric shock must be displayed in all workplaces covered by the Factories Act where electricity is used. Workers can make this regulation more effective by asking for a placard in every workroom.

When someone's breathing has stopped after an electric shock or other accident their chances of survival are improved if a mechanical aspirator can take over from normal artificial respiration. This equipment should be available in all industrial workplaces.

This is not the place to give instructions in first aid. All first aid boxes must contain a leaflet giving advice on first aid. You can get information and training from the St John Ambulance Brigade, the Red Cross or industrial safety organisations. As many as possible should be trained, in the firm's time and at the firm's expense.

Medical services:

Half the population spends a third of its waking hours at work, exposed to physical and mental stresses which not only produce the recognised occupational diseases but also cause or contribute to a bewildering variety of physical and mental disorders.

You might expect that specialist doctors would be an everyday sight in industry, working to identify and root out the causes of so much illness. In fact industrial medical services vary from nonexistent to inadequate. Apart from a few obviously hazardous processes, such as handling lead and radioactive substances, where medical examination is required by law, the employer has no statutory duty to provide medical supervision.

Workers do not have any legal right to industrial health services as they do to the National Health Service.

Employment Medical Advisers:

The old system of medical supervision by 'Appointed Factory Doctors' – hundreds of GPs appointed on a part-time basis to carry out statutory medical examinations – was replaced in February 1973 by the Employment Medical Advisory Service (EMAS).

A ridiculously small force of under 100 doctors specialising in occupational medicine is spread out through regional offices so as to 'cover' the whole country.

As well as carrying out the statutory functions of the old AFDs, under the Factories Act, the service is supposed to extend its supervision to hazardous trades not covered by special regulations, and to the psychological stresses of industry. In addition it is supposed to advise employers, trade unions, workers and general practitioners on the medical aspects of any employment problem. Any employed person, not just those in factories, has a right to consult the Employment Medical Adviser.

This right is most important and should be used to the full whenever an individual or collective health hazard is suspected. Any doubts about the usefulness of the service may be justified, but by using it extensively workers will demonstrate that the Medical Adviser is supposed to be their servant as much as management's. Industry produces enough health problems to overload a service ten times the size of EMAS; continued pressure should force continued expansion and it may one day be big enough for the job. (The example of the Factory Inspectorate, overloaded from the beginning and still hopelessly undersize, is a warning against putting too much faith in this process. Such institutions are tools which can be made more serviceable by workers but they can never be more than pruning knives, trimming off symptoms without threatening the economic roots of disease.)

If your workplace comes under the Factories Act, your employer must display the name and address of the local Employment Medical Adviser at the main entrance to the works.

Industrial medical officers:

Doctors working full time in industry are mostly employed by the larger companies and by nationalised industries like the National Coal Board. Most firms do not have their own medical officer. Where they are employed they should be able to provide a more comprehensive service than outside agencies but all too often their time is taken up with statutory examinations, the pursuit of 'malingerers' or collection of evidence to defeat compensation claims. Because they are part of the management, there is inevitable distrust from workers. But co-ordinated pressure from the shop floor may help the more conscientious doctors win management approval for better prevention methods.

Industrial health schemes:

These have been established in eight or nine centres where a lot of small industrial firms are concentrated in a relatively small area. These voluntary schemes are financed by premiums from the firms which join, and it usually costs about £3 per worker per year.

In return the firm hopes to achieve a reduction in sickness absence by the prompt treatment of injuries at the workplace. Many subscribers hope that their quarterly cheque will tidy up all medical problems in one neat package and they don't welcome suggestions from the service that say £10,000 should be spent on new ventilation. The service knows that if it is too critical it risks losing a premium.

The best hope for making these services work is a militant shop floor which demands action on hazards. Management will then be forced to use the health scheme to the full.

Group industrial health schemes operate in Rochdale, the West Midlands, Dundee, Slough, Central Middlesex, Manchester, Newcastle, Harlow and Peterborough. Any employers in these areas without their own medical department should be pressured into joining.

o The world famous industrial hygiene service run as part of the Slough scheme was closed in 1964 when the Government refused £35,000 a year to keep it going.

General practitioners:

Most GPs have little idea of their patients' working conditions, let alone the diseases they may cause. Many an appendix has been whipped out of workers suffering from lead colic when one simple question, 'What is your work?', would have indicated the most likely cause and one simple injection would have relieved the acute symptoms.

A mercury worker had mercury poisoning for a year without his doctor or dentist recognising it. The dentist removed all the man's teeth. (For other examples see pages 3 and 171.)

Even when the diagnosis is correct there may be no attempt to find the cause – a step that might help prevent further cases. It is important to tell your doctor when you think that any condition may be related to your work. If he agrees ask him to refer your case to the local Employment Medical Adviser.

None of this adds up to a system for *preventing* occupational disease. Advanced techniques for screening workers for sensitivity to particular chemicals *before* exposure and for detecting normally imperceptible physical and mental changes among exposed workers remain largely unused. The resources for carrying out detective work to catch new health subversives (or even keep track of the 'old lags' of occupation disease) are scattered through numerous institutions with little co-ordination.

There should be a national Occupational Health Service, integrated with the present National Health Service, to which all workers have right of free access at all times of day. There would be doctors at local health centres with special training in occupational medicine; specialist doctors and nurses would cover large factories and groups of smaller factories. Rehabilitation of workers after injury or illness would be part of a service whose emphasis would be on health and its preservation rather than disease and its treatment.

An essential part of the OHS concept is that it should be firmly rooted in shop floor organisation. Elected safety delegates would have statutory powers to inspect the workplace and order a stoppage of production pending further investigation by the OHS. In larger workplaces a full-time, safety, health and welfare delegate elected by the workers would be paid by the OHS.

A comprehensive occupational health service is now official TUC policy. The Labour Party has promised to set up an OHS if it is returned to power. It promised the same thing in 1958 and again in 1966.

The employers have successfully resisted the concept of compulsory joint safety committees for nearly 50 years. It is easy to see that the far more radical idea of a worker-based occupational health service will not be won without a struggle.

7.

Accidents

If you work a lifetime in industry you can expect to have at least one serious injury that will keep you off work for more than three days.

If you work in construction you can expect three or four before you retire, if you live that long. One in 50 building workers dies in a site accident.

The risks are even greater for miners and trawlermen.

Any manual worker can expect many injuries needing first aid during a working life; for the average industrial worker there's a one in three chance of having one this year.

As mechanisation and high speed work methods spread, fewer workers can afford to take the risk of accidents lightly. Even in the apparently safe entertainment industry five performers are killed each year by electrical equipment on stage.

The typical injury at work involves none of the complex hazards described in previous sections. It is more likely to be inflicted by some everyday part of the work system that is not as safe as it seems.

The injury will go down on the forms – on your death certificate if you are unlucky – as an 'accident'. The word is a convenient label for industry to put on its long roll call of dead and wounded. All it means is that the employers did not actually plan to maim or kill. And it preserves the myth that workplaces are basically safe and that 'accidents' are caused by the carelessness of workers.

Workers are carefully educated to believe this myth. These are the opening words of a booklet for workers issued by the Royal Society for the Prevention of Accidents (RoSPA):

o 'Everything possible is done to enable you to work in safety but your co-operation is essential.'

The message from the British Safety Council, a rival organisation which uses American methods to sell safety to industry, has the same flavour.

o 'This responsibility for blame may be due to carelessness, thoughtlessness, ignorance, tomfoolery, or bad practice . . . Rather than state in a few words that employees are the root of the trouble, we have listed many of the causes that are produced by this human failure.'

According to these specialists dedicated to your protection: It's your own stupid fault when you are injured!

It is surprising how many workers have been taken in by this line in safety propaganda. It's not at all surprising that the injury toll continues to rise.

This section shows that most accidents are caused by badly designed work systems which will eventually injure anyone exposed to them for long enough. Carelessness is seldom the cause – unless you are talking about the carelessness of the employer. The time has come to turn the propaganda around and force the employer to plan *not* to injure people.

The 'attitude of the worker to safety' is no more the cause of industrial accidents today than it was in the days when little children were mangled by unguarded machinery in the cotton mills. Machines, buildings and arrangements of work are still designed to the cheapest specification that will produce goods at the greatest profit. Engineering design concentrates on the product and excludes the operator until the last possible moment. Safety, health and, last of all, comfort are treated as bolt-on goodies.

Accidents hang on the end of long chains of neglect produced by this attitude. We have already seen some of the dangerous links: noise, vibration, high and low temperatures, shift work, speed-up, stress, fatigue and narcotic chemical fumes. Any one of these can reduce your 'accident-resistance' but there has to be some hazard ready and waiting to deliver the actual injury.

These hazards are present in almost every system of work in almost every occupation. They will not be eliminated by posters from the accident-prevention organisations – unless the posters are used to stuff up leaky roofs that cause slippery floors or are wrapped round sharp corners on workshop machines.

They will be eliminated when workers realise that accidents are built into the workplace like holes in a pin table. The need is for anger, not the guilt-ridden 'safety-consciousness' of the safety posters.

The traditional attitude:

Most accident prevention work starts when it is already too late. Exhortations and posters start to fly after the ill-conceived work system has been set up and accepted as quite normal.

This is a sample question from a training syllabus for young people published by RoSPA:

Printing
(a) Place – Any work area.
Demonstrate how you would stack awkward shaped objects on to a trolley, then show how you would manipulate this trolley through a confined work area.
(b) Place – Any room with an article placed somewhere above ordinary reaching height.
Show how you would improvise a standing platform to reach this article. Demonstrate the stepping on to this platform, the retrieving of this article and the stepping down.

Manipulating trolleys loaded with awkwardly-shaped objects through confined work areas is a certain formula for accidents, no matter how long the young innocents practice the art and however many certificates they get for their efforts.

Workers who regularly use improvised standing platforms to reach inaccessible objects will eventually have a fall. (Perhaps there should have been a third question for the young print workers: 'Show how to improvise a stretcher from a broken ladder and a bundle of safety posters.')

Having accepted industry's own low standards the accident-prevention missionaries start to build a similar attitude in the worker. The same RoSPA syllabus has this entry under 'Human Factor':

> o Faculties; reasoning, judgement, consideration, understanding. Accidents do not happen they are caused; horseplay and tomfoolery, carelessness and thoughtlessness, lack of concentration, lack of respect for oneself and others, familiarity, drinking, fatigue, haste, working conditions, frustration, irritability and boredom.

They might just as well have added excessive masturbation and poor church attendance. Economic factors and the attitude of the employer are not mentioned.

Under 'falls of objects and persons', construction work is identified as a particular hazard area but the syllabus does not list 'lack of toe boards and guard rails' which although illegal, is one of the commonest reasons for falls on site.

While industry continues to take its heaviest toll among young workers, it is right that they should receive pre-entry training – providing it spells out clearly that they will face needless danger at work. RoSPA-style training ('There is inestimable value in coaching youngsters from the beginning of their careers while their minds are still malleable and receptive') which skips over the real facts of life and death in industry will certainly not reduce the accident figures.

More important, it will help to put off the day when a new generation of workers demands that industry adapts *its* standards to them rather than the other way round.

RoSPA and the British Safety Council cannot go too far in questioning the priorities of industry. The first lives by donations and grants, the second makes management pay for its services. Neither kind of support would last long if these voluntary bodies made real links with workers and started to point out the true causes of accidents. Who would buy the safety posters if they were designed for the boardroom wall, with slogans like **'Lives before Profits'**, or **'Stop Killing People'**?

Safety officers:

Safety officers working within industry suffer from the same limitations. As servants of management they are sel-

dom given power to order real changes in work methods. In some firms their role has more to do with minimising claims for damages by injured workers than preventing injuries. Few show up regularly on the shop floor, where the hazards are, and so they are not known or respected by workers.

Like Factory Inspectors (see Section 10, Safety Law), voluntary safety organisations and industrial safety officers are most useful as sources of information. It is unwise to rely on them for real protection or drastic accident-prevention measures.

Most firms do not have safety officers – **there are less than 15,000 for the whole of industry** – and the voluntary safety organisations admit their failure to reach the medium-size and small employers.

BSC has only about 13,000 member firms. RoSPA's industrial safety division reaches even fewer firms. There is considerable overlap between firms using one or more safety organisations and those having safety officers.

Counter-attack by workers:

The traditional approach to accident prevention – carried out on management's terms – is bankrupt. Workers will have to build their own safety organisations in each workplace and the union movement must provide the backing, information and skills needed to impose completely new standards of safety.

The attack on accidents must be based not on traditional 'safety consciousness' but on 'hazard consciousness' in which workers examine very critically the whole system of work to find the real roots of their accidents.

It is not possible to list these causes, even in a book twice this size. The broad categories of injury and parts of the body affected are well known but each workplace has its own individual mixture of risks which must be identified and rooted out on the spot.

Take eye injuries for example. Flying swarf in machine shops and chips of concrete on building sites are well known hazards – **but what about the man who lost an eye changing the oil on a car?** His special hazard appears in no textbook, but to him it is the most important eye risk in the world. If it happens again he will be blind.

Most people would put his injury down to carelessness or stupidity ('Lost an eye, changing the oil? Must be daft') but it was only possible because of the way work is done in the motor trade, grovelling around in the dark, confined space under cars.

Equipment.

A ramp or inspection pit would have given him enough space to keep his head away from the spanner. Good lighting would have helped him see the job.

Tools.

A ring spanner would probably not have slipped.

Training.

The man could have been taught always to exert force away from his body.

That was just one injury in one occupation. The permutations are almost limitless. All we can do in this handbook is show that accidents can be prevented if workers no longer accept them as inevitable and if managements are forced into a completely different attitude towards work systems.

The careless employer:

There is now plenty of evidence to swing the accident prevention offensive away from the 'careless worker' to the careless employer.

The most important document is a report called: *2,000 Accidents: a shop floor study of their causes*, published by the National Institute of Industrial Psychology in 1971. It is based on more than 2,000 accidents which occurred in four different types of industrial workshop and is different from any previous research. Observers studied what actually happened on the shop floor, working normal factory hours and clocking up a total of 42 months continuous observation.

Not surprisingly their findings challenge many of the old and convenient myths about accidents:

1. Risks were so much an integral part of work systems as at present arranged, that the more work was done, the more accidents occurred.

2. The risks which accompanied each task were specific and could be changed by changing details of the task.

3. People reduced their accident rate by gaining experience; ie they learned to avoid risks. But this experience was also highly specific and became blurred after time spent on other tasks. – In other words they had to re-learn to avoid the particular risks in a particular task when they had not done it for a while.

4. Serious accidents were often the result of an unusual situation.

'It must follow,' the report continues, 'that the two main lines of successful accident prevention policy must be a method of **design and layout** which will eliminate hazards currently being built into systems of work, and **training** to reduce the effects of inexperience.'

The NIIP team proposed a new approach to training and safety in which 'shop-floor trainers' would help overcome the effects of unsatisfactory work systems. They stressed that this was only a partial solution in the absence of systems design.

Although the firms studied were 'probably among the best' in terms of attitude and safety record, existing knowledge of accident prevention methods was not getting through to the shop floor – let alone a design approach to hazard removal.

'In three of our shops, the presence of a safety officer, a plant engineer or a designer was an event. In the fourth shop, we did not see it at all.'

'The Factory Inspectorate, the employers' federations and RoSPA all publish pamphlets about particular risks in particular trades but none of our observers ever saw any of this literature in any part of any of our workshops.'

The general pattern of training was haphazard and most commonly consisted in 'sitting with Nellie', with intermittent instruction from chargehand, machine setter or foreman.

Only one workshop had an injury records system that could have been used to locate accident blackspots but even there the warnings did not appear to be drawn out and acted on.

One shop recorded only half its 'reportable' accidents – accidents causing more than three days absence which must, by law, be reported to the Factory Inspectorate and entered in the official register.

None of the firms seems to have had a system for identifying areas where protective equipment like gloves, goggles and ear plugs should have been worn. Where equipment was issued and accepted there was no follow-up to make sure that protection became a habit.

The list of failures in engineering, design and, above all, communication, exposed in these 'good firms' could go on for pages.

Again and again the point emerges that work must be designed to use the abilities of human beings to the full while taking the fullest account of their limitations.

> 'People were expected to repeat complex actions with perfect consistency, time after time. And were expected to avoid danger by instant reaction to warning stimuli. When they failed at either of these activities, they laid themselves open to injury. Yet these are both activities at which people are known to be unreliable and slow.'

Some of the dangers had nothing to do with the function of the machine. Power presses had needlessly sharp edges on which workers cut themselves. Men were hurt by impacts from moving guards and one static guard had a razor edge.

The lesson for workers is clear: don't adjust your mind, there is a fault in the system. Yet the workers, supervisors, and management in these four workplaces accepted the explanation of carelessness as the cause of most accidents. This belief prevents the changes in attitudes that are needed to change the injury record. The report says that two things are required:

> 1. Management must be induced to take an interest and to look at what is really happening on the shop floor.
> 2. Workers must be encouraged to feel that something ought to be done.

Pressure on management:

Clearly the two go together like boot and backside but who is to encourage the workers to feel that 'something ought to be done?' Not the management. As the report says,

> 'A general social pressure to do something about risks might embarrass industrial management because it can see itself as the executive of the action required.'

Social pressure is clearly long overdue.

The initiative must come from a militant campaign throughout the trade union movement. **It must reach into the smallest and worst-organised workplaces.** As the NIIP observers found, the unions have their own communications gap: they recommended unions to improve their information services so that information reaches those who need it.

They also recommended that unions will need to train safety representatives in accident prevention.

The examples which follow show how accidents are built into common work situations.

Built-in accidents – example 1:

Problems: In the despatch department studied by NIIP, workers suffered a surprising number of cuts and falls, some causing absences of several weeks. It did not take long to find that the work method and not the workerforce was accident-prone.

Men were cutting their hands on the metal reinforcement of old packing cases and on the metal banding of parcels. Falls occurred in several areas but the worst ones were concentrated at the vehicle loading point where metal plates were used to bridge the gap between loading bay and vans. There were also several accidents inside the vans.

Solutions: The decrepit packing cases were quite unsuitable for the job: too big for comfortable lifting, they forced the workers to put their hands at the corners where the reinforcement was jagged. They could have been replaced with purpose-designed plastic containers. Metal banding on parcels could have been replaced with plastic. The men should have been given gloves.

Inside the building floors were uneven and would not have come up to Factories Act standards.

At the loading point, vans and platform could have been arranged to fit closely so that bridge plates became unnecessary; or they could have been arranged at the same height so that the plates would not slope. The plates could have been widened to the full width of the van door and they could have been ribbed to give better grip. The whole department could have been equipped with non-slip boots for less than the cost of injury absence. The roof could have been mended to stop the floor getting slippery. Vans could have been properly lit so that workers would not stumble in the gloomy interiors. Training could have been given in lifting and handling methods.

Ergonomics.

This job had never been designed as a work system and the men were paying the price. Most observers would have blamed them for carelessness but the study showed that the more goods they handled the more accidents they had. (The traditional, superficial approach would have identified the men who handled most packing cases as the most careless, or as 'accident-prone'.)

The suggested modifications would still not give the despatch department a designed work system. To do that would have required examination of all handling methods, including mechanical equipment, and the development of a system that integrated men, machines, building and vans into a single safe process.

This is where the experts in ergonomics really come into their own and where many managers start slithering towards the door. Ergonomists have an expensive habit of telling management that the everyday tools of industry are unsuited to human beings.

Example 2 – machine tools:

The controls of one lathe were evaluated and it was discovered that the ideal operator would have to be 4ft 6in tall, 2ft across the shoulders and have an 8ft arm span.

A walk around the average machine shop is likely to reveal many of the following faults or omissions:

o **Controls that are poorly positioned, uncomfortable to use, require excessive force to operate under load or can only be engaged after a long wait for parts to line up.**

o **Knobs on operating levers retained by circlips, a cheap piece of engineering which leaves the knobs free to rotate in such a way that your hand could slip and be injured.**

o **Stop switches inaccessible in an emergency.**

o **Foot stop bars not fitted.**

H

o **Emergency braking systems, which inject DC current into the motor windings for almost instantaneous stopping, not fitted.**

o **No protection for operator (or machine) from swarf and suds.**

o **Change-speed covers that have to be removed completely to get inside, with the result that the machine will be left in the wrong speed or the cover will be left off. (There are alternative hinged covers with microswitch cutout devices.)**

Many devices essential to safe and convenient operation have not been fitted because they are expensive optional extras rather than integral to the design. Under this heading come feed stops with positive and accurate cutout. Some lathes have no cutout device but rely on mechanical arrest of the saddle and operation of the feed shaft overload clutch. Others, without overload clutch, stop when a shear pin fails in the drive.

A design engineer who has actually worked in precision machine shops points out that this list is far from complete even in hard safety terms, let alone factors causing inconvenience and fatigue:

> The list and its permutations are embarrassingly long and are more in keeping with mechanisms in their first decade of development or only intended for very occasional use. It is almost impossible to believe that most people responsible for lathe design have ever had to use their product for more than brief periods.
>
> Apart from uprating various parts to cope with increased feeds and speeds, there has been no coherent evolution to meet present needs. One of the results is that gear tooth speeds in most main drives are now excessive in relation to the accuracy of the gears used, and noise levels are uncomfortably, sometimes dangerously, high.

Example 3 – mobile cranes:

If the lathe emerges from ergonomic examination as unfit for humans, a basic tool of the construction industry, the mobile crane, comes out even worse.

An ergonomic survey of 57 cranes and drivers by Glamorgan Polytechnic's Department of Civil Engineering and Building came up with the following results:

5 per cent of drivers had had accidents when leaving the
cab
68 per cent of drivers had difficulty getting in and out
There were 34 different controller layouts among 57
cranes
Only two layouts included 'dead-man' control systems
87 per cent of drivers would like standardised controls
95 per cent of machines could be accidentally set in
motion
72 per cent of drivers sometimes forgot that controls
were different from previous machines
76 per cent confessed to controller movement error.

o Heating systems are dependent upon the engine speed,
no ventilating systems exist in cabins and during the
winter months the drivers' clothes become damp due to
the high humidity of the atmosphere, causing condensa-
tion to form on the walls of the cabin.

o It is significant that one driver met on this survey was
over 50 years of age. Older people will not or cannot
occupy these jobs because of the arduous conditions.
The drivers consider that health and physique are affected, eg overweight, stomach ulcers, haemorrhoids and
hypertension. 67 per cent of drivers experience stiff
necks, cramp in legs, aching back, pains in arms and
legs, either after completing a specific task or after the
changeover from one crane to another . . . Headaches
are a common occurrence and assumed to be caused by
viewing high lifts with the bright sky in the background,
also pains in the stomach which, it is reported, although
not confirmed, are caused by inhaling carbon monoxide
fumes from the exhaust outlet which is often adjacent
to the cabin. 67 per cent confessed to getting tired whilst
sitting at their controls although this was considerably
affected by boredom.

A noise survey of 37 of the cranes found
the following levels:

71- 80dBA	2 machines
81- 90dBA	13 machines
91-100dBA	13 machines
101-110dBA	8 machines
111-120dBA	1 machine

A sample of operators aged between 22 – 49 was found
to have an average hearing level about 10dB higher than a
non-exposed control group in the 'speech frequencies' of
500, 1,000 and 2,000Hz. This means that some of them must
have been experiencing real difficulty following conversation. See Section 3, Noise.

These mobile workplaces, probably costing tens of

thousands of pounds each, are clearly accident-prone and a danger to health. Again, they have been designed to do a job without including the operator in the definition of 'job' – and the verdict must be 'unfit for humans'.

Example 4:

o Ideal specification for overhead crane operator

Arm length: 4ft

Neck length: 1ft

o Failure to meet these requirements will result in back-ache and fatigue.

Operator modification:

In the examples above the modification of man by machine is gradual. A more dramatic example is provided by the woodworking machine demonstrator who had most of the fingers of his right hand missing. The manufacturer was proud of the man's great skill and said that, because of his injury, he could get much closer to the cutters than other people.

Whose error?

The examples that have been given may not apply to your workplace but the principle of built-in accidents applies to nearly all situations. The more work you do the more accidents you have.

If other factors like heat or cold, noise or fumes, stress or fatigue are also involved, accidents become even more likely.

A few employers get near to recognising this, like the Volvo engineer who said: 'Our philosophy is that any operating or handling mistake that can be made, sooner or later will be made. So we have every safeguard against human mistakes.' Even this ambitious statement puts the emphasis on human *error*. As the NIIP study showed, you don't have to make a mistake to have an accident in many quite normal work situations.

This extract from the 1970 report on the Offices, Shops and Railway Premises Act reinforces the point:

'Fractured limbs from falls on wet or greasy floors were not uncommon; one man died following a thigh fracture caused by catching his foot in a loop of string on the floor'. The errors were in the floor, not the workers, but most local authority inspectors attributed the worst accidents to carelessness.

Safety and profits:

The myth of the careless worker lives on, convenient for industry and for the inspectorates who have to explain the appalling accident figures on their 'beat' each year. o In 1968 the Chief Inspector of Factories suggested it would not have been reasonably practicable to prevent more than half of a sample of accidents studied.

The American safety expert, H.W.Heinrich, has said that 98 per cent of accidents can be prevented. The difference lies in the words 'reasonably practicable'. These words tend to mean 'reasonably economical'.

> 'Accidents in factories and the home are usually the result of cheap engineering.'
> Professor M.W.Thring, Queen Mary College, London, at Society of Environmental Engineers symposium, June 1971.

It should now be clear that the worker's drive for safety is in direct economic conflict with the employer's drive for economy. Talk of an 'identity of interest' between the two sides on safety is waffle. Workers and their families are paying dearly in lives, limbs and lost earnings for substandard work systems. For the employer on the other hand accidents are cheap. The NIIP report suggested from its findings that the cost to a large factory was 'peanuts . . . no doubt one of the reasons why accidents are not regarded as a serious problem.' The report went on:

> 'However, the cost of accidents is not simply accountable and is not a burden on the factory so much as on the community . . . the community has a hospital service, a national insurance scheme, and a legal service to pay for, thus relieving the factory of further responsibility for the people it maims. The factory produces goods and injuries; the community at large pays for both.'

The double subsidy:

As a large part of the community and as the only victims of industrial injuries, workers are paying twice over.

The time has come for workers to refuse the double subsidy and to demand of employers the investment in systems and skills that will make work safe.

Action:

This represents a fundamental challenge to the supremacy of profit and it will not be won unless it is backed by the full power of the working class.

The essentials are:

Anger:

Two thousand men and women are killed each year by accidents at work. o Tens of thousands of lives are ruined. o Hundreds of thousands of families are thrust into hardship and worry.

This is British industry's small contribution to an obscene human sacrifice which demands from workers throughout the world 100,000 bodies a year – a demand which steadily grows as industrialisation (and 'carelessness') is profitably exported to the developing world.

Organisation:

Every workplace must organise to fight hazards. The realisation that accidents (and diseases) are built into work systems will turn sour unless it can be channelled into successful action. Some safety battles may be won by a spontaneous protest like a walk-out. The deep-seated hazards will only be beaten by solid organisation, backed and serviced by the whole union movement. The TUC and trade union leaders must be pressed into declaring war on industrial hazards instead of mouthing platitudes about 'disturbing figures' each time the Chief Inspector of Factories issues his annual catalogue. (See Section 13, Organising.)

Information:

This is one of the missing links. Workers desperately need facts on accident risks and health hazards in their particular occupations. Only a few unions are generating any kind of information; much of it uncritical of present standards in industry. It is not produced in sufficient volume to reach more than a few in each workplace.

Information must also be collected in the workplace if hazards are to be properly identified and if workers are to be confident in their demands.

Accidents cannot be tackled in isolation; the workplace safety group needs to build up a comprehensive picture of all the hazards – slippery floors, dangerous machines, noise, fumes and so on. Different factors may be causing injury and disease in their own right and contributing to other dangerous situations. (As when noise causes deafness in one area and adds to general stress in the next.)

An approach to workplace inspection, official or unofficial, is suggested in Section 8, Action.

Even careful and critical inspection may not reveal all hazards. Comprehensive *accident records* can often point to unsuspected danger areas. Management must not only keep proper record of *all* injuries but also make them available to workers.

Records should show: the nature of the injury; the part of the body injured; what actually inflicted the wound; the exact part of the works where it happened.

All injuries, however minor, should

1. Receive first aid

2. Be properly recorded for accident prevention analysis. (Recording of an injury can also be important in later claims for damages – see Section 11, Winning damages.)

First aid and accident records are best handled at the same time by a permanently-staffed surgery. If the workplace does not have a surgery this could be added to the list of demands in a safety campaign.

If this is clearly not realistic, the trained first aiders on the shop floor will have to keep records (and not lose money through the extra work time lost). This would have the advantage that information would be held by a worker.

The Industrial Health and Safety Centre run by the Factory Inspectorate in Horseferry Road, London SW1, should provide ammunition for workers when management claims that 'it can't be done'. The place is crammed with equipment for doing jobs safely and comfortably. Judging from the comments of visiting workers and managers, many of the exhibits have never been seen on the average shop floor or building site.

The location of the Centre in London of course guarantees that it is inaccessible to the majority of industrial workers. Joint visits organised by management overcome the problems of distance and finance, but such outings tend to be inhibited. On your own, you can get down to hard comparisons between the best of current safety engineering and what you actually use at work. Tours are usually conducted by a factory inspector. Group visits need to be booked in advance. Individuals can look around at any time without booking.

Booklets on hazards and accident prevention are noted in the back of this handbook.

Skills:

The TUC and unions, having campaigned for the creation of workers' safety representatives, will have to intensify their training effort, especially where complex hazards are involved. Training needs to be conceived from a shop floor point of view.

Sometimes problems will be beyond the skills of both safety reps and management. Workers may have to insist that management brings in outside experts – for example an ergonomist to redesign a work system. (Watch out for any management attempt to introduce work intensification in the guise of ergonomic redesign.)

Management's responsibility:

It should be made quite clear that, however extensive the knowledge and skill built up on the shop floor, responsibility for hazards and prevention rests firmly with the employer. The aim is to force management to accept this responsibility.

The individual worker:

Without the backing of shop floor safety organisation

individual action is restricted. Apart from working towards this objective you can safeguard your own safety by reporting all hazards and defects and, if possible, refusing to work until they are put right. Such refusals can lead to victimisation so, again, solid organisation is essential. But you may have to be the one who makes the first move.

Personal checklist:

The idea that some workers are 'accident-prone' because of some basic mental deficiency is well-loved by accident researchers who would rather find faults in the worker than the employer. More conscientious investigation of the relationship between workers and their job tends to reveal much simpler reasons for high accident 'scores'. The high scorer in a warehouse where workers handle large objects without proper lifting aids may turn out to be shorter than his mates; he may be the one who gets through most work; he may be the one who does the biggest variety of jobs and has to learn (or re-learn) each one as he does it.

Other factors are now emerging which may increase your vulnerability to built-in dangers:

Eyesight:

Research has shown that three-fifths of accident-prone workers in a metal works had poor vision. See also p 185.

Breakfast:

The accident rate among a group of steelworkers who did not eat breakfast was double that of those who did. Those who didn't eat before coming to work were physically and mentally below par by about 11o'clock. After lunch the accident rates levelled up.

Tranquillisers:

Research on driving performance has shown that tranquillisers affect vision and reflexes, making people more liable to accidents. One type does not have this effect so if you have to take tranquillisers ask your doctor to prescribe this type.

NB: Eagle-eyed and stuffed with breakfast, you'll still have an accident if the work system is not safe.

8.

Action

Previous sections have dealt with hazards and the steps that should be taken to protect you from them. This section is to help you find out which ones are present in your own workplace so that you can begin a systematic campaign for improvement and achieve standards you consider safe and comfortable.

This will be difficult without strong shop floor organisation. Some suggestions for organisation are made in Section 13, but the form of the organisation doesn't matter too much, as long as it works and confronts the employer with absolute solidarity on any threat to health or safety.

Getting the facts:

The main problem is going to be getting information, especially about chemicals or highly technical hazards like radiation. It will be very useful if you can make contact with members of scientific and technical unions employed in the same organisation, for example in the laboratories.

Links with other workers in a combine can be used to find out, for example, what substances go into the materials you use and what safeguards are provided during manufacture.

Other people in the works may be able to find out a great deal: storemen or clerks in the order department may know the names of raw materials and where they come from. Delivery drivers may carry Transport Emergency Cards when a load is toxic or corrosive. (For their own safety and that of firemen and general public, they should insist on Tremcards – see Section 4, Chemical Hazards, p100.)

The value of a workers' information network is speed.

Official union channels are slow because enquiries pass through many hands before, in most cases, ending up at the TUC or the TUC Centenary Institute.

Unions with their own safety departments (see page 319) should be quicker, providing they don't have to pass the enquiry on.

If you are really worried about something, don't let district offices hang about writing letters. Make sure they telephone the TUC Medical Adviser or the Centenary Institute information service straight away. Or forget the procedure and do it yourself.

The same applies if union officials dismiss your fears and you are still not happy.

If you think anyone is in immediate danger and management won't take action, stop the process and call the Factory Inspectorate or whatever inspectorate is supposed to police your employment. (See pages 240-242.)

The Factory Inspectorate and Employment Medical Advisory Service will also answer enquiries and advise on problems.

Various voluntary organisations may also be useful, though mainly as sources of literature.

Organisations and publications are listed at the back of this book.

Don't be put off by bald management statements that something is safe. If that is so, they will be able to prove it quite easily.

Wherever you send an inquiry it is important to give the fullest possible information. For example if you want to find out if a chemical is dangerous, include as many of the following as you can:

o What it is, its trade name, or code number
o The name and address of manufacturer
o How it is used and how much is used
o What you think it is doing to workers, eg headaches, skin rash
o What precautions are taken, eg type of respirator

Don't accept that nothing can be done to improve conditions.

This is the oldest argument: noisy machines have been replaced ten times over since the first workers were told it was impossible to silence them. Many new ones are actually more noisy.

The following is a suggested sequence of action for a systematic attack on hazards. (If one hazard sticks out like a sore thumb ignore the sequence and tackle it straight away.)

1. Obtain accident and sickness records from management. Look for pattern, eg hand injuries in one particular area.

2. Inspect the workplace. If management won't let safety stewards have freedom of movement, workers in each area should do their own hazard checks and report back. Look for hazards that could account for sickness and injury patterns. The checklist which follows may help in getting a complete picture.

3. List all machine and process risks and how serious you think they may be in each area.

4. Make a separate list of all chemicals used. Find out what they are and what they could do to health by using the Directory of Toxic Substances at the back of this book. Check in the Index for fuller details or make enquiries.

5. Compare precautions being taken with those that should be taken.

6. Decide priorities for action, eg major hazards (or ones where further, expert, investigation is needed); the ones that are causing most concern; or the ones that are quickest and easiest to solve. It may be a good idea to go for something easy first, for example a rough floor that people keep tripping on. Success will convince everyone that things can be changed.

7. Press management for elimination of known hazards.

8. Press for investigation by outside experts, eg industrial hygienists, where level of risk is not known. Demand full disclosure of any report.

9. Set programme for improvement to standards well above the minimum for survival.

10. Go on for standards of comfort, until work is as pleasant as it can be.

Checklist:

The checklist which follows may help you look at your workplace in a systematic way but it cannot cover all the risks of different occupations. You may be able to construct a much better list from your own experience. In either case don't let the list get in the way of common sense.

You can tell a lot about a place by just looking around, listening to noise levels, using your nose to sample the air, and your finger to check the amount and colour of dust on ledges. Don't ignore your senses: it is best to put them to work first thing on each shift when they are still fresh. Strangers often notice faults you have become accustomed to: opinions from young workers whose ears, noses and expectations have not yet been dulled by industry are particularly valuable.

Organisation:
o Do you have a safety steward or stewards? ☐
o Do you have a workers' safety committee? ☐
o Is there a joint safety committee with management? ☐
o Do you elect your own representatives to it? ☐
o Can it get anything done, or is it a talk-shop? ☐

Management:
o Is there a works doctor? ☐ or industrial health service? ☐
              nurse? ☐
              safety officer? ☐
              industrial hygienist? ☐
o Are proper accident and sickness records kept? ☐
o Do they obey the law? ☐

Workplace – general:
(with apologies to miners)
o Is it: a fit place to spend half your waking hours? ☐
      clean? ☐
      well-lit? ☐
      well-ventilated? ☐
      comfortably-heated? ☐

Major hazards:

o Could any of these be a risk: noise? ☐
vibration? ☐
radiation (all kinds)? ☐
extreme heat? ☐
extreme cold? ☐
chemicals? ☐

Accidents – housekeeping:

o Are gangways kept clear? ☐
all surfaces non-slip, level and well-maintained? ☐
floors kept free from oil, spillages and obstructions? ☐
materials stacked safely? ☐
light bulbs and neon tubes replaced promptly? ☐

Accidents – stress:

o Is it noisy? ☐
too hot? ☐
too cold? ☐

o Does equipment cause vibration? ☐
o Are narcotic chemicals used? – eg trichloroethylene? ☐
o Is work pace too fast for safety? ☐
o Can you work comfortably – ie without stooping or stretching? ☐

Machinery:

o Are guards fitted to all dangerous parts (round the back as well)? ☐
o Are they good enough? ☐
o Do they really: keep you out? ☐
keep the hazard in? ☐
o Do automatic guards 'fail safe'? ☐
o Can you reach the stop control in an emergency? ☐
o Is DC injection braking fitted to machine tools? ☐
o Are machines spaced: far enough apart for safety? ☐
far enough from gangways, fork trucks, etc? ☐
o Can machines be isolated when guards are off? ☐
o Is there a 'permit to work system' which prevents start-up during machine maintenance? ☐

o Are noise and vibration levels safe? ☐
o Is the cutting oil: clean (dermatitis)? ☐
refined (skin cancer)? ☐

Transport:
o Is there a properly designed traffic system? ☐
o Are routes marked off with white lines? ☐
o Is there a: rule of the road or one-way route? ☐
speed limit? ☐
o Do fork trucks cause fumes? ☐
o Are drivers trained? ☐
o Are loads kept small enough for them to see where they are going? ☐

Electricity:
o Is all equipment earthed? ☐
voltage reduced wherever possible? ☐
equipment regularly maintained? ☐
work done only by electricians? ☐
o Are overhead wires, crane conductors, etc, protected from contact, eg by metal ladders, vehicles? ☐
o Are workers trained to treat shock victims? ☐
o Are 'permit-to-work' systems operated? ☐

Cranes:
o Is the safe working load clearly marked? ☐
o Is there a load indicator? ☐
o Are there safeguards for anyone working near overhead tracks? ☐
o Is proper lifting gear available for different loads? ☐
marked with the safe load? ☐
examined every six months? ☐
o Are drivers of overhead cranes protected from: fumes from the shop? ☐ radiation? ☐
o Can they hear instructions or see signals? ☐
o Has two-way radio been considered instead of signalling? ☐

Compressed air:
o Are air lines, vessels and pressure relief valves tested regularly? ☐

o Have workers been instructed in the hazards of compressed air jet hitting eyes or other body openings? ☐

Chemicals:

o Do workers complain of: irritated eyes, nose and throat? ☐
coughing or wheezing? ☐
headaches, dizziness, sleepiness? ☐
nausea, vomiting, diarrhoea? ☐
skin rash or irritation? ☐

o Do these symptoms appear with any particular materials? ☐
in any particular departments? ☐

o Is there any pattern of disease – eg, lung cancers – among retired workers? ☐

o Are dangerous substances used? ☐

o Toxic? ☐

o Corrosive? ☐

o Inflammable? ☐

o Explosive? ☐

o Are they labelled to show contents, danger, precautions and first aid? ☐

o Are there warning signs in danger areas? ☐

o Will management identify all chemicals? ☐

o Can safer materials be used? ☐
the process be sealed off? ☐

o Is there local exhaust ventilation to extract dust and fumes? ☐

o Does the employer, or a consultant, test the air regularly? ☐

o Are permanent monitoring devices installed to detect very dangerous substances? ☐

o Are they set to warn of the smallest concentrations? ☐

o Are medical tests carried out regularly? ☐

o Are results made available to workers? ☐

o Is emergency breathing apparatus readily available? ☐

o Could bulk storage, fumes or dust be community hazards? ☐

o Could your products endanger other workers? ☐
o Do they know? ☐
o Are waste chemicals disposed of safely? ☐
o Are washing/showering facilities good enough? ☐
o Is there a free overalls service? ☐
o Can you take toxic materials home on your body or clothing? ☐

Fire:

o Could you get out quickly? ☐
o Are all gangways, staircases clear? ☐
o Can all escape doors be opened from inside? ☐
o Has everyone been instructed in escape drill? ☐
o Could you raise the alarm easily? ☐
o Is there a telephone nearby? ☐
o Has the fire alarm been tested recently? ☐
o Can you hear it everywhere, even in the toilets? ☐
o Are extinguishers plentiful? ☐
                  regularly checked? ☐
o Is there an automatic sprinkler system? ☐
o Has the Fire Brigade made an inspection recently? ☐
o Do local firemen know of any substance that could endanger them? ☐

Fire and explosion risks:

o Are flammable materials used in smallest possible amounts? ☐
o Are any materials liable to spontaneous combustion? ☐
o Would spilled liquids run into other areas? ☐
o Is waste material cleared up and removed? ☐
o Could dust cause an explosion? ☐
o Do any machines run hot? ☐
o In high risk areas, is there anything to cause:
        sparks? ☐
        flames?
        excessive heat? ☐

Confined spaces, vessels and silos:

o Have you been taught safe methods for entry? ☐

o Is breathing apparatus and life-line available? ☐
                                       accessible? ☐
                                       maintained? ☐
o Are spaces always tested before entry? ☐
o Do people always work with a mate standing by? ☐

Protective equipment:

o Is everything possible done for safety before equipment is issued? ☐
o Is the right equipment issued for the hazard? ☐
o Is it individually issued? ☐
o Does it fit properly? ☐
o Is it comfortable for the length of time it has to be worn? ☐
o Does it really protect you? ☐

9

The Legal Machine

This section explains the main machinery of the legal system as it affects safety and compensation. It examines some of the historical, social and economic factors which influence it.

- o The structure of the law
- o Statutory safety standards
- o The failure of enforcement
- o The Robens Report
- o Common law compensation
- o State benefits
- o History of legislation

The law serves best the interests of those who have a hand in making it. We should not be surprised that it is at its weakest when it deals with workers' health and safety.

All the same, it is important to understand how the law works because it can be used more effectively to protect health and secure compensation when health is damaged.

The first step is to shake off the awe in which most of us hold the law, whether we think of it as wearing a helmet or a wig. Professor K.W.Wedderburn puts it nicely in the preface to *The Worker and The Law* (Penguin):
'law is not a mystery; it only uses long words'.

The structure of the law:

The law breaks down into two main divisions:
1. Criminal law:

This deals with wrongs against society where some authority takes the initiative to prosecute. The police and public authority and inspectorates generally enforce the criminal law.

2. Civil law:

This deals with the private rights of individuals and groups. It is the individual who decides whether to do anything about a wrong that has been done to him.

There are two main kinds of law which operate in the two parts of the system:

1. Common law:

The ordinary law of the land as developed over the centuries. It is 'judge-made law'.

2. Statute law:

The body of laws made by Parliament. When an Act of Parliament is passed it goes onto the Statute Book and the common law on that subject is displaced.

Civil and criminal law are administered separately by the civil courts and the criminal courts, though they overlap to a certain extent – for example in the courts of appeal.

The civil courts decide their cases on the basis of both common law and statute law.

The criminal courts deal almost exclusively with the laws made by Parliament.

The same *event* can lead to a criminal law prosecution and to a civil law action. Suppose a man has his fingers amputated in a power press which was not properly guarded:

1. The employer stands to face a **criminal** prosecution because, by not guarding the press, he has clearly broken one of the requirements of the Factories Act. Enforcement of this **statute** is handled by the Factory Inspectorate. If it decides to prosecute it brings its case in the lowest **criminal court,** a magistrates court.

2. The action of the state against this **crime** has not done the injured worker much good. He wants compensation for his lost fingers. He brings a **civil action** against his employer claiming damages for loss of earnings. His case will be based on the employer's breach of a **statutory duty** under the Factories Act and of his **common law duty** to take reasonable care for the safety of his workers. The case will be heard in a **civil court** – the county court when the damages sought are less than £750 or the High Court, for any greater sum.

The next part of this introductory section on the law goes into more detail on statutory safety standards, the way they have developed and the low priority that the State gives to their enforcement. The practicalities of using statutory standards in the fight for safety are dealt with in Section 10, Safety Law.

Other aspects of common law and compensation, including state benefits are dealt with later in this section.

The practicalities of winning damages are described in Section 11.

The practicalities of getting National Insurance benefits are explained in Section 12.

Statute law:

Statutes are the same things as Acts. They start as Bills which are put before Parliament, usually by the Government of the day and sometimes by individual MPs (when they are called private-member's bills). After various stages of debate and procedure in both houses of Parliament they may be passed as Acts, whereupon they 'go onto the Statute Book'.

Government legislation usually passes almost intact through the parliamentary machine; private member's bills have a high mortality rate but they have produced some of our more enlightened social legislation, like abortion law reform and help for the disabled.

Important private bills on compulsory workplace safety committees have consistently failed to reach the Statute Book.

Ministers may have powers to make special regulations under certain Acts.

Statutes oust common law:

When a new law is enacted it displaces the common law on that subject in a way that is best shown by an example. Suppose an Act is passed laying down minimum health and safety standards for deep-sea fishermen, the employers will still have a common law duty to take reasonable care. But standards that might previously have been accepted as reasonable – for example, trawlers without de-icing equipment – might actually become illegal under specific sections of the new act.

Statutory safety standards:

Safety legislation:

The statutes that concern us are the ones applying to safety, health and welfare at work. The best known is the Factories Act which reached its present form in 1961, more than a century and a half after the first factory legislation attempted to curb the abuses of the Industrial Revolution. (See short history at the end of this section.)

Other non-factory occupations have gradually been brought under statutory control but it is a major weakness of the present system that some six million workers are still not covered by legislation. For them there is no protection; only the right to claim common law damages if the employers fail to take reasonable care.

Statutory safety standards are potentially the most powerful method for preventing injury and disease at work. This is because they not only lay down precise requirements for hundreds of work situations but they also provide for inspectorates to police industry and ensure compliance.

That is the theory. The practice is rather different because the punch is pulled at almost every stage:

1. The acts do not cover all the working population.

2. Many of the regulations are weakly drafted; that spirit of 'reasonableness' which characterises common law standards often infects safety statutes with such qualifications as 'so far as is reasonably practicable'.

3. The enforcement agencies vary from ineffectual to almost non-existent. Although laws in this field have exactly the same status as other criminal law like the Road Traffic Acts – rigorously enforced by the police – the inspectorates treat the law as negotiable.

4. When, occasionally, offending employers are finally brought to court, their offences are usually treated as being in a different class from other crimes. Fines are purely nominal – an average of £40 under the Factories Act, for example.

5. The law is designed to restrain employers and, to some extent employees, from hazardous conduct. With the exception of mines and quarries legislation, it does not confer rights of positive action, such as the right of workers to inspect the workplace.

Official policy on enforcement:

The official policies on enforcement serve to castrate safety law.

When the police stop a motorist who has been doing 90mph on the M6 they do not tell him they'll be back next week to see if he's sticking to 70. They do not advise him on the technical advantages of a brighter speedometer. They book him.

Yet the biggest enforcement agency for safety law in industry, the Factory Inspectorate, has adopted just this 'advisory' role. The employer who breaks the law can expect several advisory sessions before prosecution is even threatened.

Can it be that the consequences of breaking this kind of law are less serious? Hardly. In 1971 the Inspectorate itself reported that nearly one in three deaths in factory processes was due to the employer's criminal act. In construction, the employer broke the law in more than half the cases where a man was killed.

It is hard to see how such crime can be regarded as open to friendly discussion, yet the quotes and examples which follow confirm that this is indeed official policy.

o 'Our strong impression is that routine visits tend to be brief, superficial and usually unproductive.'
Robens Report.
o '. . . the responsible government departments and inspectorates tended in their evidence to describe their primary function in terms of improving standards of safety and health at work, rather than in terms of law enforcement as such . . . in practice they find that in most cases advice and persuasion achieve more than duress.'
Robens Report.
o 'Originally conceived as law-enforcement agencies, the style and nature of the activities of the inspectorates have changed over time as the scope of their work has grown in volume and complexity, and as society's ideas

and expectations about authority and behaviour have
changed.'
Robens Report (our bold).
The Robens Report does not define 'society'.
o 'The Factory Inspectorate has never attempted (and
has certainly never achieved) rigorous enforcement of
the Factories Act such as a Teutonic country might
attempt.'
Mr W.J.C.Plumbe, former Chief Inspector of Factories.
**No doubt workers will be happy to lay down more lives
in the cause of keeping the Teuton threat from our
shores.**

Enforcement of the Offices, Shops and Railway Premises Act is played to the same rules:

o 'Most authorities preferred to rely on persuasion, particularly with regard to environmental requirements
such as heating and lighting, as they considered that a
higher standard was more likely to be attained by securing the co-operation of occupiers. Prosecution action
was taken where, for example, there was a **continued**
failure to fence dangerous machinery.' (Our bold.)
The Offices, Shops and Railway Premises Act 1963, Report by the Secretary of State for Employment for the
year ended 31 December 1970.

What do these attitudes mean in practice? Workers at
the Enthoven lead works at Darley Dale have first hand experience:

Ken Fletcher Jnr:
o 'The Factory Inspector is never there when we are
drossing the pots. They should come at night. When they
come it's never working: it's closed down. They have a
day cleaning up before the Factory Inspector comes
round.'
Ken Fletcher Snr:
o 'The foreman says "clean this up, clean that up because the Factory Inspector is coming round".'

o 'Factory inspectors who visited a works were horri-
fied to see that the metal press machine had no guard,
magistrates were told.
There had been an accident on a press at the same firm
a few months previously but on that occasion there had
not been any prosecution because of assurances that
such an accident would never happen again. However
there appeared to have been no action taken to follow
this up.
For the firm it was said that when the inspectors visited
the premises the machine was being operated without
their knowledge.' The firm was fined £100.
RoSPA report

Statutes and the judges:

When the preventative role of safety legislation fails the injured worker may find the statutory standards strengthen his case in a claim for damages.

The judges made such inroads into the Factories Act during the 1950s that some sections had no more strength than the common law duty to take reasonable care. Professor Wedderburn refers to this as 'the wreckage of judicial interpretation'.

It was decided, for example, that the worker who met with an accident whilst walking *from* his bench to the toilet was not covered by the Act because Section 26 specified safe means of access *to* an employee's place of work. This childish interpretation, which ignored the *intention* of the law, was corrected by inserting the words 'and from' in the Factories Act of 1961.

Various explanations have been advanced for such decisions. It has been said that they represent no more than a scrupulously objective interpretation of the law but in that case why has this approach produced so few decisions which *strengthen* the law?

In spite of these many weaknesses, the statutory system works just well enough to give us a glimpse of how effective it could be. The Power Press Regulations made under the Factories Act provide a classic example.

o There were 498 accidents on power presses in 1964, 159 in 1971. The only thing that changed between those two dates was the law. The Regulations became operative in 1965. The fact that other types of accident increased in this period makes the reduction doubly significant.

If the regulations are obeyed it should be physically impossible to have an injury. Yet out of a total of 245 amputations at power presses in 1969 only 98 led to prosecutions. Real enforcement of the regulations could bring a further transformation.

The inspectorates are so conditioned by their advisory role that they sometimes surprise themselves with the effectiveness of their powers.

The 1970 report on the Offices, Shops and Railway

Premises Act tells of one local authority which found that final notices before legal action was taken 'have a-remarkably galvanising effect upon a situation which, up to that point, would best be described as one of monumental inactivity'.

It must be a comfort to employers to know there is a final notice *before* legal action is taken.

The system of law and its enforcement clearly does not work properly. Three thousand deaths each year make the point that it is not meant to work.

The Robens report:

The government committee on Safety and Health at Work, chaired by Lord Robens, also found that existing arrangements were not working. But, after two years study, it came to the amazing conclusion that the fault lay in the statutory approach rather than in the particular system it was looking at.

Instead of recognising that a proper statutory system has never actually existed in Britain it decided that there was *too much law* and this led to 'apathy' about safety. What was needed, according to Robens, was less law and more voluntary self-regulation by industry itself, guided by flexible codes of practice rather than slavish compliance with minimum standards.

This 'revolutionary' approach amounts to little more than a recognition of the existing situation in which most employers can choose whether to obey the law.

The report does not make it clear how apathy is to be dispelled or what would make employers meet the higher standards of codes of practice when they currently fail to meet the minimum requirements of the statutes.

Rigorous enforcement is rejected. The one element that might make such an approach work – compulsory workplace safety committees and workers' inspectors – has been rejected.

Instead Robens gives us a watery formula which places on employers a duty to *consult* employees on measures for promoting safety and health.

A more responsible attitude on the part of employers is also supposed to stem from the requirements that they draw up a written safety policy and include information about accidents, occupational disease and prevention measures in the Company's annual report.

Other main proposals in the report:

1. A single Act covering virtually all workers. This would not be a detailed statute like the Factories Act but would make provision of a safe and healthy system of work a statutory duty on all employers. Detailed regulations could be made under the Act but Robens suggests making more use of voluntary codes of practice for different trades and hazards.

2. A national authority for safety and health at work.

3. A unified inspectorate able to issue improvement notices and prohibition notices without reference to a court. (Employer able to appeal and, in the case of an improvement notice, carry on as before until appeal is heard.) Less prosecution but bigger fines available for really bad cases.

4. More prevention work by both TUC and CBI and more collaboration between them on health and safety.

The report contains a lot of useful information laboriously brought together from the watertight compartments of the bureaucracy. Some of its proposals, like unified legislation and inspection and 'instant' prohibition orders, are obvious and sensible. It all seems quite plausible. It did not fool the industrial lawyer Anthony Woolf who has described it as 'dangerous nonsense'.

In an article in the magazine *Manufacturing Management* he points to the central fallacy:

'The fact is,' says the Robens Report, 'that the traditional concepts of the criminal law are not readily applicable to the majority of infringements which arise under this type of legislation. Relatively few offences are clear-cut, few arise from reckless indifference to the possibility of causing injury, few can be laid without qualification at the door of a particular individual.' I wonder who told them that? But I wonder more what they thought their next sentences mean. 'The typical infringement arises rather through carelessness, oversight, lack of knowledge or means; or sheer inefficiency. In such circumstances the process of prosecution and punishment is largely an irrelevancy.'

But if the manager of a factory breaks the law because of 'lack of knowledge or means, or inadequate supervision or sheer inefficiency', why should prosecution and punishment be irrelevant? . . . If he breaks the law through 'sheer inefficiency', why is that less criminal than forgetting to have his tyres or brakes checked?

Woolf finds the answers to these questions in 'the canker of corruption of the body politic and industrial, which has always made real enforcement of the law unthinkable. It takes the form of a tacit or overt agreement, by successive governments, by legislators, by magistrates and by a series of supine inspectorates, never to challenge seriously the logic of competitive free enterprise.'

Special actions:

There are three types of legal action which could be used by workers or unions to enforce compliance with statutes. They do not seem to have been used yet but they could make a powerful impact in a campaign for safety by the union movement.

1. A worker can bring a criminal prosecution against his employer for breach of a safety statute.

2. Workers could take out a high court injunction against an employer restraining him from illegally exposing them to a danger. This could be a costly action but if it succeeded the dangerous process would be stopped until made safe.

3. Perhaps an injunction could be obtained requiring the Factory Inspectorate, or some other inspectorate, to enforce the law; or damages could be claimed for injury resulting from its failure to do so. This would cost too much for a worker to attempt without union support or legal aid.

The rest of this section deals with some general aspects of the common law, compensation and National Insurance Injury Benefits.

The practicalities of using statutory safety standards are dealt with in the next section.

Common law compensation:

Common Law is the ordinary law of the land. It has developed over the centuries as a result of decisions made by the courts. Case law and precedent are therefore at the heart of it. When the two parties in an action, the plaintiff and the defendant, appear before the judge they will try to persuade him that previous cases favourable to their arguments fit the present circumstances. (As we have seen, a claim for damages may also be based on breach of a statutory duty but millions of workers will have only the common law to rely on if they are injured, and the precedent system applies to *interpretations* of statutes in just the same way.)

The judge may decide the case on the basis of such previous decisions or the case may be so unusual that he is forced to give a judgement which will itself become a *precedent* for any similar cases which follow.

The common law is therefore constantly adapting itself to new types of case and, after a considerable time-lag, to new social attitudes.

It is the job of the civil courts to adjudicate wrongs between individuals. These wrongs are known as 'Torts' and the one that concerns this book is the tort of *negligence*. If you take your employer to court in an attempt to win compensation for injuries you will have to prove not only that the injuries resulted from your work for him, but that they were caused by his negligence. Proving your case means convincing the judge that, on balance of probability, your story is the true one.

To prove that your employer was negligent you have to show that either:

1. He knew of the danger and **failed to take reasonable care** to protect you from it

or

2. As a responsible employer he **should** have known of the danger and protected you from it. This can be difficult when the effects of a particular hazard are not widely known in a particular industry. A construction worker who claimed damages because of deafness caused by a stud gun lost his case when it was held that, at the time, a reasonable employer in the industry would not have known that noise could deafen. The man had complained about the noise; if he had also said 'I think it is damaging my hearing', he might not have lost his case.

Moral: Complain about all hazards and spell out what you think they could do to you. Put it in the accident book. (See Section 11, p257.)

As a means of preventing accidents and disease the common law duty to take reasonable care leaves much to be desired;

1. There is no agency to enforce these standards. (One of the better proposals in the Robens report would correct this. The duty to take reasonable care, as presently defined by the courts, would become a statutory duty.)

2. The law is only activated **after** the event and then only if the worker has not only a 'good' case but the will to pursue it. Only 10-20 per cent of injuries result in a claim for damages. Only about 20 per cent of claims are settled in the worker's favour.

3. The definition of 'reasonable care' is subject to interpretation by individual judges. The normal standards of 'responsible employers' in any particular trade are generally taken as the yardstick. A backward industry like construction is therefore judged by its own low standards and those standards are perpetuated.

4. Damages do not impose a direct burden on the employer. The insurance company pays out and any adjustment in the annual premium will be small.

5. There is no link between common law compensation (or state injury benefits) and accident prevention. The authorities do not make employers pay into an injury fund in proportion to their toll of injured and dead.

> o When the English railway contractors took their navvies to France to build railways in the 19th century the terrible rate of deaths and maimings fell dramatically. The French courts were forcing the contractors to pay compensation to the injured and the widows, without proof of blame. Suddenly it became cheaper to care for the men than to disregard safety in the pursuit of profit.

6. The 'penalty' of damages is unrelated to the scale of risk to which workers are exposed. It is cheaper to kill three young men who have no dependants (about £500 each for their 'estates') than to maim one man, whose loss of earnings and other damages might run to £50,000.

Damages and the judges:

Only 20 per cent of cases are successful in spite of the fact that most of the 'intake' has been screened by trade union legal departments. The attitudes of the judges to the claims of workers must have something to do with this.

In *Accidents and Ill-Health at Work*, John Williams describes the social and professional filters through which barristers pass on their way to the bench:

> 'The processes of legal practice and the traditions surrounding the profession tend to withdraw the individuals concerned from practical appreciation of the problems of the mass of ordinary people and to establish their acceptance of existing economic arrangements. This background will inevitably tend to influence judgement on standards of behaviour.'

Whether or not this social and professional isolation results in a deliberate bias towards the employer, you can usually be sure that there will be no bias in your direction. You certainly cannot assume that the benefit of doubt in a difficult case will swing your way. On the other hand the victim of an accident, his or her workmates and the union can do a great deal to ensure that doubts do not arise. The 'legal first aid' applied after an accident can make the difference between a solid case and a shaky one – just as medical first aid can make the difference between permanent disability and swift recovery.

The practical steps to follow, on matters like preserving evidence and making statements, are described in Section 11, Winning Damages.

State benefits:

Compensation for industrial injuries and disease is also provided by the State under the National Insurance (Industrial Injuries) Act of 1946. If you are injured at work or contract one of the diseases that are recognised as being industrial (the 'prescribed diseases'), you have a right to a whole range of benefits. **Negligence by your employer does not have to be proved, but you do have to prove that the injury happened at and arose out of your work.**

The advantage of this system should be speed and

simplicity, whereas common law compensation is slow, complicated and uncertain.

Unfortunately the system is not the fount of universal justice it should be. The benefits rarely match the financial losses you suffer and securing them can be slow and uncertain, particularly in cases of disease. The system does not provide for the self-employed and fails to recognise some conditions as industrial diseases, notably bronchitis caused by dust, deafness caused by noise, and 'whitefinger' the disease caused by vibration.

Most important is the gap through which anyone can fall if they do not know they are entitled to benefit. The system does not seek out the injured, they must go to it.

Workers are therefore, once again, faced with a complicated system. The system that, above all, should be designed for the ordinary man or woman has become another paper labyrinth where you often need a lawyer for guide.

The system is described in Section 12.

Common law compensation and national insurance benefits are entirely separate systems. The iniquitous rule under the old Workmen's Compensation Act that you had to choose to pursue one or the other was abolished in 1948. You can now take your employer to court *and* claim injury benefit. There are still some points of contact, one of which arises from the different status of diseases as defined in the Industrial Injuries Act. If a disease or condition is prescribed it may be easier to win damages from your employer whose lawyer might otherwise claim that your condition cannot be 'industrial'. (This doesn't mean that you *will* get damages if it's 'prescribed' or that you cannot if it is not ; but one helps the other.)

Full pay for the injured:
It is a disgrace that most workers are cut off without wages the moment they are injured in the pay of their employers. A full-pay clause should be written into every agreement on wages and conditions.

For most workers the aftermath of an accident is financially difficult. The average spell off work is four weeks but the combination of lost wages and extra expenses can get you into financial difficulties which can take months to sort out. **No-one should try going it alone.** Shop stewards, district officials and union lawyers can do more than the individual; the union may have its own injury benefit scheme and its lawyer may be able to write to your HP company or landlord explaining your situation and asking them not to chase payments until you are straightened out again.

History of legislation:

Mid 18th century: Industrial Revolution gathering momentum. Cotton mills built on water power are hungry for cheap labour. Pauper children from the workhouses of the south are exported to the new mill areas to serve as free labour. Men, women and children work all hours in terrible conditions which are completely unregulated by law.

1802: Health and Morals of Apprentices Act. Designed to curb some of the abuses of child labour. Very limited standards of heat, light and ventilation. Working hours limited to 12 a day. Sleeping quarters of boys and girls separated and some form of education provided. The emphasis on the morals of the children in a society which approved the gross immorality of child labour is revealing. Enforcement by local magistrates did not work. Magistrates not interested, or too friendly with the mill owners.

1819, 1825, 1831: Patches stuck on the Act of 1802 in abortive attempt to make it work. 12-hour day for young persons in cotton mills.

1830s: Workers and reformers begin their long campaign for shorter hours.

1832: Sadler Committee investigating child labour reports: 'Stunted, diseased, deformed, degraded, they pass across the stage, each with the tale of his wronged life, a living picture of man's cruelty to man . . .'

1833: Royal Commission appointed to investigate child labour in factories. Set up as a result of agitation and to apply some whitewash. The new Act which resulted in the same year was a victory for the reformers. First four Fac-

I

tory Inspectors appointed because magistrates had failed to do anything to enforce the 1831 Act and to check hours of work of young people: 10-hour day for those between 13 and 18. Coverage extended to woollen and linen mills. Still no legislation for those outside textile industry.

1834: Tolpuddle Martyrs. Six Dorchester labourers sentenced to seven years deportation for administering union oath. Old Act of 1797 was dusted off in order to get them.

1837: First common law action by worker claiming damages for work injury fails.

1840: Royal Commission set up to examine the employment of women and children in mines and manufacturing, still not covered by legislation. The squalid exploitation of men, women and children in the secret depths of the mines had existed long before the Industrial Revolution. First successful compensation claim. Girl injured by revolving shaft in mill awarded £100 and £660 costs.

1842: Mines Regulations Act. Mineowners forbidden to employ women and children underground. Six more acts between now and 1911.

1843: First Mines Inspector appointed.

1844: Limited requirements introduced on 'fencing of shafts in textile mills in response to terrible injuries suffered by women and girls whose clothes got caught in them. Enforcement of factory legislation not working in spite of the inspectors and their increasingly critical attitude.

1848: Hours of women as well as young persons restricted to 10 a day. Cotton bosses devise 'relay system' to dodge this law and magistrates turn blind eye.

1850: Maximum hours actually **extended.**

1855: Manchester textile manufacturers form the Factory Law Amendment Association to fight 'undue restrictions and mischievous interference' with their profitable trade. Later merged with the National Association of Factory Occupiers. Dickens called it the Association for the Mangling of Operatives.

1856: The 'Manglers' score a victory. Sympathetic Parliament passes the Act which they promoted to **reduce** the duties on guarding to those parts which women and children were likely to pass.

1860s: Factory legislation gradually extended beyond textiles.

1862: Parliament makes it even easier for shipowners to operate 'coffin ships' and Plimsoll begins his 30 year campaign.

1964: Potteries and match industry covered by Factory Act.

1867: Larger manufacturing and heavy processes like blast furnaces now covered by law.

1871: Third Trades Union Congress supports Plimsoll after he has been rejected by the establishment. Demonstrations and protests by workers all over the country against overloading of ships lead to formation of Plimsoll Committee. Legislation and the Plimsoll Mark on ships were to follow.

1878: The first Act that looks like real factory legislation. The law on fencing is reinstated. The law is consolidated and duties of certifying surgeons defined. Inspectorate gets Chief Inspector and district organisation.

1886: Hours worked in shops regulated for the first time. Physical conditions in offices and shops will remain unregulated for another 78 years.

1891: New powers enabling Home Secretary to make regulations for dangerous trades.

1898: First Medical Inspector of Factories appointed.

1900: Safety Act gives some protection to railwaymen.

1901: The Factories and Workshops Consolidation Act. For the first time there is a comprehensive code for health and safety. Act remains in force until 1937. This legislation was won by the Trade Union movement, especially miners and cotton workers, in alliance with radicals and in the face of Government proposals that would have weakened statutory controls.

1911: Mines Act codified all mines regulations in comprehensive safety system. In force for 43 years without amendment.

1937: Factories Act. Not greatly different from that of 1901.

1946: National Insurance (Industrial Injuries) Act.

1949: Gowers Committee proposes extension of statutory standards to agriculture and offices. Government continues long opposition to inclusion of office workers.

1952: Agriculture (Poisonous Substances) Act.

1954: Mines and Quarries Act.

1956: Agriculture (Safety, Health and Welfare Provisions) Act.

1963: Offices, Shops and Railway Premises Act brings eight million under cover. Pressure from new white collar unions an important factor in success.

1967: Labour Government publishes proposals for extending statutory safety standards to new areas. Discussions drag on through 1968 and '69 until, in face of criticism and practical difficulties, Robens Committee is set up to find new formula in 1970.

1971: Mineral Workings (Offshore Installations) Act 1971. Covers safety and health of workers on oil and gas platforms, etc.

1972: Robens Report published. Early action promised, but proposals do not get into the new programme for Parliament.

10

Safety Law

The previous chapter dealt with the machinery of the law as it affects health at work and compensation for injuries.

This section is concerned with the practical aspects of statutory controls and the ways in which you can use them to improve working conditions.

The whole mass of statutory safety standards is too big to summarise here. This section is intended as a guide to the present legislation and the ways in which you can ensure that the particular regulations for your workplace are enforced.

Booklets which explain the different Acts in more detail are listed at the end of the book.

o Workers covered by statutory standards
o The different Acts
o Enforcement – the inspectorates
o How to make use of the law
o How to make use of the inspectorates
o Enforcing your own standards:

Statutory safety standards:

Coverage:

There is no single law covering the health and safety of all workers. A rag bag of different Acts and subsidiary regulations has been thrown together to deal with the abuses of employers in different fields; government has not sat down to draw up a master plan based on the needs of all workers.

The result is an extraordinary variety of provisions which often lay down different standards even when the

risk is common to all occupations. The rules on ladders, for example are different under the Factories Act, the Construction Regulations (which come under the main Act) and the Agriculture (Safety, Health and Welfare Provisions) Act. Women workers in offices and shops must be provided with means for disposing of sanitary towels but there is no such provision under the Factories Act.

The strength of the different Acts also varies. The Factories Act is considerably weakened by numerous qualifications which allow the employer to comply 'as far as is reasonably practicable'. The Mines and Quarries Act of 1954 would have been emasculated in exactly the same way if objections from the NUM had not won the removal of nearly all qualifications at the drafting stage.

The different Acts, the workplaces they cover and the strength of enforcement agencies are set out in the following tables:

The Factories Act 1961 and supporting regulations:

Approx. coverage: 8,500,000
Covers: factories, construction sites, shipyards, docks and warehouses with mechanical power, brickworks, potteries, cement works, paper making and printing, laundries and dry cleaning, garages, power stations (except nuclear), gas works and slaughter houses, railway workshops.
Enforced by: Factory Inspectorate, local authorities and fire authorities.

Offices, Shops and Railway Premises Act 1963:

Approx. coverage: 8,000,000
Covers: offices, shops, warehouses without mechanical power, wholesale departments, public catering, canteens, fuel storage depots, railway buildings.
Enforced by: local authorities.
Factory Inspectorate enforces where the office is in factory, local authority and railway premises. Mines and Quarries Inspectorate enforces in offices at mines and quarries. Fire authorities enforce fire provisions of the Act.

Mines and Quarries Act 1954:

Approx. coverage: 345,000
Covers: mines and quarries.
Enforced by: Mines and Quarries Inspectorate.

Agriculture (Poisonous Substances) Act 1952:
Agriculture (Safety, Health and Welfare Provisions) Act 1956:

Approx. coverage: 340,000
Covers: farms where labour is employed.
Enforced by: safety inspectors and field officers of the Ministry of Agriculture, Fisheries and Food and, in Scotland, Department of Agriculture and Fisheries for Scotland.

Total covered by Acts	**17,185,000**
Total not covered	**approx. 6,000,000**

Enforcement agencies:
Factory Inspectorate:

Number of places to be inspected under the Factories Act	250,000
Including places to be inspected under the Offices, Shops and Railway Premises Act	400,000
Size of Inspectorate ('authorised establishment' 1971)	714
Size of general inspectorate in field	450
Number of *visits* (not necessarily inspections)	300,000
Number of prosecutions 1971 (firms or individuals)	1,330
Maximum fine under Factories Act	£300
Average fine	£40
Cost of Inspectorate + work on occupational health	£5,500,000

Local Authorities:

Number of places under OSRP Act	755,800
Size of inspectorate: no centralised inspectorate; some local authorities have full-time specialists, most have unqualified staff on part-time inspection	
Approximate total	5,000

Number of general inspections claimed in 1970	214,580
Number of inspections by HMFI under OSRP Act	about 60,000

Note: some workplaces have not been inspected once since Act introduced in 1964

Number of prosecutions 1970	432
Maximum fine under Act	£300
Average fine	about £30
Cost of inspection:	Not known

Mines and Quarries Inspectorate:

Number of workplaces under Mines and Quarries Act	4,946
Size of inspectorate 1971	135
Number of visits and inspections 1971	
coal mines	17,264
other mines	825
quarries	6,042
Number of prosecutions	None*
Maximum fine under Act: plus maximum 3 months prison for owner or manager in certain cases	£200**
Average fine	—
Cost of inspectorate, plus research, etc	£2,350,000

* In 1970 the NCB brought five prosecutions and the Procurator Fiscal in Scotland brought 11. ** For first offence likely to cause death or serious injury.

Agricultural safety inspection:

Number of places covered by safety act	112,660
Number of full-time inspectors (1971)	44

Plus part-time inspection by 425 agriculture field officers in England and Wales

No full-time inspectors in Scotland but part-time inspection by 11 agriculture wages and safety officers.

Number of full-scale inspections claimed in 1970	24,500
Number of prosecutions (cases) 1970	184
Maximum fine under Acts	£50
Average fine	—
Cost of inspection, research, etc	£744,000

Some totals (rough estimates)

Total number of workplaces covered	1,200,000
Total number of full-time inspectors	1,000
Total number of visits (not necessarily inspections)	500,000
Total number of prosecutions	2,000
Total cost to Government of occupational safety and health work	about £10,748,000
Total cost of industrial accidents is believed to be	more than £500,000,000

The unprotected:

Nobody knows how many people work in places not covered by statutory safety standards. There are thought to be about six million in this situation.

If your work is not covered it does not mean that it is safe. On the contrary, some of the most dangerous jobs are outside any safety law, for example, civil engineering work on railway tunnels and bridges, and deep sea fishing. Others not covered include workers in transport and aviation, education, hospitals, hotels, pubs, entertainment, postal services, post office engineering, electricity transmission line engineering, parts of the water supply industry, and many others.

The definition of a factory under the Factories Act includes any premises (whether or not within a building) in which one or more persons are employed in manual labour in any process for, or incidental to:
1. The making of any article or part of an article;
2. The altering, repairing or ornamenting, finishing, cleaning or washing, or the breaking up of any article; or
3. The adapting for sale of any article; where the work is carried on by way of trade or for purposes of gain or by a local authority or on behalf of the Crown.

The quality of present coverage can be likened to a large wall whitewashed by a five-year-old. Parts have been missed altogether, parts have been done twice or more and in some places you can't really tell as in this example:

o Dudgeons Wharf, Isle of Dogs, E.London, July 17 1969: six men died when an oil storage tank exploded during demolition.

Two weeks earlier the fire brigade had been asked for advice on demolishing tanks which had contained myrcene oil. The fire brigade had a look and decided the tank farm 'was or might be' a factory and thus the responsibility of the Factory Inspectorate.

The factory inspector had a look and couldn't make up his mind if it came under the main act or the Construction Regulations. His superior was still considering this fascinating demarcation issue when the six men died.

The administrative rag-bag did not kill those men – the cause, as usual, could be traced back to economic factors in the reluctance of the tank farm owner to pay the full cost of doing the job properly – but a system based on human need would have saved them.

Five of the dead men were firemen. Firemen are among the millions for whom there are no statutory safety, health and welfare standards.

Is your workplace covered?

It is important to find out if your place of work is covered by one or more of the Acts and regulations.

If it is, your employer must by law display an official notice summarising the main provisions.

o It should be in a place where you can easily see and read it, not in a supervisor's office.

o If there is no notice, this does not mean the place is not covered. Many employers do not display these abstracts and this applies particularly to shops, offices, construction sites and small workshops.

o If your workplace obviously falls into one of the categories that have been listed, make the management get whatever official abstracts cover the workplace and put them on display. This can be a good point with which to start a safety campaign because it is simple to carry out and it focusses attention on the fact that the employer has legal obligations to protect your safety, health and welfare.

o He should also display the addresses of the relevant inspectorate and of the Employment Medical Adviser.

o If your work is covered by special regulations under the Factories Act – eg The Carcinogenic Substances Regulations 1967 – the employer is obliged by law to give you a printed copy of the regulations, if you ask. All workers should get a copy and ensure that regulations are obeyed.

First aid boxes and thermometer:
While checking the walls for official abstracts look for
first aid boxes which must be provided under all main acts.

Check also that there is a thermometer to show the
temperature of the workplace. (This obviously does not
apply in outdoor activities like agriculture and construction,
but it does apply in a site office under the OSRP Act.)

Is the workplace registered?
Sometimes the lack of an abstract may indicate that
the workplace is not registered with the relevant authority.
This means it will not be inspected until the appropriate inspectorate tracks it down.

o Most of the 46,249 new premises registered under the
OSRP Act in 1970 had to be 'discovered' by local authority
inspectors because the employer had not complied with his
duty to register straight away. Only five were prosecuted.

If your employer understands that you can easily
check with the Factory Inspectorate, the Mines and Quarries Inspectorate, the Local Authority or Ministry of Agriculture inspectors, he will quickly register the workplace.

The object is not just to score a point but to secure as
much protection as can be gained from statutory standards.

Using the law:
In making use of statutory standards it is important to
get the fullest protection from the strongest parts of each
act. Most of the legislation imposes limited duties on the
employers and confers few rights on the worker. There are
two exceptions:

1. The Mines and Quarries Act: has the best safeguards
of any workplace safety legislation. It lays down that:

o Workers have the right to appoint Workmen's Inspectors and Accident Site Observers.

o Workmen's Inspectors may inspect the workplace
once at least in every month.

o Serious accident sites should not be disturbed until
inspected. These rights should be available to all workers
and it is important that those in mines and quarries use them
to the full.

2. The Construction Regulations:

These specify that any contractor employing more than 20 workers must appoint a 'suitably qualified' person to advise him on his legal duties and generally supervise the safety of the work.

The name of this safety supervisor must be entered on the abstract of the Factories Act or the abstract of the Construction Regulations, both of which must be posted on the site.

The safety supervisor cannot be doing his job properly unless he is on site regularly. The regulations specify a range of regular inspections that must be made and entered in a register. Excavations, lifting appliances and scaffolds are among the items covered.

The **health and welfare** provisions of the Construction Regulations lay down much higher standards than you might imagine from looking at the average site.

Requirements to check are those dealing with:

o first aid boxes and the person in charge of boxes
o appointment of persons to summon ambulance
o protective clothing
o shelters and provisions for taking meals and drying clothes
o toilets, washing facilities and drinking water.

The health and welfare requirements are frequently broken and seldom enforced fully. Construction inspectors give contractors much latitude in this area especially on remote sites, because they sympathise with the employer's problems in complying. These regulations are not, as some contractors and inspectors seem to believe, luxuries. They are important safeguards for health. Organised workers can ensure that they are enforced.

The lump and the law:

The cancerous growth of the 'Lump' in construction, agriculture, and an increasing number of factories, is weakening the already feeble protection of safety statutes.

These men have signed away most of their rights as workers. They get very little protection from the construction regulations; they are not eligible for Industrial Injury Benefits when injured. They will usually have no-one to claim against for damages. More important, they undermine the safety of their workmates. Their activities may result in rickety scaffolds or unshored trenches which would be illegal if they were *employed* workers. Others may be endangered by the hazards they create or by going to rescue them from trouble.

A large proportion of lump workers may dilute the number of *employed* workers on any job to the point where parts of the regulations do not apply. For example where there are less than five people employed (in the legal sense) first aid boxes are not required under the Construction Regulations.

Deaths and injuries to self-employed workers do not have to be reported under the Construction Regulations so the true record of the industry is hidden by the lump.

Looking at the whole industry, the lump serves to undermine union organisation, which is already weak. It is no use just dismissing lump workers as 'a load of scabs' and hoping they'll go away; the Lump is a symptom of the industry's approach to labour – not its cause. Organised sites have shown the way by refusing to work with lump labour or insisting that the main employer takes on the lump workers and that they join the union.

Only when sites are 100 per cent organised can safety demands be enforced. (See Statistics, p100 and other effects of the Lump, p28.)

Other trades:

Regulations for the **pottery industry** also require the employer to appoint a supervisor to carry out 'systematic inspections' to ensure compliance throughout the factory.

Regulations for **shipbuilding** require the employer to appoint a full-time safety officer in yards employing more than 500.

Go for the absolute duties:

Very little will be achieved by using the law for its own sake but it can be one weapon in the shop floor attack on hazards. If this attack is concentrated on the main causes of danger and concern to workers you can use the law on these points as one of the arguments in getting management to operate safely.

Most of the regulations place two kinds of duty on the employer:

1. Absolute duty: where the law says the employer shall, will or must comply.

2. Qualified duty: where he must comply 'wherever possible' or 'as far as is reasonably practicable'. If it *is* practicable then the employer has an absolute duty to do it.

The first kind is easier to use because you can demand compliance. Some of the most important hazards are covered only by qualified duties but you can still use them successfully. For example, tripping or slipping accidents due to poor housekeeping are among the most common cause of injury. Bad housekeeping giving rise to hazards must nearly always constitute a breach of the qualified duties under sections 28 and/or 29 of the Factories Act. Any shop steward who knows these duties should be able to spot breaches and be a match for the boss when it comes to arguing the toss about whether it is reasonably practicable to do anything about them.

One of the most important absolute duties covers the guarding of dangerous parts of machines. Although the wording is different, this protection is given under all the Acts, whether the risk is a power press in a factory, a bacon slicer in a shop, a conveyor in a mine or a power-take-off on the farm tractor.

Using the Inspector:

There is so much wrong with the enforcement system and the attitudes of those who run it that many workers have written off all inspectors as stooges of the employers.

This is not the way to change the attitudes or methods of the stooges and it overlooks the many inspectors who are battling not only callous employers but also restrictive policies on prosecution and stifling bureaucracy which hamper their job. Most of them probably start off with a sense of commitment and it is more profitable to assume good intentions and put them to the test than write anyone off as a time server.

Workers can do a great deal to make inspection and enforcement work properly. Here are some suggestions:

1. Make contact with the local factory inspector and try to arrange that he or she meets union representatives on the next visit. The Factory Inspectorate has already launched a policy of making contact with union representatives so that they can prepare themselves for an inspector's visit (see 1971 annual report).

2. The inspectorates make great claims for their advisory role (usually for the ears of management). There is no reason why you should not use this service and ask the inspector's advice on hazards, regulations, publications, etc.

3. Arrange for an inspector to come and talk at union or safety group meetings. (Ask him to talk about the particular problems of your trade or occupation rather than general themes).

4. When the employer is breaking the law on some hazard and will not put it right, you can ring up the local inspector. He will keep your name secret if you want him to. A visit usually follows quickly on such complaints. (But if you cry 'wolf' too often on trivial problems, the quick reflex may be gone when you need it in an emergency.) The first and only prosecution of Central Asbestos in 13 years of criminal activity followed a telephone call from a worker.

5. Never agree to clean up before an inspector's visit. The place should be in its usual state with all processes running as normal. If you hide the evidence of hazards you may be signing your own death warrant. The workers at Cape Asbestos at Hebden Bridge, Yorkshire, cleaned up and concealed the illegal tools they were required to use. Several have died from their exposure to asbestos and more are now struggling through the last days of the death sentences that were imposed on them by a criminal employer.

6. Ask management to let a representative go round with the inspector. This may be refused, especially where stewards have not established clear rights, but there is no legal reason for refusal. Inspectors come to inspect the workplace, not the management, and to enforce Acts written for your protection. It is hard to see how this job can be done properly *without talking to workers.*

> o The powers of factory inspectors are considerable. They can:
> **1.** Enter the workplace at any time, day or night, without warning
> **2.** Talk to any person and take a statement
> **3.** Take samples of any substance for analysis
> **4.** Apply to a magistrate under Section 54 for a prohibition order on any part of a plant which cannot be used without risk of bodily injury. Eleven orders were made in 1971 and the Chief Inspector's annual report said that increasing reliance might have to be placed on this method. (The Robens proposals would make it even easier to use.)

Getting inspectors to play a more positive role is not so easy for **farm workers.** The Ministry of Agriculture has very few full-time inspectors and there are none in Scotland. But they do undertake public education work on problems like the growing toll of child deaths on farms and they can hardly refuse advice to workers. The isolation of many workers and the lack of a 'shop floor' organisation may make it difficult to call an inspector when hazards are suspected.

The need for this kind of action is less pressing for those in **mines and quarries.** Workers already have rights of inspection and official inspection is generally more frequent than for other workplaces. The relationship between workers' inspectors and the M&Q inspectors is often well established. But inspection on its own achieves nothing, and there is some evidence that both M&Q and workers' inspectors will put up with unsatisfactory conditions if jobs are at risk.

For those covered by the **OSRP Act,** the usefulness of any links with the local authority may depend on whether the Council employs a qualified, full-time official. Isolation of workers in small offices and shops can again inhibit complaints. If you are worried about victimisation, check that your name will not be mentioned to your employer before giving it to the inspector – or complain anonymously by letter or phone. Union organisation in this area, which was a key factor in winning legislation in the first place, is vital if the standards laid down in the Act are to be enforced.

Hundreds of thousands of workers are not in fact getting the protection of the Act. Some of the most common infringements are listed here.

Common infringements of the Offices, Shops and Railways Premises Act:

Temperature: High as well as low; computer rooms have been measured in the upper 80s Fahrenheit. Shops with very brightly lit displays may also become far too hot.

Thermometer: Not displayed on wall.

Ventilation: Often inadequate, particularly in internal rooms and telephonists' cubicles.

Lighting: Frequently inadequate, particularly passages, stairs and WCs. Many brand-new offices fall short of recommended standards. (Note: light bulbs lose 10 per cent of their power, fluorescent tubes 20 per cent during their life.)

Dirty conditions.

Unsafe floors or floor coverings.

Waste materials causing fire risk and obstruction.

Fire protection: no fire alarms or testing of alarms, no fire drills, escape doors locked.

Dangerous stacking of goods, particularly in supermarket storerooms.

First aid boxes not installed or not fully stocked.

Sanitary conveniences not conveniently accessible.

Abstract of OSRP Act not displayed.

Organisation:

It is a delusion to think that a new relationship with the inspectors can solve all your problems.

But exposure of really persistent and dangerous operations in a particular workplace may force a prosecution and get the hazard eliminated.

None of this is much help for the six million not covered by any form of statutory safety standards.

Ultimately the rising tide of injuries and disease will turn when every workplace has built its own shopfloor safety organisation and decided what standards it finds acceptable. The strength of organised workers is the best enforcement agency.

11.

Winning Damages

Some general principles of common law compensation are given in Section 9. This chapter is concerned with the practicalities of winning damages at common law.

If you are injured at work, any claim for damages is usually against your employer. But it may be against a third party; for example the firm who owned the place where you were injured.

Self-employed workers – those on the 'Lump' in construction and agriculture – are not **employed** in the legal sense and will often find it difficult to claim damages from anyone when they are injured.

In fact many of them would be able to win a legal action if they had an organization and lawyers determined to fight their cases.

Another group is often forgotten: the widows (or dependant widowers) and other dependants of people killed at work. They too may have a claim against an employer but they are frequently unaware of their rights, and do not themselves have the facts to show who was to blame.

They need maximum support from the dead worker's former workmates and union in securing compensation.

Many other potential claims for damages are not pursued because an injured worker does not know his rights. Perhaps he or she does not return to the old workplace after an accident and loses contact with the steward who could set the ball rolling. In casual industries like construction contact (where it exists) is often lost in this way.

If you know of anyone injured at work who may have suffered any of the losses described on page 255, track them down and make sure they know they may have grounds for a claim.

There are other reasons why cases never get as far as a solicitor:

1. The injured person is afraid the boss will victimise him or her. This fear is usually unfounded but it can apply in small firms where the boss says 'We're all mates together'.

2. The case is headed off by management who make an offer direct to injured person, widow or other dependant. There *are* small firms where a paternalistic boss will set a disabled person up for life with a house and pension. Such settlements are extremely rare and might not prove to have been so generous if they had been tested in court. More often these private settlements – paid as a once-and-for-all sum which robs the victim of any right to further compensation at common law – are totally inadequate.

Never settle direct with your employer unless you have taken legal advice. If the boss really has your interest at heart he will be quite happy for you to see a lawyer.

Most of these problems can be overcome by achieving full union membership at every workplace and organising so that all possible cases are passed to the union's legal advice department. (If the organisation is geared to prevention as well as compensation, many cases will not arise in the first place.)

From now on, this section assumes that you do not slip through any of the gaps and have workmates and union with you all the way.

Grounds for claim:

Your claim for damages will be based on the employer's breach of his common law duty or of a statutory duty – or both. The employer's common law duty is to take reasonable care in providing:

1. Safe plant and equipment

2. Competent fellow workers

3. Adequate supervision and instruction

4. A safe place of work and a safe system of work.

The defence:

Although your claim is against your employer, any damages are going to be paid by the firm's insurance company. It is no use expecting a generous approach from the employer because the insurance company is calling the tune. It is interested solely in profit, which means paying out as little as possible. You may be faced by various lines of defence:

1. Guided by the insurers, the employer's first move is usually to **deny liability,** often in cases where they would be almost certain to lose. There are good reasons for this. It is up to you to prove that the employer was to blame for your injury and the insurance company often sits back in the hope that you'll find it too difficult and just give up, or settle for less than your lawyer thinks you should.

2. Contributory negligence. Even if the employer's fault is easily proved, a most popular line of defence is to argue that you were partly to blame for your accident. If successful this cuts down your damages in proportion to your share of blame. Employers can nearly always use this argument — but it is up to them to prove it this time.

3. Employee's consent. This used to be a common defence. The employer has to prove that you consented to run the risk of injury — as a circus performer or stunt-man does — and not just that you knew of it, so it's not often used. But don't accept danger money if you can get safety; that could be taken as evidence of consent.

The employer can no longer use the defence of 'common employment' in cases where your injury is caused by the negligence of a fellow worker. Under this defence, which had its roots in judges' decisions in the first half of the 19th century, you were presumed to have agreed to run the risk of injury by the negligence of your workmates in 'common employment' with you. This disgraceful rule – designed to thwart a threatened flood of actions by workers – was not fully abolished until 1948.

The employer is now responsible for negligent actions by his employees in the course of their duties.

Under a later reform of the common law, an employer

is also responsible for the negligence of a third party who supplies him with machinery that causes an accident. You do not have to sue the supplier as well.

Damages are awarded for:

1. Actual loss of money or goods, eg loss of wages or damage to clothing.

2. Loss of earning power. This is an important class of damages. If an injury means you can't earn as much as you did before you can claim the loss of earnings at so much a year.

3. Damages for pain and suffering and loss of expectation of life.

4. Loss of amenity – that is, the hobbies and pleasures which may not cost you any earnings but which can be quite as important in making life worth living.

Legal first aid:

Speed is the key to success in an action for damages. In law you have three years from the time of the accident (or from the time of diagnosis of an industrial disease) in which to begin proceedings, but evidence and witnesses may have disappeared long before the time is up.

The crucial period for later success may be measured in days rather than years. Many victims believe they cannot start an action until they have either returned to work or recovered from the injury. This delay can be disastrous; the injured worker who shouted to his mates 'stuff the doctor, get a lawyer' had the right idea. But if you **have** delayed, that doesn't necessarily mean that it's no use claiming; only that you should now get on with it as quickly as possible.

Because the victim will seldom be in a state to safeguard his own interests the role of workmates and stewards is crucial. Immediately after the accident someone should:

1. Make a sketch of the accident area before anything is moved. A photograph would be even better but unless special arrangements are made for such events you are unlikely to be able to get a camera quickly. Perhaps a flash camera should be part of every shop steward's stock equipment.

2. Check any equipment or tools for defects which might have caused the accident. A steward can legitimately demand that these should be preserved for later inspection and not 'lost' or taken off for reconditioning. (Under the Mines and Quarries Act the scene of a serious accident must be undisturbed until inspected by workmen's inspectors and the Mines Inspector.)

3. Collect names and addresses of witnesses. This means anyone who

    (a) saw the accident;

    (b) knows something of the events leading up to it or;

    (c) came on the scene soon afterwards and can describe what they saw.

Most accidents result from a dangerous situation that may have existed or been building up for a long time and any information can be valuable. If in doubt, tell the lawyer and let him sort it out.

In the case of **industrial disease**, collection of evidence may be more difficult. The sections on chemical hazards and industrial diseases will provide clues to possible causes. Samples of suspect materials, such as cutting oil from the victim's machine in a case of dermatitis, should be put in a bottle. A label should give the date and the signature of a witness. Do not take samples of dangerous substances unless you are absolutely certain how to handle them safely or you may end up in the next bed to the victim. Just make a note of such materials and how they are used; copy carefully whatever is written on the label, especially if it contains any warning.

The names and addresses of other workers who have suffered the same disease or who have similar symptoms could be vital evidence. This is because the employer may claim that a chemical or process is perfectly safe and the victim's condition is caused by abnormal susceptibility or some exposure not connected with work.

This kind of vigilance on the shop floor can help in spotting industrial diseases early. It should be a standard part of shop floor activity, regardless of any legal issues – see Section 8, Action.

Returning to the immediate aftermath of an accident, there are still several stages to be completed, to ensure that the fullest evidence will be available in preparing any action for damages.

1. **Any accident, however small or apparently insignificant, should be reported at work.** You should see that a brief and accurate entry is made in the accident book, and make a copy of the entry. If you think someone or something you can identify was at fault, make sure that goes into the book as well.

A small cut might turn septic and keep you off work for a long time. A pain in the back or a lump in the groin can go on for weeks before being diagnosed as a 'slipped disc' or hernia (rupture). Without an entry in the book you would have a job to prove the injury was caused by heavy lifting at work.

2. **Get proper medical treatment.** If you are sent to hospital this should be automatic, but for smaller injuries you should consult your own doctor and not rely solely on the works first aid system. Give the hospital doctor or your GP a full account of the accident so that full medical evidence will be available *outside* the workplace. This will greatly assist your lawyer who may have difficulty getting the facts from your employer.

Get your doctor to tell you exactly what you are being treated for and, in the case of back trouble that persists, insist on definite diagnosis, by a specialist if necessary. Most patients are reluctant to demand such things of their doctor but many GPs are not familiar with occupational disease or the implications of diagnosis in claims for National Insurance benefits and damages.

Doctors and surgeons should be asked to preserve any objects or particles removed from wounds. Metallurgical examination of a chunk of metal could show where it came from or that there was a flaw in a tool, casting or workpiece. By the time the case comes up this could be the only specimen available.

3. **Report the accident to the Department of Health and Social Security's local office.** Claim injury benefit if you

are obviously going to be off work for more than three days. You may be eligible for other benefits. See Section 12. The insurance officer will check with your employer that you really have had an injury at work.

4. Get legal advice as soon as possible. Most unions have legal aid departments and the shop steward or branch will get you a form which should be filled in and returned as quickly as possible.

If for some reason – perhaps you are out of benefit with the union – you cannot use its legal service, you should find your own solicitor. Choose one who specialises in injury claims: the firm in the High Street may be red-hot at house conveyancing but it is unlikely to have had much experience of industrial injury cases. If you don't know the name of a specialist firm, your union should be able to recommend one even if you are out of benefit.

Unless you have a very large income or a big chunk of savings you should be able to get legal advice free in the first place, and get state legal aid, either free or subsidised, if you wish to sue for damages. Your solicitor will help you with the forms.

If you have successfully followed the previous steps your lawyer should have a useful collection of evidence but he may want more. You may have to be examined by a specialist so that exact medical evidence can be presented. An engineer may also be brought in to prepare technical evidence on the cause of the accident.

Your employer will usually give him access to the workplace and it is important that any meeting 'on site' is not shared by anyone from the employer's side who might gain from knowing the strength or direction of your technical evidence.

Statements:

Meanwhile the employer, and the insurance company are collecting their evidence (or hiding yours). Because they and their experts have free access to all parts of the job and to all workers they start with a big advantage. Good shop-floor organisation can ensure that this advantage is not abused. Work that would cover up evidence can be blacked.

The employer will want to get statements from the injured person and from witnesses. Workers often fail to recognise the significance of such statements, especially when they are collected by the safety officer. His action may be genuinely in the cause of accident prevention but that will not stop management using statements for 'damages prevention'.

Methods used to get statements are often quite shameful: injured workers are interviewed in hospital while still confused or shocked. Workmates are called into a manager's office and a 'statement' is built up by question-and-answer. The witness is asked to sign it there and then.

Statements obtained in this way from witnesses, who may be under the impression that the evidence is to help a workmate, are unlikely to be accurate and can actually destroy a justifiable claim. The bits left out can be as damaging as inaccuracies put in; if there was something wrong which was not the victim's fault, make sure this is clearly stated in any document.

Here is a checklist on giving statements:

1. The employer does not need a **signed** statement to help him prevent accidents in future.

2. A formal statement is therefore going to be legal ammunition. The employer's side hope it will help them defeat a claim.

3. You are under no duty whatsoever to give a statement to your employer. Witnesses may choose to give a statement to one side or the other, neither or both.

4. If you are already in the hands of a solicitor any request for a statement should be referred to him.

5. If you choose to give a statement make sure you know who you are giving it to.

6. Never sign anything unless you have had ample time to consider it and make any alterations.

7. Never sign a statement for the employer or insurance company until you have a copy to keep and show to the injured worker's lawyer.

8. If an official Inspector asks you for a statement you must give it to him. This may be used in later **criminal** proceedings but it won't affect a **civil** claim for damages.

Progress of a case:

The dealings between your solicitor and your employer and his insurance company will probably be more like a poker game than a process of human justice. Your solicitor makes a claim against the employer. The employer passes the claim to his insurance company which then collects its evidence. It may want its own specialist to examine you to check the extent of any disability for which you are claiming.

The sequence of events may then go something like this:

1. The insurance company begins negotiations with your solicitor and makes an offer. The first offer will probably be too low.

2. Negotiations may continue for some months, with further offers. Your financial state is steadily deteriorating and the insurance company may make an offer just before Christmas when it will be difficult to refuse.

3. At any stage your solicitor may recommend that you accept the latest offer. Some solicitors are known to the insurance companies as 'settlers'; others prefer to fight it out in court for a higher settlement.

4. If your solicitor is not satisfied with the offer he will ask for your or the union's authority, to start proceedings. He passes the papers to a barrister who prepares a legal document, the writ, setting out the facts and allegations. The writ is then served on the employer or his solicitor.

5. The employer's side enters a defence or, occasionally, admits liability.

6. Even at this stage the insurance company may make you another offer. They sometimes do this at the door of the court when, they hope, you will accept almost anything not to go through with the ordeal. All offers should be referred to your solicitor.

7. This final offer may be 'paid into court'. You then face one of the hardest gambles in the poker game. If you accept, the case does not go to court and you get the money. If you don't accept the case goes ahead. The judge does not know of the money 'paid in'. If he awards bigger damages the gamble has paid off; if he awards less, then you get whatever he awards and your side will have to pay all the costs incurred by both sides from the date the money was paid into court. He may award nothing. Clearly the insurance company cannot lose by this manoeuvre which reduces an injured worker to the level of a contestant in 'Take Your Pick'.

8. Either side may appeal against the judge's decision. The appeal goes to the Court of Appeal and, if either side is still not satisfied, the case can be taken to the House of Lords. The original decision can therefore be reversed and then reinstated.

One of the biggest problems in court will be to convey to the judge a complete understanding of the accident. The judge is at the end of a line of communication which starts when you give the story to your solicitor. He has to make the barrister understand and the barrister has to convince the judge.

If you start with an experienced solicitor he will know about the hazards of work and will be able to pass his understanding up the line. He will know the type of evidence and expert witnesses needed to clinch a case.

Although you depend very heavily on the experience of your lawyer, don't be afraid to insist that he gets on with the action and does not spend months in negotiations.

Although this section is about winning compensation, the main aim of shopfloor organisation is to prevent accidents and disease. By organising for safety, rejecting dangerous equipment (like the building workers who chopped up all the rickety ladders on a site) and complaining about hazards you can begin to achieve this goal. At the same time you deny the employer his defence of contributory negligence.

Check now!

Is your employer insured? To comply with the Employers' Liability (Compulsory Insurance) Act he must be insured so that, regardless of his own financial state, workers or dependants can be fully compensated for injury or death. He must display a certificate to this effect where workers can see it.

12

Industrial Injury Benefits

This section is to help you or an adviser to obtain the fullest possible benefits for any incapacity or disability caused by your work.

Most claims are settled without difficulty at the first stage; but it is still a good idea to absorb as much as you can of this section before making even a simple claim.

In other cases, life can become very complicated for a claimant and this section must unfortunately reflect that complexity if it is to help in the difficult cases.

Don't forget that the union can help at every stage, from the first form to the High Court.

Action summary:

Steps to take if you are injured at work and are likely to be off for more than three days.

1. Report the injury at work, or get someone to do it for you.

2. Tell your shop steward and ask what benefits, advice or legal assistance are available from the union.

3. Make a claim for benefit to the insurance officer, an official at the local office of the Department of Health and Social Security.

The advice given under 'Legal First Aid' in Section 11 may also be useful at this stage.

If a case gets complicated and you can't get help from the union for any reason, get advice from one of these:

The local branch of the Claimant's Union

A law centre

The Citizens Advice Bureau

The charts on the next page will help you find your way around the system.

1.

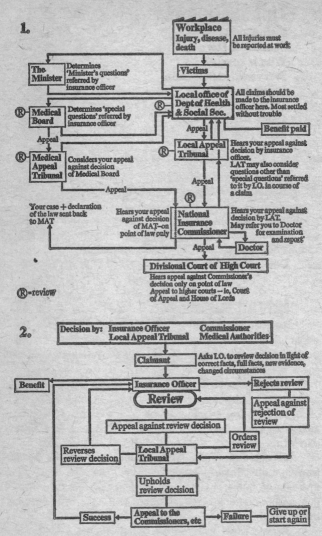

Chart 1 shows the main parts of the system. Chart 2 shows the review procedure.

This section has:

Introduction:

This section is not an exhaustive statement of the law on industrial injury benefits. It is a guide to the kinds of problems which can arise in the course of a claim, and to some of the ways of getting round them.

Information in the earlier parts of the section should enable you to obtain full benefit at the time of your initial claim to the local insurance office. You can then avoid the anxiety of going through the appeals machinery. **The later part of the section** is a guide to the appeals procedure.

To obtain the full benefit of the law, and to avoid its traps in a difficult case you have to understand in detail the meaning of numerous long, obscure passages of legal jargon, and the different interpretations that have been put on them.

Bear in mind that you are claiming a legal and not a moral right; the law, and not commonsense, must therefore be quoted as authority.

Officials whose daily lives are ordered by a series of

obscure regulations tend to acquire great respect for the small print and will readily accept claims which appear to be based on it. A claim based simply on commonsense is more likely to be refused (regardless of whether it is right or wrong in law) than one dressed in the language of the regulations.

If you want to argue about the law of industrial injury benefits you must therefore familiarise yourself with the law at its sources. You shouldn't rely only on this chapter – and certainly not on those parts of it which appear to be clear. They may be clear because they are a deliberate simplification of a complicated law.

The law stated is as at May 1973: The rates of most benefits are changed in October each year. Some of those given may already be out of date by time of publication. You can find out current rates from your local insurance office.

Sources of law:

Acts of Parliament:

The main source of all law on industrial injury benefits is Acts of Parliament and in particular the National Insurance (Industrial Injuries) Act 1965. This Act, with amendments made by later Acts of Parliament, states the basic law. Its provisions are in some parts easy to understand and in others impossible. (This Act is referred to in this section as 'the Injuries Act'.)

Regulations:

While the Acts of Parliament set out the framework of the scheme, the various sets of regulations made by the Secretary of State (formerly the Minister of Pensions and National Insurance) under these Acts also have the force of law.

You can find all the relevant Acts of Parliament and Regulations in a blue loose-leaf collection published by H.M.Stationery Office and available in most good public libraries.

Commissioners' Decisions:

Many decisions of the Commissioner of National Insurance covering important questions of interpretation of the law are also available through HMSO. Each type of benefit is assigned a letter:

U: unemployment

S: sickness

P: retirement pensions

G: maternity benefit, widow's benefit, guardian's allowance and death grant

I: *industrial injuries*

F: family allowances

A: attendance allowance.

These decisions are published both individually and in bound volumes.

In addition there is the *Index and Digest of Decisions* given by the Commissioners, normally referred to as 'The Digest'. This is a valuable collection of extracts from published decisions in loose-leaf volumes kept up to date by sporadic issues of supplements. It is quite expensive but for those who regularly fight tribunals and appeals well worth having. Otherwise you will find it in the reference section at good libraries.

The Commissioners decide which decisions are important enough to publish. Important decisions in favour of claimants are often not published. If you know of these decisions their value as precedents is as good as published decisions. Local offices often have copies of unpublished decisions. Ask to see them.

The Commissioners' decisions can be used as authoritative statements of the law. It is a great help in any case where the insurance officer is wavering if you can produce a decision by the Commissioners on the very point. You should certainly use the decisions in appeals.

Note that if a court has made a ruling on a particular point, that overrules any contrary decision by a Commissioner in a similar case. If there are two conflicting decisions on a point, usually the later one is preferred. If a later decision specifically *disapproves* an earlier one, it can be taken that the earlier one no longer has any authority.

K

Law Reports:

These are useful if, on a point of law, you are appealing to the courts, against a Commissioner's decision. Usually these are published as an appendix to the Commissioner's decision.

Who is covered:

The Industrial Injuries compensation scheme is basically an insurance scheme. Contributions – the weekly National Insurance stamp – are paid into the *'Industrial Injuries Fund'*. The Government also contributes (out of ordinary revenue from taxation) an amount equal to one fifth of the money provided by workers and employers. All the benefits described here come from this fund.

Insurance under the scheme is compulsory for certain types of workers. Others are excluded.

1. Persons in 'employment in Great Britain (Northern Ireland has a separate but similar scheme) under any contract of service or apprenticeship, whether written or oral and whether expressed or implied'.

Sometimes it is difficult to distinguish whether a person is engaged under a contract of service (an employee) and therefore obliged to participate, or under a contract for services (a self-employed person) and therefore excluded. The oldest test is whether your employer has the right to control exactly how you do the work (you're an employee) or whether you decide how it's done (you're a 'contractor'). In fact it's not as simple as that. The distinction was first made in the days when a master had the right (and the skill) to control the smallest actions of his servants, and it's now unworkable in practice. Other relevant questions are to ask whether you can be dismissed (employee) and whether you get a wage (employee) or a price for the job (contractor).

As explained in previous sections, self-employment seriously weakens your right to protection under statutory safety standards and your right to claim compensation under common law.

Employees get far better insurance benefits than the self-employed (they also get unemployment benefit). Their weekly contribution is smaller than the 'self-employed' stamp.

Even if you are not insured for other benefits, such as sickness and unemployment – either because your earnings are too small or your hours are too short – you still have to contribute (at special rates) to the scheme. And you can, of course, then claim benefit from it.

2. While employees are the main class of workers covered by the scheme others are specifically included. They include crew members of British ships and aircraft ; public and local authority employees, taxi-drivers and others. In doubtful cases, study the *First Schedule of the Injuries Act*. Part II of the Schedule prescribes employments which are outside the scheme.

Unlike unemployment benefit there is no qualifying contribution period for injury benefit. If you are injured on your first day at work you can claim benefit.

Preconditions for claim :

There are three main types of benefit payable under the Injuries Act – Injury Benefit, Disablement Benefit and Death Benefit. To obtain benefit you must show that you are an insured person who has suffered a 'personal injury caused after 4th July 1948 by accident arising out of and in the course of his employment'.

'Personal injury' means injury to the living body of a human being It does not include damage to an artificial appendage like spectacles or a wooden leg, even if the damage stops you working (see R(I) 7/56). It also includes a disease. In any case where an industrial accident causes a disease which is not a prescribed disease for your occupation you can claim benefits as though the disease were an injury. Diseases held to be injuries have included: asthma (CSI 2/48); ringworm (CI 46/49); malaria (CI 6/49); poliomyelitis (CI 159/50); tuberculosis (CI 195/50); typhoid fever (CI 401/50); fibrositis (R(I) 3/51). Any attempt to show that a disease fits the definition of personal injury is likely to raise the question of whether it resulted from an 'accident' or a 'process' – (see page 272).

In some parts of the Injuries Act – and in common language – the terms 'injury' and 'accident' are interchangeable. It is not necessary to show two separate events – an injury and an accident. For example, in CI 5/49 an injury to arm muscles through extra strain imposed by shovelling sand was held to be an injury caused by accident. (See also CI 52/49, R(I) 71/51, CI 27/49). All that is needed is that there be a particular moment when the accident/injury occurs (R(I) 52/51). (The problems of interpretation which arise from this lack of precision in the law are discussed at length by the House of Lords in the appendices to decisions R(I) 16/66 and R(I) 3/69.)

It is often difficult to say whether it was the accident or some other factor which caused the injury. The test laid down in R(I) 12/52 para 7 and CI 27/49 is that *it is not necessary for the accident to be the main or sole cause of the injury.* It is enough if the work contributed to the injury *to a material degree.*

This has led to much argument in cases where a worker suffers a slipped disc in the course of his work. It is apparently medically possible to have a slipped disc for some time without feeling it. There can come a moment in your work when the disc suddenly becomes painful. In many cases benefit has been refused on the grounds that the injury (the slipped disc) was not caused by an industrial accident. Decisions in which it has been successfully claimed that a slipped disc is an injury caused by industrial accident are CI 94/50; R(I) 53/51; R(I) 19/63. In CI 94/50 the worker had a slipped disc in 1946. It slipped again in 1948. It was held to be immaterial that the 1946 injury made him more likely to suffer a further one. (In fact the earlier injury made it easier to prove his claim.) Other decisions involving slipped discs have gone against the claimant (R(I) 20/56; R(I) 35/59; R(I) 12/60; R(I) 33/60 and R(I) 4/65).

To succeed in such a case the medical evidence must show that the work caused the injury and not that the sudden pain was merely a symptom of a pre-existing condition. For this purpose it is usually necessary to show an unusual strain.

In other cases, not involving slipped discs, claimants have been more successful. In CI 147/50 the accident caused an ear condition which made the claimant more susceptible to infection. While in this state he contracted influenza. It was held that the flu was caused by the accident. The principle is clearly set out in R(I) 3/56 that as long as an industrial accident is an *effective cause* of the injury then, even if the injury would not have occurred but for some non-industrial event, the injury is caused, for the purposes of the law, by an industrial accident. (See CI 5/49). This principle does not depend on the order in which the industrial accident and the non-industrial event occur.

Decisions on this point often include the words 'chain of causation'. There is little consistency in the decisions.

Example. The claimant was not yet fit to return to work after an industrial accident in which he had injured his sacro-iliac joint. He persuaded his doctor to allow him to return to work. On his way to work he slipped in the street and in saving himself from falling, suffered a further injury to the same joint. It was held that the incident in the street merely demonstrated and prolonged the incapacity caused by the original accident (R(I) 3/56).

Example. The claimant sustained an industrial injury to his foot which did not render him incapable of work. Later, away from work, he trod on a pebble which pressed on the injury to the foot, causing him to turn over on his ankle and break it. It was held that the resulting incapacity was caused not by the original injury but by a new interim cause – the 'chain of causation' was broken. (R(I) 16/55.)

Similar decisions unfavourable to claimants are CI 114/49 ; CI 384/50 ; R(I) 33/53 ; R(I) 27/58 ; R(I) 4/58 ; R(I) 2/61 and R(I) 5/61. In any claim where the question of the 'cause' is likely to be an issue, it is essential to produce arguments to show that the chain of causation is not broken.

Note that similar problems about causation arise where you have to show that your incapacity for work was caused by an industrial accident as opposed to some other event.

Accident:

The word 'accident' has produced difficulties. It has not been precisely defined – different decisions have highlighted different characteristics. Some have emphasised that an event, to be an accident, must be unexpected by the person who is injured. Thus in Joint District School Board of Management v. Kelly (1914) the death of a schoolmaster murdered by his pupils was held to be an 'accident'. (See also CI 18/49; CI 51/49; CSI 63/49 and CI 123/49.)

Other decisions (in which the injury and the accident are indistinguishable) have emphasised the need for a physiological change for the worse occurring at some point in time (CI 5/49; CI 27/49; CI 52/49; R(I) 52/51; R(I) 71/51; R(I) 20/56; R(I) 19/60).

Another characteristic of an accident is that it must be an identifiable event or series of events as opposed to a process. There is no explicit formula for distinguishing a process from an accident. But there comes a time when the 'indefinite number of so-called accidents and the length of time over which they occur take away the element of accident and substitute that of process'. (CI 257/49.) Cases decided against the claimant on the ground that the injury was caused by process, not by accident, include CI 257/49 ('Raynaud's phenomenon' developed from operating a grinder for five years) CI 125/50. Contracture from gripping of hacking out knife and chisel); CSI 21/49 (Tuberculosis from unhealthy working conditions over a period); CSI 25/49 (incapacity resulting from series of sprains sustained while shovelling coal in a confined space); CI 244/50 (bus driver's conjunctivitis caused by continuous draught in his cab); R(I) 42/51 (strained chest muscles from lifting 700 blocks weighing 50lbs); R(I) 25/52 (disease caused by wearing wet gumboots over a long period); R(I) 19/56 (osteo-arthritis of fingers developed after three days of hand stitching leather); R(I) 7/66 (sudden death after 18 years' exposure to ethylene glycol dinitrate and nitro glycerine).

Decisions favourable to claimants can generally be divided into three categories:

1. Those where a repeated event is held to be a series

of accidents eg, C(I) 29/49 (where the claimant's work involved lifting a 15lb counterbalance weight many times a day); R(I) 77/51 (hernia, the result of repeated operation of an exceptionally stiff lever); R(I) 24/54 (cysts from frequent burns and pricks) and R(I) 43/55 (psycho-neurosis and skin condition caused by nervous shocks inflicted by sound of repeated explosions).

2. Those where in the course of a continuous process a particular event can be picked on as the accident, eg, R(I) 18/54 (sustained pressure on knee culminating in a lesion of a popliteal nerve. The accident was held to have happened at that point).

3. Those where the process is so short that it can still be treated as an accident eg, R(I) 43/61 (claimant worked on a job for nearly three days before feeling a sudden pain), and R(I) 4/62 (claimant worked from 4 to 31 January 1961). It has been held that a 'process' is generally reckoned in years rather than days.

Within the limits mentioned above, many different events have been held to be accidents, including: shock caused by seeing a fatal accident to a workmate (R(I) 49/52), sunstroke and exposure to heat (R(I) 4/61), exposure to cold and wet (CI 123/49. CI 3/51). Merely because the event which causes the injury is not sudden and violent, it does not follow that there has not been an accident.

Arising out of and in the course of employment:

Industrial injuries insurance is limited to risks of employment. If you are injured by an accident unconnected with your employment you have no claim. (You will have to claim sickness benefit.) The two expressions 'out of' and 'in the course of' have different meanings.

The test of whether a man is acting 'in the course' of his employment is not the strict test of whether he is at the relevant time performing a duty for his employer. He may be 'in the course' of his employment when he acts negligently, even disobediently, so long as it is something reasonably incidental to his contract of employment (R(I) 3/69).

'Arising out of his employment' signifies that not only was the claimant engaged in his employment, or something incidental to it, at the time of the accident, but that his employment, or something incidental to it, actually caused the accident (R(I) 10/52).

Example. The claimant worked in a shed which was not sufficiently heated and where a draught was frequently caused by open doors. He got influenza which developed into bronchitis. It was held that the influenza (a virus infection) did not arise out of the employment, nor did the bronchitis which resulted from it. (R(I) 32/57.)

If there is any evidence that the accident was caused by something other than the employment it will be up to the claimant to prove the contrary. (Proof and evidence are dealt with on page 296.)

The course of employment is limited in numbers of ways. The following are some of the more common ways in which it has been sought to disallow a claim as not arising in the course of the employment:

1. Travel to and from work: In general your employment does not begin until you reach your place of work and does not end until you leave it.

But if you are injured in a vehicle provided by your employer, you are in the course of your employment.

If the employer merely arranges with the local bus company for extra buses (which are also open to the public) to enable his employees to get to and from work, an employee travelling in such a bus is outside the course of his employment. (In case of doubt, see Section 8 of the Injuries Act.)

If you provide your own means of transport (including walking), you will not normally be covered before you reach or after you have left your employer's place of business (R(I) 45/52; R(I) 48/52). If, however, you are off the public road (eg on a private road belonging to your employer) and no longer subject to the same risks of accident as the general public you are in the course of your employment (R(I) 5/67; R(I) 1/68).

In some cases, it has been held that an employee's duties started at the time he left home eg where his home is his business headquarters (R(I) 38/53; R(I) 59/53). Of course when you are travelling on duty you are in the course of your employment (R(I) 4/49; R(I) 64/54; R(I) 34/59). But note the adverse decision defining when duty starts in R(I) 2/67.

It is not possible to deal in depth with all the cases covering travel to and from work (see Index and Digest under 'Travelling to and from work'). You are more likely to succeed if you are on an emergency call (R(I) 21/51), or are obliged by the terms of your employment to take something (R(I) 17/51) or someone (R(I) 8/51) with you.

2. Activity outside working hours: If you arrive early at your place of work, you are not outside the course of your employment simply because the working hours have not started. The test is whether you are there (a) for your own convenience as in (R(I) 43/55) where a laundry worker, before clocking in, deposited her own personal washing in the sorting room of the laundry and there sustained an injury (Claim disallowed) or (b) for that of your employer as in (R(I) 3/62) where the employee arrived early to avoid the rush hour and so conserve her strength for work. (Claim allowed.) (See also R(I) 1/59.)

When you are injured at your place of employment after working hours, the test is whether being there was incidental to your employment.

Example: A miner who remains to use a pit-head bath is still in the course of his employment (CI 22/49, CI 23/49, CI 24/49, CI 26/49, CI 34/49, CI 211/49) but if he remains in order to use the canteen he is doing an act for personal reasons. (CI 120/49, R(I) 52/52.)

Sometimes a person can be in the course of his employment when he is not on his employer's premises and not in normal working hours.

Example: A nurse on call, staying at a hotel booked for her nursing team (CI 374/50), and a resident cook who, though she had finished her work was still subject to her employer's orders (R(I) 49/51) were in the course of their employment. So were a sub postmistress working at home after hours (R(I) 64/51) and a driver who, on a Sunday, rescued his employer's van from a burning garage (R(I) 63/54).

3. Meal Breaks and Intervals: Generally if you take a meal in a canteen provided by your employer during working hours (but not after working hours) you are in the course of your employment (CSI 6/49, CI 120/49, R(I) 11/53, CI 34/50, R(I) 11/53). You are similarly in the course of your employment when going to and from such a meal (CSI 6/49; R(I) 17/60) so long as the journey does not involve going out on to the highway (R(I) 74/52; CI 282/49; CI 456/50). The reason for this distinction between meals taken during a break and meals taken after work seems to be that it is in the employer's interest for employees to be well-nourished in working hours.

Acts for personal purposes during a break, other than eating in an employer's canteen, will generally not be in the course of employment (R(I) 27/53, R(I) 45/53, R(I) 80/53).

4. Non-working acts during working hours: If you have an accident during working hours, and at the moment of the accident are not actually working, it will be difficult to show that you were in the course of your employment. The decisions are almost uniformly against claimants. Probably you will only succeed if you can show that the things you were doing were 'natural to the worker, are not (or would not be) objected to by the employer, and do not to any significant extent interfere with the performance of the worker's duty' (R(I) 1763). Using a lavatory will often, but not always, be in this category.

Claims arising out of non-working acts do not always fail:

o **A labourer injured his hand while attempting to retrieve a tin of tobacco he had dropped. It was held that he was in the course of his employment (R(I) 32/53).** Other attempts to recover property have been held to be outside the course of employment (R(I) 78/52, R(I) 20/54). It appears that one of the relevant matters is how much time is used in retrieving the property.

Accidental sleeping during employment is in the course of it (R(I) 36/59) but not deliberate napping.

Smoking is generally outside the scope of employment (R(I) 9/60) but where smoking is permitted and it is not the smoking but an employment risk which is the *cause* of the accident then the accident is in the course of employment (R(I) 2/63 – an important decision. See also R(I) 4/64).

Acts done out of curiosity such as tampering with machinery (R(I) 77/54) and wandering on the employer's premises (R(I) 71/52) and R(I) 45/59) are outside the course of employment.

Taking a breath of fresh air by leaning out of a window (see R(I) 24/63, drying clothing (R(I) 6/55) and conversation (R(I) 21/53) during a lull in work can be in the course of employment, but not always. Making and drinking tea can undoubtedly be in the course of employment (R(I) 21/ 53, R(I) 16/61) but not if it is made at what might be regarded as an unreasonable time (R(I) 34/53).

5. Trade Union meetings: In R(I) 63/51 an apprentice injured during a meeting held with the employer's permission – in the workshop where he worked and limited to employees – was held to be in the course of his employment (see also R(I) 9/57). On the other hand where the meeting was held after working hours and employees of other establishments were invited, an opposite decision was reached (R(I) 46/59). See also R(I) 36/54. The reasoning behind the distinction is obscure.

Breach of regulations:

Section 7 of the Injuries Act provides:

Accidents happening while acting in breach of regulations, etc. An accident shall be deemed to arise out of and in the course of an insured person's employment, notwithstanding that he is at the time of the accident acting in contravention of any statutory or other regulations applicable to his employment, or of any orders given by or on behalf of his employer, or that he is acting without instructions from his employer if:

a. the accident would have been deemed so to have arisen had the act not been done in contravention as aforesaid or without instructions from his employer, as the case may be; and

b. the act is done for the purposes of and in connection with the employer's trade or business.

This provision appears to be of great help to employees. In practice the requirement that the act be done for the purposes of and in connection with the employer's trade or business has ensured that its benefit is very restricted. You can test whether this section is going to help a claim by asking the following questions:

1. Did the accident arise out of and in the course of the employment? If the answer is 'yes', stop worrying as the section does not affect such a claim. If the answer is 'no', go on to next question.

2. Were you acting in contravention of a regulation or without instructions? If the answer to this is 'no', Section 7 does not help you. If the answer is 'yes', go on to next question.

3. Was the act for the purposes of and in connection with the employer's trade or business? If the answer is 'yes', the claim will succeed.

The interpretation of this section has become confused in practice by judges at the highest level who have taken the view that a dangerous act by an employee can be outside the course of his employment, independent of regulations or orders. If a person is injured in the course of such an act Condition (a), above, cannot be satisfied. The claim is bound to fail.

The decisions concerning this section are confusing. They can be examined in the Digest under 'Breach of Statutory Regulations, etc'. The reasoning behind them is not explained in this section because the author cannot understand it. A well-prepared claimant might be able to use the confusion in this area to his advantage.

Emergencies:
Section 9 provides:

Accidents happening while meeting emergency. An accident happening to an insured person in or about any premises at which he is for the time being employed for the purposes of his employer's trade or business shall be deemed to arise out of and in the course of his employment if it happens while he is taking steps, on an actual or supposed emergency at those premises, to rescue, succour or protect persons who are, or are thought to be or possibly be, injured or imperilled, or to avert or minimise serious damage to property.

The Digest has a section headed 'Emergency' which quotes claims made under this section. The word 'premises' seems to be fairly widely defined.

Section 10 of the Injuries Act provides:

Accidents caused by other person's misconduct etc. An accident happening after 19 December 1961 shall be treated for the purposes of this Act, where it would not apart from this section be so treated, as arising out of a person's employment if:

a. the accident arises in the course of the employment; and

b. the accident either is caused by another person's misconduct, skylarking or negligence or by steps taken in consequence of any such misconduct, skylarking or negligence, or by the behaviour or presence of an animal (including a bird, fish, or insect), or is caused by or consists in the insured person being struck by any object or by lightning; and

c. the insured person did not directly or indirectly induce or contribute to the happening of the accident by his conduct outside the employment or by any act not incidental to the employment.

Again there are sections in the Digest under the headings 'Animals', 'Insects', and 'Skylarking'. The section headed 'Misconduct' does not specifically refer to this section though the definitions given in it might be relevant.

In any claim where Section 9 or 10 may be of assistance, it will be necessary to look up how the sections have been applied in practice.

Injury Benefit:

Accidents:

After any but the most trivial injury it is important to take immediate action to ensure that a future right to benefit is not lost. If you suffer a personal injury and you believe it was caused by an industrial accident the law – Section 48(2)

– entitles you to have that question determined and a *declaration* made and recorded accordingly – *whether you make a claim for benefit at the same time or not.* This can be important when you have no immediate claim for injury benefit – perhaps you are not incapacitated for work – and there is a possibility that the injury could have serious consequences (resulting in a claim for disablement or even death benefit), years after everybody has forgotten how the injury was caused. You should consider obtaining a declaration even if no claim for injury benefit is made. A symptom occurring years after a trivial accident can often be related to it. As medical science progresses, such situations are likely to become more common. (The declaration procedure does not apply in the case of a prescribed industrial disease.)

The first step in any claim should be to report the accident to your employer. (The law requires you, or a representative, to do this.) The notice should be given either to the employer, or to a foreman or some other official appointed for the purpose. Noting the particulars in an accident book is sufficient.

The procedure for reporting varies from shop to shop. Whatever the procedure, make sure that the information has been taken in by the person you report to. It's no good if the person is so busy that he immediately forgets all about it. Whenever possible, the information should be written down.

Failure to report the accident need not destroy your claim (eg, R(I) 2/51, R(I) 59/62) **if you can show a good reason for not reporting it** – for example its apparent triviality or the lack of any proper procedure for reporting.

It's a good idea to note the names and addresses of any witnesses. They may be of value in the future if the claim is disputed. If, several months later, they have left that job, you will still be able to trace them. Employers may not be keen to help you trace witnesses, particularly where there is a possibility of an action for damages. (See Section 11, Damages.)

Even if the accident has not been reported and there are no witnesses, the claim is not bound to fail. But the clearer the evidence, the better is your chance of success.

The fact that there is not evidence of all the particulars of the accident will not in itself prevent a claim succeeding. In R(I) 18/54 the claimant could not pinpoint the exact date of the accident. In this case the accident was not a single definable event. But in a case where the accident was sudden and identifiable, your claim might be disallowed if you couldn't remember the date.

If there is a chance that the existence, circumstances or relevance of an injury will be disputed, ask the doctor who first examines you to make a note of whether or not he thinks the injury could have been caused in the way you say it was. If the doctor agrees with your explanation, this will be helpful later on.

If there is a chance of a dispute, evidence on how the accident happened should also be obtained from witnesses as soon as possible.

Claims for injury benefit:

The procedure for making a claim is clearly described in various leaflets available free from the local office. In the first instance your claim should be made in writing on the appropriate form. (Forms are obtainable, free, at the local office.)

It is probably easiest at this stage to give comparatively short particulars and offer to supply any further information needed. The insurance officer will make enquiries about any matters on which he is not satisfied. Don't withhold any material evidence – you might land yourself and your advisers with the trouble of an appeal (see R(I) 6/51). The powers of the insurance officer under the Claims and Payment Regulations (and particularly under Regulations 3, 4 and 9) should be noted.

Apart from the accident itself, the insurance officer dealing with a claim for injury benefit needs to be satisfied that you are really incapacitated for work.

The Digest includes a large number of decisions on this matter. Incapacity for work is defined the same way for industrial injuries benefit as it is for sickness benefit (CI 99/49).

A person is incapable of work if, having regard to his age, education, experience, state of health and other personal factors, there is no work or type of work which he can be expected to do. (R(S) 11/51.)

The type of work which you can be expected to do varies with the length of your incapacity. If the incapacity is for a short period, at the end of which you can expect to return to your usual job, or a similar one, then you will be incapable of work for that period. On the other hand, after a longer period of incapacity, the authorities would expect you to look for a different kind of work (see R(S) 7/60). In practice, where the claim is for injury benefit (which is limited to 26 weeks), you will not normally be expected to do a different kind of work.

If you are actually working, this is evidence of your capacity for work (CI 8/49) but the fact that you have worked does not itself prove that you are *capable* of work (You may only have worked because of very compelling circumstances as in R(S) 8/55 and CG 30/49). But you cannot usually claim injury benefit for the days when you actually work.

Medical evidence:

Normally in a claim for injury benefit, the certificate from your own doctor (which is sent with the claim) is sufficient medical evidence. It will state that in the doctor's opinion you were incapable of work at the time of the examination; the reason for the incapacity and either: the day on which you will be fit to resume work (this is called a 'final certificate') ; or the period during which you will remain incapable of work ('intermediate certificate').

Get the doctor's certificate on the earliest possible day. If you are still incapable of work when the certificate runs out, go back for a new one so that the certificates are consecutive.

If the doctor knows about your work, it is useful to get him to note on the certificate those aspects of the job which make you unable to do it.

Neither you nor the insurance officer are obliged to accept your doctor's opinion of your capacity for work

(R(S) 4/56). If the insurance officer is not satisfied with the certificate he will refer you to another doctor, usually the Regional Medical Officer, for an additional report on your capacity for work or the relevance of the injury to your incapacity. The insurance officer may or may not prefer the Medical Officer's report. The insurance officer may decide a claim for injury benefit (other than from a prescribed disease) on his own assessment of the medical evidence. When injury or disablement benefit is claimed for a prescribed disease the insurance officer is obliged to refer certain questions to doctors or to a Medical Board (see pages 284, 285).

If you have obtained a letter from a doctor, you are not obliged to produce it to the authorities if it is unfavourable (R(S) 1/58). But if you have informed the authorities that you intend to produce a particular piece of evidence, your position will not be improved if you then fail to produce it. It might be better not to mention it at all.

It is very difficult for a layman to question the decisions of doctors. All you can do is to see that they (whether they are your own doctor, a specialist, a Medical Officer, a Medical Board or a Medical Appeal Tribunal) are in possession of all the facts and hope that they will conclude in your favour. You cannot tell in advance whether a fact is favourable or not, so you should see that they have any evidence that could be relevant:

a full account of the accident,

up to date records of medical treatment,

earlier medical history,

other existing disabilities or handicaps,

psychological effects of the accident,

the kind of work which you do.

You may be able to convince an insurance officer that an adverse doctor's report was made, for example, on incomplete knowledge of your work. But it is much better to provide the doctor with the full facts in the first place.

Other evidence:

In addition to medical reports, the insurance officer can consider other evidence of incapacity:

a statement by an employer that he would not employ you,

the fact that you have applied for jobs and been rejected.
(See R(S) 10/54 where a claimant was thought by doctors to
be 'capable of some type of restricted employment'),

the opinion of an employment exchange on your chances of
finding work,

evidence on the nature of your job (this would normally
be relevant only in claims for injury benefit),

your previous work record (if it shows you are not the kind
of person to malinger).

Medical attendance and treatment:

Where you are an in-patient in a hospital it is presumed that you are incapable of work (see R(S) 1/58). Similarly if you have to attend hospital for treatment, you are
likely to be incapable of work on the days when you have to
attend (though not necessarily on other days). But if you
go to your own doctor to be examined and are found to be
capable of work, you are not regarded as incapable for
work on that day (see CI 40/49) – even though you had to
miss work to go to the doctor!

Prescribed diseases:

When injury benefit is claimed for a prescribed disease, and there is any doubt whether you are actually suffering from it the insurance officer must refer the question to
a doctor or doctors. This is known as a 'diagnosis question'.
If there is some doubt whether or not a prescribed disease
is a continuance of a prescribed disease contracted earlier,
he must refer such questions to a doctor or doctors (a 'recrudescence question').

Injury benefit will be paid in respect of days of incapacity for work in the period of 26 weeks beginning with the
day of the accident or any part of that period for which disablement benefit is not available.

This rather complicated provision should be studied in the original (Section 12(2) of the Injuries Act).

Injury benefit is a flat rate benefit assessed according
to the number of dependants you have. There is an earnings
related supplement. The rates are higher than for sickness
benefit – so where possible a claim should be made for injury benefit rather than sickness benefit.

Disablement Benefit:

Disablement benefit is available when an industrial accident or prescribed disease leaves you with a loss of physical or mental faculty great enough for your resulting disablement to be assessed (according to the law) at not less than 1 per cent (Injuries Act S12). It is payable whether or not you have claimed injury benefit and regardless of your capacity for work.

An office worker who sits all day at a desk will receive the same benefit for a disabled foot as, say, a postman who is forced by the disability to give up his job.

A separate claim has to be made for disablement benefit and in the first instance it is made to the local insurance officer. He must refer some questions, such as the degree of your disablement ('disablement question'), to a medical board for decision. In some restricted circumstances such questions can be referred to a single doctor. (Determination of Claims and Questions (No.2) Regulations 1967). Other questions are determined by the Insurance Officer, with appeals to the Local Appeal Tribunal and from there to the Commissioner.

The principles governing assessments by medical boards are set out in Section 12 of the Act, Schedule 4 to the Act and Regulation 2 of the Benefit Regulations. An assessment must state the degree of your disability as a percentage (these percentages are arbitrary figures set out in the second schedule to the Benefit Regulations). The assessment must specify the period it has taken into account and whether the assessment is provisional or final. If you suffer from a disability which is expected to change for better or worse over the years the Medical Board should make a provisional assessment. Before the end of the period of the provisional assessment the case must be referred back to the Board for a further provisional or final assessment. In cases of permanent disability an assessment can be for life.

You can't collect disablement benefit for the three days immediately after the relevant accident or while you are drawing injury benefit.

If you are not incapable of work for the whole 26

weeks after the accident, but have some disability from it, it is usually financially better to claim disablement benefit as soon as you become capable of work, or, if you are not incapable of work, some days after the accident. In most cases this will result in your receiving higher benefits, should you later become incapable of work, than if you claim injury benefit only for the days of incapacity.

Your likely entitlement to different benefits should be carefully thought out because:

Injury benefit is not payable for any period in which disablement benefit is received, sickness and disablement benefits can be paid at the same time.

In some cases you may decide to claim disablement benefit during the first 26 weeks. If, before the claim is finally determined, you find you would be better off receiving injury benefit, you can withdraw the claim.

Some people continue their work in spite of considerable disabilities caused by an industrial accident. They are nevertheless entitled to disablement benefit and should be encouraged to claim. Sometimes people don't claim because they are unaware that under the legal definition they are disabled. The loss of a kidney or a tooth for example may not prove to be much of a handicap but it's a disability all the same. Other disabilities not readily identifiable as such include impairment of your senses (of smell, for example), psychological effects of shock and susceptibility to further injury or disfigurement.

Assessment of disability can become complicated, and sometimes unjust, if your disability results from both an industrial accident and a non-industrial cause. (The rules, set out in Regulations 2(3) and (4) of the Benefit Regulation, have to be read several times in order to be understood.)

There are two situations:

1. A non-industrial disablement (say a permanent disability of a knee valued at 5 per cent) exists before the accident. The Board must take into account the whole disablement, less the proportion of disability you would have suffered had there been no industrial accident.

Example.

Non-industrial disablement of knee:	5 per cent
Industrial injury to foot on same leg:	8 per cent
Total disability (mobility seriously affected by the combination):	17 per cent
Less original, non-industrial disablement:	−5 per cent
Final assessment	12 per cent

2. The *cause* of non-industrial disablement arises *after* the industrial accident. A similar calculation is done but only if the disablement which would have existed without later, non-industrial disablement is 11 per cent or more. In the example above, therefore, if the knee injury happened after the industrial accident (damage to foot, assessed at 8 per cent) no additional benefit could be claimed, even though the combination of injuries totalled 17 per cent. An assessment cannot be reversed simply because of a subsequent accident: if you lose a toe in an industrial accident and then lose the whole foot in a later, non-industrial, accident, your assessment for the lost toe remains unchanged even though you no longer have the foot from which you lost the toe.

Where the medical board is satisfied that 100 per cent disablement resulted from an industrial cause, they are not required to make a deduction in respect of a non-industrial cause (Benefit Regulation 6).

Medical Boards may not deviate without good reason from the degrees of disablement set out in Schedule 2 of the Benefit Regulations.

Occasionally a Medical Board has to assess a disability which no longer exists at the time of its examination – for example if you make a late claim for a disability which has been cured.

The Board must not decide any questions which can only be decided by the determining authorities (insurance officer, Local Appeal Tribunal and Commissioner).

Benefits:

Disablement benefit is paid either as **a.** a weekly pension or, **b.** where disablement for the period taken into account is assessed at under 20 per cent, as a gratuity. (The amount of gratuity is calculated in accordance with Regulation 3 and Schedule 3 of the Benefit Regulations.) The maximum amount, for an assessment of 19 per cent for seven years or more, is £740. In certain cases (see Claims and Payments Regulation 17) a gratuity can be paid by instalments. In a period of inflation this may not be very wise.

In calculating the pension payable, disablement assessed at over 20 per cent is rounded to the nearest 10 per cent. (For full details see Injuries Act Schedule 4, para 4.) For a single adult the weekly rate ranges from £2.24 at 20 per cent assessment to £11.20 at 100 per cent.

Note that if a claimant has died from a cause unconnected with the accident before the claim is dealt with, it could be advantageous to his widow if the disablement were assessed at below 20 per cent and a *gratuity* obtained, rather than the back payment of a disability pension from a higher assessment for the period up to the claimant's death.

Additional allowances:
Unemployability supplement:

Section 13 (1) of the Act provides for your weekly rate of disablement pension to be increased if, as a result of the relevant loss of faculty, you are incapable of work and likely to remain permanently so. (A person is treated as being incapable of work and likely to remain permanently so if the loss of faculty is likely to prevent his yearly earnings exceeding £104.)

Note first that this benefit is not available to you if you are receiving a disablement gratuity (R(I) 48/59). But if you are eligible for a gratuity you may convert it into a pension under Benefit Regulation 6(2) and so qualify for unemployability supplement.

A finding by a medical board on whether or not you are incapable of work and likely to remain so may be considered as evidence by the determining authorities; but it is for them, not the medical board, to decide the question (see CI 4/49 and CI 44/49).

Favourable decisions on the question of whether or not a person is likely to remain permanently incapable of work are CI 44/49, R(I) 58/52. Adverse decisions are CI 99/49 and R(I) 43/54.

The current rate of unemployability supplement is £6.75 per week.

Increase of Unemployability Supplement:

You may be able to get an increase of the unemployability supplement according to your age on the 'qualifying date'. The qualifying date is usually the beginning of the first week in which you qualified for unemployability supplement. Section 13A of the Injuries Act defines it more fully. The maximum ages to qualify for this are 60 for a man and 55 for a woman. The weekly amounts vary between 0.35p and £1.15p.

Special Hardship Allowance:

This is another supplement to Disablement Benefit. It is payable if you are:

a. incapable and likely to remain permanently incapable of following your regular occupation;

and:

b. incapable of following employment of an equivalent standard which is suitable in your case,

or;

c. if you are and have at all times since the end of the injury benefit period been incapable of following that occupation or any such employment (1965 Act S14 (1)).

Special Hardship Allowance is not limited to persons receiving disablement **pension.** Benefit Regulation 6 (1) lays down that it is available to a person who is entitled to a disablement **gratuity** as if the gratuity had been a pension.

Special Hardship Allowance and Unemployability Supplement are alternatives. You cannot be paid both in the same period.

Claimants should note the circumstances set out in Benefit Regulation 5. This says you are not to be treated as capable of following an occupation or employment merely because you work in it during a period of trial or for rehabilitation or training. This regulation also applies in cases where you are waiting to undergo surgery.

The Digest contains numerous cases in which a claimant's right to Special Hardship Allowance has been challenged and argued about. It is worth studying them if you are claiming SHA. The main points covered under the section include:

1. What is meant by regular occupation and how to determine if a person is working in it.

2. How a person's prospects of promotion or advancement in his employment are taken into account.

3. The meaning of 'employment of an equivalent standard'.

4. Assessment of a person's capability of following such employment.

5. The period and amount of the award of Special Hardship Allowance.

In making a claim for Special Hardship Allowance there is no substitute for being familiar with previous cases. Their number and difficulty can work in your favour when you know all the arguments and, if necessary, how to answer them.

A claim for Special Hardship Allowance will usually be based on evidence of facts from the following sources:

1. The employer

2. Medical evidence

3. Independent persons (eg, workmates) with experience of your employment or of any other employment which has been suggested as suitable in your case.

4. The claimant himself.

The maximum amount of Special Hardship Allowance is £4.48 per week with an overall maximum (together with Disablement Benefit) of £11.20.

Constant Attendance Allowance:

This allowance is available if you have been assessed as 100 per cent disabled and, as a result of the relevant loss of faculty, you need somebody to look after you all the time. (Section 15(1) 1965 Act.) The allowance may be made in addition to Unemployability Supplement or Special Hardship Allowance. There are several rates:

1. where you are to a substantial extent dependent on constant attendance for the necessities of life and likely to remain so for a prolonged period, the maximum rate (reducible if the attendance required is part-time only) is £4.50 per week.

2. where the greater attendance is required because of exceptionally severe disablement – up to £6.75.

3. where your disablement is so exceptionally severe that you are entirely – or almost entirely – dependent on full-time attendance for the necessities of life, and are likely to remain so dependent for a prolonged period – £9.00 per week (Benefit Regulation 7). This allowance is limited if you are a hospital in-patient. (Benefit Regulation 26.)

Hospital Treatment Allowance:

If you are receiving disablement benefit (including a gratuity) assessed at less than 100 per cent and you receive in-patient hospital treatment for the relevant injury or loss of faculty, the disability is treated as though assessed at 100 per cent during the period in hospital. (See Section 16 and Benefit Regulation 8.) Note Benefit Regulation 26A and Section 33(1) of the Injuries Act.

An in-patient is a patient who occupies a bed in a hospital (see R(I) 27/59). Anything less is unlikely to qualify. (See R(D) 2/52; R(S) 28/52; R(I) 27/59.)

Dependant children:

If you have a family which includes a child or children, you are entitled to increased benefits:

a. for any period during which you are entitled to injury benefit

b. if you are entitled to disablement pension, and are either entitled to unemployability supplement or receiving, as an in-patient in a hospital or similar institution, medical treatment for the relevant injury or loss of faculty. (Section 17/1.) The children in respect of whom a claim can be made and further conditions of entitlement are defined by Section 17(2) to (6).

In most cases it is relatively easy to determine when this allowance is payable, but if you live apart from your children or they are partly or wholly maintained by someone else difficulties may arise.

Benefit Regulations 13 and 14 provide for such an event in language which must be carefully studied to be understood. **Note** that the definition of a child (Section 86(2) and Family Allowances Act 1965 S2) is a person under the compulsory school age limit; or under 19 and receiving full-time education; or under 16 and incapable of regular employment.

The allowance is £3.30 for the first child, £2.40 for the second and £2.30 each for the third and subsequent children.

Dependant Adults:

You are entitled to an increase in respect of certain dependant adults if you are:

1. Receiving injury benefit; or

2. Entitled to unemployability supplement; or

3. Receiving, as an in-patient, medical treatment for the relevant injury or loss of faculty.

The adult dependants are:

a. A wife (this does not include a woman to whom you are not married) with whom you are residing;

b. A wife to whose maintenance you are contributing;

c. A husband incapable of self-support to whose maintenance you are contributing or with whom you are residing;

d. Certain relatives (defined in Schedule 5 to the Benefit Regulations) whom you are wholly or mainly maintaining;

e. A woman having the care of your children.

This increase is given by Section 18 of the Injuries Act and is further defined by Benefit Regulations 9, 10 and 11. The current allowance for any such dependant is £4.15 per week but it can be valued according to the dependant's income. This increase can be paid only in respect of one adult.

Death Benefit:

If you die as a result of an injury or disease that would have entitled you to injury or disablement benefit if you had lived, there are six classes of person for whom death benefit may be available.

As usual the burden of proving the facts is generally on the person making the claim.

The evidence of the victim (often the most important witness in proving an accident and its consequences) will not be available but this makes no difference to the standard of proof required. Whoever makes the claim will have to use other witnesses.

Once again questions of causation will arise in proving that death resulted from the injury or disease. Again the test is not whether the injury was a direct or indirect cause. For the claim to be proved it must be shown that it was an 'efficient' cause, not a mere condition (R(I) 14/51). A claim will not fail simply because it is possible or conceivable that death was due to another cause. But it must be shown that it *probably* resulted from the injury.

The three propositions on causation set out in R(I) 3/56 should be studied. Note that an accident can be the effective cause of a death even if:

a. The dead person has a pre-existing condition rendering him or her susceptible to death from it; or

b. The accident causes susceptibility to a fatal disease which he or she then contracts. (See also R(I) 54/52.)

There are a number of decisions in which it has been held that where the accident or disease produces a mental or nervous state which causes someone to commit suicide then the death is a result of the accident or disease. (See CI 172/50, R(I) 2/57 and R(I) 36/60.) Note also the cases reported in the Digest under the heading 'Suicide' where the necessary connection between the accident or disease and the suicide was held not to be established.

Certain kinds of injury and disease have given rise to numerous death benefit decisions – and in particular cancer, heart disease and injuries to the head. (See Digest under 'Tumour', 'Heart – diseases of' and 'Brain – diseases of'). Most of the decisions go against claimants, usually because of the rules on burden of proof and because of difficulty in dealing with medical evidence. The claimant must show that, on balance, the medical evidence points to death as a result of the accident. In many cases doctors are not able to say that there is a connection between the accident (eg, a blow on the head) and the disease causing death (eg, a brain injury), even though the start of the disease coincides very closely with the accident. This kind of difficulty can be overcome. It can be argued:

a. That the doctors, or even the injured person have underestimated the extent of the injuries;

b. That doctors, when they are uncertain, may decline to give an opinion even if on balance they favour the claimant.

(A doctor must be fairly certain before giving a positive opinion but claims should be decided on the balance of probabilities.) The Digest lists all the various ailments dealt with in different parts of the volume under the heading 'Medical Cases'. You should look up any cases that may be relevant before making a claim.

The six classes of person for whom a claim for death benefit can be made are as follows:

Class of person	Entitlement defined in:	
	Injuries Act	Benefit Regulations 18 and 19
1. Widow of insured	Section 19	
2. Widower of insured	Section 20	
3. Children of insured's family	Section 21	14 and 14A
4. Parents of injured	Section 22	
5. Relatives of insured	Section 23	21
6. Woman having care of insured's children	Section 24	

Death benefit is usually payable in periodic amounts, known as a 'pension' or 'allowance' according to the category of person who receives it. In certain cases a widow or a parent receives a gratuity. The rates vary according to the relationship.

Prescribed diseases:

You can claim benefits for two types of disease:
1. A disease caused by an industrial accident.
2. A prescribed disease (a disease prescribed by regulations in relation to certain types of employment). In a situation where you would be certain to claim benefit both because a disease is prescribed and because it is caused by an accident then you are entitled to benefit only on the basis that it is prescribed.

The first thing you must show is that the disease is prescribed in relation to your work. Part I of the first schedule to the Prescribed Diseases Regulations sets out the diseases in the first column and the related occupations in the second. You have to show not only that you were required by your contract to work in the occupation but also that you have *actually* worked in it. (CI 59/49, CI 60/49.)

The occupations listed in the second column of the schedule as 'involving' certain actions or exposure to certain substances and processes. 'Involvement' means something more than just very occasional involvement. In a case where your involvement was not sufficient, it might be held that the disease was contracted by an industrial accident, providing you can show the necessary connection.

Where 'handling' is described as being part of an occupation this includes the use of tools on the relevant material (CWI 26/49). It can include sweeping (CWI 26/49) and shovelling (CSI 69/49) – see also (CWI 13/50), (CI 114/50).

Occasionally it may be difficult to show that you encounter the substances and processes in the course of your occupation. In any case where disagreement may arise over analysis or identification of substances, samples should be collected with care (see page 256). You or your representative should be there when samples are taken. It is even better if an expert can do this. The union might agree to employ one; or a workmate in a scientific or technical union might assist.

Note that the list of prescribed diseases has been altered and increased since 1959.

The date of development of a disease depends on the type of benefit claimed.
In a claim for injury benefit it is the first day on which you became incapable of work.
In relation to disablement benefit it is the day on which you first suffered the relevant loss of faculty;
or, in relation to both injury and disablement benefit, it is the first day on which benefit could be paid under the Claims and Payments Regulations.

In relation to death benefit it is the date of death. (Regulation 6 of the Prescribed Diseases Regulations.)

If you suffer from a condition which resulted from a prescribed disease you are treated as if suffering from a prescribed disease. (Regulation 3 of the Prescribed Diseases Regulations.)

Regulation 7 lays down how the recrudescence of a prescribed disease is to be treated.

Note that different procedures apply in relation to pneumoconiosis, byssinosis, Farmer's lung and diffuse mesothelioma. These are laid down in Part VI of the Prescribed Diseases Regulations. (See also page 146 of this book where assessment of disability in pneumoconiosis victims is described.)

The procedure for claiming benefit in respect of a prescribed disease is only slightly different from that in accident cases.

You claim in the usual way to the insurance officer. But he cannot determine all questions as he can in a claim for injury benefit. He must refer some questions to a doctor or doctors:

a. whether you are or have been suffering from a prescribed disease (a 'diagnosis question')

b. whether you have contracted a prescribed disease afresh ('a recrudescence question') (Prescribed Diseases Regulation 25).

Only in restricted circumstances can he dispense with the report (Prescribed Diseases Regulation 26).

Having obtained the report the insurance officer must decide the diagnosis or recrudescence question himself or refer it to a Medical Board. (Prescribed Diseases Regulation 27.) If the insurance officer determines it himself you may appeal against his decision to a Medical Board. (Regulations 28 and 29.)

If you disagree with a Medical Board's decision on a diagnosis or recrudescence question you have a right of appeal to a Medical Appeal Tribunal. (Regulation 30.)

There are provisions for review of decisions on diagnosis and recrudescence questions. (Regulations 31 and 32.)

Proof and evidence:

In most cases it is up to you to show that you are entitled to the benefit claimed. The 'burden of proof' falls on you.

Accidents:

If your claim involves an accident you will have to

produce evidence to show that:

1. There was an accident (your own account of what happened and that of any witnesses)

2. the accident arose **out of and in the course of** your employment

3. the employment was insurable employment

4. the accident caused the personal injury (or disease), disablement or death for which the claim is made.

Prescribed disease:

If your claim is for a prescribed disease you must produce evidence that:

1. The prescribed disease is prescribed in relation to your work,

2. You have, or have had, the disease; and

3. You developed it as a result of the employment.

In addition to the above, you have to prove certain facts to get each type of benefit:

Injury benefit. To get this you must show that, **a.** as a result of the injury or disease, you are or were incapable of work for the period for which you are claiming and **b.** that this period is within the injury benefit period.

Disablement benefit. You must provide evidence showing that you suffer the relevant loss of faculty, as a result of the injury or disease.

Special hardship allowance:

You must provide evidence that, as a result of your loss of faculty, either **a.** you are incapable of following your regular occupation (or suitable employment of equivalent standard); or **b.** you have at all times, since you became eligible for disablement benefit been incapable to that extent.

Death benefit:

It must be shown that the victim died as a result of the injury or disease.

In all these types of claim you must satisfy the determining authority (insurance officer, appeal tribunal, etc.) that, *on the balance of probability,* the circumstances entitle you to benefit (R(I) 32/61). If various witnesses produce conflicting accounts of a particular accident, the determining authority will consider the different stories and decide on balance which it thinks is nearest the truth. (R(I) 32/61.) Where there is a dispute about the facts you should see that the determining authority has all the evidence which supports your claim.

There are two main exceptions to the rule that a claimant has to prove his case:

1. Accidents:

By Section 6 of the Injuries Act, if you can show that your accident arose *in the course of* your employment then it is presumed that it arose *out of* your employment. Only if there is evidence (which must be more than mere speculation – (R(I) 1/64) that the accident was caused by something not connected with the employment will you have to prove that the accident arose both in the course of and out of your employment (CI 3/49, R(I) 21/58). Cases of this kind are listed in the Digest under the heading 'Presumption'.

2. Prescribed diseases:

If you can show that you were employed in a prescribed occupation at any time within one month immediately prior to the date you developed a disease prescribed in relation to that occupation, it is presumed to be due to the nature of your employment, unless proved otherwise. (Prescribed Diseases Regulation 4(1). Note: this does not apply to Prescribed Diseases 38, 41, and 42.)

This does not completely remove the burden of proof from a claimant. You still have to prove the main facts on which you rely before the presumption arises. These are usually not very difficult to prove.

There are instances throughout the Injuries Act where if one matter is shown to be true then another is 'deemed' to be true (Section 9) or is treated as being true (Section 10).

It is very rare that you will have to prove every single matter. In most cases there will be no dispute at all about your right to benefit.

The rules of evidence:

In ordinary law courts, rules of evidence lay down what weight to give to various accounts of an event and even whether the court is entitled to consider those accounts at all. The determining authorities in industrial injury cases are not bound by these rules but they may attach less weight to evidence which would not have been admissible in an ordinary law court. If you are up against a lawyer he will certainly quote rules of evidence to get a tribunal to give particular weight to, or to disregard, a particular piece of evidence. You may be able to do the same but be careful unless you are sure what you are doing.

The best evidence of a particular event is an oral account of it by someone who witnessed it. When evidence is given orally a determining authority can clear up any ambiguities by asking questions. Anyone who disagrees with the account can test it by cross-examination. Little weight will be given to evidence from someone who did not witness the event personally and only heard of it from someone who did. It is important to support a claim with the best evidence available. Official documents, such as birth certificates or entries in record books, are generally taken as true, but can be disproved by strong evidence that they are not correct. A baptism certificate, for example, could show that a birth certificate was wrong. (R(S) 15/52.)

In preparing your case, examine very carefully any evidence you intend to produce and try to anticipate any evidence which could be produced in opposition.

Example. A claim for Special Hardship Allowance.

o Your employer might state that you are capable of following your regular employment. But does he really know the extent of your disablement, the details of the work involved in your employment or the legal meaning of 'capable' and 'regular employment'? A doctor's statement can be tested by the same questions.

There is no reason why you should not give evidence in your own claim. You are usually the one who knows most about it. The determining authorities may wish to hear your story direct rather than through your representative.

You and your representative should try to get all the facts and issues clear in your minds before you start. Your representative can help by reminding you, as you give your evidence, of any points you might forget.

Remember that a skilled advocate can easily twist your words into the opposite of what you mean, eg, by suggesting you are mistaken, unreliable or short-sighted. You and your representative can do this to hostile witnesses in appropriate cases.

Comment:

It is important to understand the difference between evidence and comment. You may give evidence only of facts which are within your knowledge. Comment is the indication of conclusions to be drawn from evidence. The distinction is often blurred.

For instance, if a witness states that he saw the claimant limping that is evidence of the fact that the claimant limped – no more. The determining authority might infer from that fact that the claimant had a stone in his shoe. The claimant, by his comments on the fact of his limping, might persuade the authority that their inference about the stone was wrong.

Comment can be used, where there is no direct evidence on a point, to show what inferences can be drawn from the evidence available or, where there is a conflict in the evidence, to show why one version is more likely to be true than another.

Lying:

If you think that a witness is lying it is usually better not to hurl abuse at him. Concentrate on giving the determining authority reasons to doubt the evidence given. It may be better not to suggest that the witness is lying but that he is mistaken; the authorities dislike finding that a person is committing a fraud unless the evidence clearly shows it. They are happier to say that he is mistaken – particularly if he is someone with status. This is not to say that a witness should not be called a liar in an appropriate case. It's merely a warning to be careful.

Insurance officer:

In the first instance *all* claims are made to the insurance officer, an official in the local office of the Department of Health and Social Security. His duty is to investigate a claim and to decide all questions arising in connection with it except the 'special questions' which he must refer to other bodies.

Disablement, diagnosis and recrudescence questions have been described earlier.

The insurance officer must refer two other types of question elsewhere:

'Minister's questions'. These are:

1. Whether a person is or was employed in insurable employment

2. Whether a person is or was exempt from payment of contributions

3. Who is or was liable, as employer, for payment of contributions

4. The rate at which contributions are or were payable

5. Whether a constant attendance allowance is to be granted or renewed, and if so for what period and amount

6. How the special limitations on death benefit are to be applied.

'Family questions', for example who is maintaining a child or in which family a child is to be treated as included. These questions must also be referred to the Minister (the Secretary of State for Social Services).

Once a final decision has been reached on all special questions the insurance officer will decide any further questions and make his decision. The Insurance Officer decides claims on the basis of written evidence only.

In the course of determining a claim the insurance officer may refer any questions, other than a special question to a Local Appeal Tribunal for determination.

Such a reference should be within 14 days of the submission of your claim. You must be given notice of it. The procedure is similar to that given below under 'Local Appeal Tribunals'.

If the insurance officer has decided any claim or question adversely to you, you must be notified in writing of the decision, the reasons for it and your right of appeal. (National Insurance Act 1965 S69 – see 1966 Act S8 (1).)

Local Appeal Tribunal:

If you dispute the insurance officer's decision on any question which he has power to decide you may appeal against the decision. You must lodge a written notice of appeal at the local office within 21 days of the decision. The notice should state the grounds of appeal. (Insurance Act S69.) It should be a brief summary of reasons why the decision is disputed. They need not be detailed – often they can't because insurance officers don't always give full reasons for their decisions. You can always add new grounds after the notice of appeal has been delivered.

Advance details:

Often in advance of the tribunal hearing the parties to it will have delivered to the Tribunal full details in writing of the arguments on which they intend to rely. This is so that the disputed issues can be known in advance and time will not be wasted hearing unnecessary evidence and arguing over undisputed points. It also enables the parties to prepare their cases properly in advance. Usually, you are the one who gains most from this procedure because you are the one most likely to be put off by unexpected arguments or evidence.

There is no fixed rule about how much should be stated in writing before the hearing. Additional points can always be raised at the hearing itself. If an entirely new point is raised a party who disputes it can ask for an adjournment on the grounds that he had no reason to believe it would be brought up and that he needs additional time to deal with it. If you apply for an adjournment it is likely to be granted only if the new point is one for which you could not have been expected to be prepared.

The Tribunal:

The local tribunal has three members. One is from a panel of persons representing employers and one from a panel representing employees. The third member is an 'independent' chairman.

The Tribunal must give notice to interested parties of the time and place of the hearing.

The parties:

At the hearing itself the following people are entitled to be heard:

claimant,

insurance officer,

Secretary of State;

any interested person – for instance another claimant whose right to benefit may be affected by the decision (Determination of Claims and Questions Regulation 9).

The parties need not be present in person and may bring or send a representative (*legally qualified or not*). Any party may introduce evidence and question witnesses. The public is generally admitted.

Witnesses:

Where facts are in dispute you should ensure that any witness on whose evidence you rely is at the hearing. If the witness cannot come, get a signed statement from him.

Be careful of witnesses who are able to give evidence in support of a claim but are reluctant to do so. Often such witnesses do not take care about what they say; it can be better not to call them at all.

Procedure:

The normal procedure is for each party in turn to produce his evidence – by giving it himself, by calling witnesses and by producing written evidence such as doctor's reports. Each party has a chance to cross-question each witness.

When all the evidence has been called the parties get an opportunity to make a speech to the Tribunal. A speech should cover the facts – for example what conclusions you think the tribunal should draw from the evidence. It should also cover the law – for example the meaning of a particular word or phrase in Acts or Regulations and how it applies in the present case.

Sometimes the legal submissions will take the form of a discussion. If a tribunal member objects to a point on which you are relying, answer his objections: he is not necessarily against your arguments. He may well support you and merely wish to get from you arguments to use against points he expects to be raised by other parties · or even by other members of the tribunal.

In arguing a case it is helpful to have all the material at your fingertips. If you want to refer to a regulation, a decision or a piece of evidence you can then find it without searching through a book or a mound of papers.

In cases where only points of law are being argued, the facts are contained in an agreed bundle of documents and there is no need to produce witnesses.

Before presenting your case, make a list of the points you want to get across. Once you are sure the Tribunal has understood a good point, do not go on repeating it and don't bury it with a lot of wrong arguments. If you forget to make a point at the right time wait for a convenient moment and ask permission to make it. The Tribunal has power to vary its own procedure and it is unlikely to object.

Representatives:

If you are representing a claimant, don't do all the talking if the claimant is capable of making his or her own points, particularly where facts are disputed and the claimant can give evidence on them. If the claimant fails to mention an important fact you should bring it up, not by stating it yourself but by asking the claimant a question so that he or she can state it. Your function as a representative is to help the claimant present the case as well as possible.

Adjournments:

Any of the parties can ask for an adjournment for any reason. You would have good grounds if a witness is ill on the day or a particular piece of evidence has not yet been received. Inform the Tribunal as soon as possible so that the hearing can be fixed for a later date without everybody having to attend. If you ask for an adjournment at the hearing when you could have done it earlier you will antagonise the Tribunal and the adjournment may be refused.

The Tribunal's decision is not usually announced at the hearing. It must be recorded in writing and must include a statement of the grounds for the decision. A copy must be sent to the claimant, the insurance officer and the interested parties.

Note the points on the procedure in the Digest under

the heading 'Local Tribunals'. The procedure is very similar in non-industrial cases. Both are governed by the same laws – National Insurance Act 1965 S69 and Determination of Claims and Questions Regulations.

Note also that the local Tribunal and the Commissioner have power to receive medical evidence without a claimant's knowledge if it is thought that disclosure to the claimant would be harmful to health.

National Insurance Commissioner:

You can appeal to the Commissioner against the decision of a local tribunal, so can the insurance officer, or your trade union (National Insurance Act 1965 S70(1)). The notice of appeal must be given in writing to the local DHSS office on an approved form. It must state the grounds for appeal. Forms are available from the local office.

The Commissioner or a Deputy Commissioner normally sits alone. If there is a particularly difficult question of fact he may have an assessor, usually medically qualified, to sit with him or he may refer any question to a doctor for examination and report. In either case it is still the Commissioner who decides the question on the basis of advice or report.

Cases of particular legal difficulty and importance are sometimes dealt with by a Tribunal of Commissioners. From the claimant's point of view it makes little difference if the hearing is before a single Commissioner or a Tribunal.

Procedure:

The procedure before the Commissioner is generally similar to that of Local Tribunals but slightly more formal. Like the Local Tribunal he can hear all the evidence (including any new evidence) afresh. In a case where the facts have been contested between the parties from the beginning, and where new evidence is introduced on appeal, the Commissioner will want to know why the evidence was not raised either in the original application to the insurance officer or before the local tribunal. Whoever brings in the new evidence – whether claimant or insurance officer – will need to have an answer to this question. Otherwise the Commissioner might conclude that the evidence has been fabricated to defeat the reason given for earlier decisions.

Often the Commissioner will have to decide only a point of law – in some cases this is the only ground of appeal to him (see below). If the point is a comparatively simple one he has power to dispense with a hearing altogether and make his decision on the basis of written representations by the parties.

Points of law:

It is impossible rationally to explain the difference between a point of fact and a point of law but an understanding of some of the concepts involved is vital, particularly in cases where an appeal can only be made on a point of law. Some examples may help.

A question of fact arises when there is more than one story about an event. One witness may say that on a particular day the weather was fine, while another may say it was raining. The insurance officer, tribunal or commissioner will have to decide which story is correct. That would be a decision on a *question of fact*.

However, in deciding this question of fact these authorities are obliged to act 'reasonably'. Whether or not the decision is 'reasonable' is a *point of law*. It would be unreasonable to make a finding of fact which, if other facts found in the decision are true, cannot be true.

A decision which is based on such a finding is wrong in law and should be appealed against.

Similarly it would be a mistake of law to come to a conclusion of fact without supporting evidence. Thus if there is evidence to suggest that it was raining and none to the contrary, the insurance officer, tribunal or Commissioner would need a very good reason for rejecting this. A finding of fact that it was not raining, for which no good reason is given, would be wrong in law.

Again, where there is conflicting evidence, a reason must be given for rejecting one version and not the other. Failure to give reasons is an error of law.

The distinction between a mistake of fact and an

error of law is important in two types of appeal:

1. From a Medical Appeal Tribunal to the Commissioner.

2. From a decision of the Commissioner to the Courts.

In both cases an appeal can only be made on a point of law.

The distinction between a point of fact and a point of law is explained in Decision R(A) 1/72.

Medical Board:

Medical Boards consist of two (or sometimes more) doctors. One acts as chairman. The members are appointed by the Secretary of State.

Their main function is to determine the 'special questions' of disablement, diagnosis and recrudescence, described earlier.

Disablement questions must be referred by the insurance officer to the Medical Board. Exceptions are set out in Section 41 of the Injuries Act and DOC and Q Regulations. Diagnosis and recrudescence questions are not always referred to Medical Boards – see Part V of the Prescribed Diseases Regulations.

The decision of the Medical Board on a question properly referred to it is binding on the non-medical authorities. A board's capacity is not merely advisory.

You must be given reasonable notice of the time and place of the hearing. You have no right to be represented (DOC and Q Regulation 7), but the Board may permit a representative to be present if they think he is likely to be of assistance.

In most cases the hearing will be in two stages:

1. The Board obtains the facts on which to make their decision. A representative is usually allowed to be present – this presence can be very valuable because it is important at this stage to ensure that the Board has a correct picture of the facts behind the claim. It is often difficult to show that a Board has based its decision on false information when a mistake may be concealed beneath medical jargon.

2. The clinical examination. Representatives are only very rarely allowed to be present.

Once a claim reaches the stage of a Medical Board

hearing a determination will already have been made that you have suffered personal injury by accident. Sometimes difficulties can arise with the Medical Board, particularly where the accident and injury are one and the same event. Medical Boards have occasionally taken the view that the injury/accident was not related to the work. (Note decisions in the Digest under 'Personal Injury by Accident'.)

The *Handbook for Industrial Injuries Medical Boards* published by HMSO gives clear instructions on most of the difficult points which may emerge in the course of a Medical Board hearing. Boards will regard it as authoritative and you can save time by quoting from it instead of original regulations and decisions.

Medical Boards are required to give written notice of their findings and reasons.

Medical Appeal Tribunal :

If you want to appeal against the decision of the Medical Board notice of appeal must be given within three months of receiving notice of the Board's decision. Your notice of appeal should be made in writing to the Local Office and you must give reasons. The appeal will be heard by the Medical Appeal Tribunal, usually in public.

You are entitled to representation. The Minister also has a right to be heard. Notice of the time and place of hearing must be given. Witnesses may be called and examined in the usual way.

Before launching an appeal, bear in mind that the Medical Appeal Tribunal may reconsider *all* aspects of the Board's decision, not merely those you may complain of in the grounds of appeal. For this reason, if the Board's decision is, in some respects, unusually favourable (eg, the finding of a rather tenuous connection between an accident and a disability) though in others unfavourable (eg, a rather low assessment of the disability) it may not be to your advantage to appeal.

Grounds for appeal:

There are all kinds of grounds on which a Medical Board decision can be criticised, though it may be more difficult than criticising a decision by an insurance officer if the medical aspects of the decision are too technical. Even this difficulty can often be overcome by a little research in the public library.

The first thing to check is whether the Board has come to a wrong *finding of fact*. This could be reversed on appeal. (In contrast, where a decision has been made *in ignorance of a material fact,* a *review* may be more appropriate than an appeal.

The most common grounds for an appeal to the MAT are that the Board failed to apply correctly the principles which govern its decision, including those requiring it to give reasons. These principles can be studied in the Digest under 'Medical Appeal Tribunals'.

Note: the so-called 'Paired organs' principle of assessment was abolished in 1970. The principles of assessment substituted for it – contained in parts of Benefit Regulation 2 – are equally difficult to understand.

Evidence:

Appeals to Medical Appeal Tribunals are comparatively technical and most claimants prefer to put their observations in writing, at their leisure, before the hearing. The procedure for delivering written representations in advance is the same as for Local Appeal Tribunals.

The appeal is likely to be some time after the Medical Board hearing so it is worth providing:
up-to-date medical information,
a full statement of all relevant facts not mentioned in the existing papers,
full information on all disabilities, not simply those which affect you most.

Note: once an appeal is made it can only be withdrawn with permission and not as of right.

You can appeal to the Commissioner against the decision of a Medical Appeal Tribunal on a point of law. The Commissioner does not have the power to reverse the decision himself but he will make a declaration of the principles of law which govern the decisions of the Medical Appeal Tribunal. Your case is then sent back to a Medical

Appeal Tribunal (it may be the same one) to be decided on the basis of the law as declared by the Commissioner.

Such an appeal is only worth making if you think the Tribunal would have reached a more favourable decision if it had applied the correct principles of law. For instance, a Medical Appeal Tribunal which fails to give reasons for an adverse decision, will be found to have erred in law. The case will go back to the Tribunal, which may easily come to the same decision, this time giving reasons. If the reasons are good in law the whole exercise will have got you nothing but a load of bother.

There are a number of decisions on this kind of appeal which should be studied carefully before appealing. Little general advice can be given except to be fully aware of the difference between questions of fact and questions of law.

(Section 42 of the Injuries Act covers appeals to the Commissioner against MAT decisions.)

Review:

The Injuries Act contains extensive powers for the review of decisions made by determining authorities (insurance officer, local appeal tribunal and Commissioner) and medical authorities. (See Section 49 of the Injuries Act.)

The insurance officer may also refer a decision to a Local Appeal Tribunal for review. Any decision may be reviewed if the insurance officer is satisfied that:

a. the decision was given in ignorance of, or was based on a mistake on a material fact (in the case of a decision by the Commissioner the insurance officer must be satisfied by fresh evidence); or

b. there has been a relevant change of circumstances since the decision; or

c. the decision was based on the decision of a 'special question' which has been revised.

Certain decisions cannot be reviewed in this way. They include a decision on a point of law by the Commissioner on an appeal from a Medical Appeal Tribunal; and a decision *not obtained by fraud* that an accident was or was not an industrial accident.

You can appeal against a decision made on review in the same way as against the original decision.

It does not follow that an insurance officer who reviews an earlier decision will automatically reverse it.

Notes:

1. Where the decision for review is a Commissioner's decision, fresh evidence is needed. This means evidence which you could not reasonably have been expected to produce before the first hearing. Whether or not it was reasonable to expect you to produce evidence would depend on a number of matters including the time and resources available to produce it. In a case where an important witness (eg, someone who saw the accident) disappears, it may be advisable to note this – and the efforts that have been made to trace him – in the original claim. If the witness turns up later, it cannot be argued that his evidence is not 'fresh evidence'.

2. Where you want to show that a mistake was made, you must show that the decision was 'based' on it. Where you want to show ignorance, there is no such requirement.

3. To be 'material' a fact must be relevant to the original decision and significant enough that it might have changed the decision if it had been known at the time.

4. If an IO decides that the conditions permitting a review do not exist you can appeal to the Local Tribunal and thence to the Commissioner in the normal way. If this appeal is allowed, the Tribunal or Commissioner will go on to review the original decisions.

5. A review may take into account not only the new corrected facts (which enable the review to take place) but also other evidence, facts and arguments which were not presented originally, and which would not themselves provide grounds for review.

It is important to remember – and exploit – the review procedure, particularly if you advise claimants. Many seek advice only after several appeals have been made without success. Often this is because they have failed to produce vital evidence, which, had they produced it in the beginning, would have ensured a successful claim.

By producing this information you can get a review,

and a favourable decision, however many times the claim has been through the machinery in the past.

The courts:

You can appeal against a Commissioner's decision to the Divisional Court of the High Court *on a point of law only*.

The procedure is technical and most claimants are well advised at this stage to obtain the services of a competent lawyer. Claimants with low incomes can obtain advice on the subject under a scheme known as 'New Legal Aid'. Before choosing a solicitor make sure he is one who knows about Industrial Injuries Benefits law. Solicitors are not taught this subject in their training and few meet it in practice.

If you are thinking of conducting an appeal to the court yourself you probably do not need the assistance of a guide such as this.

Be warned that the High Court contains more – and more subtle – traps for the inexperienced than any national insurance office.

Late claims and appeals:

Claims. The Claims and Payments Regulations prescribe the time limits within which you should claim benefit. The usual effect of making a late claim is that you lose the amount of benefit that would have been paid during the delay. In the case of disablement benefit the prescribed time limit is three months from the date on which the conditions for receipt of benefit are satisfied. You cannot normally obtain benefit for a period more than three months before the date of a late claim.

But if you can show a reasonable cause for your delay you will not lose benefit. Decisions on what constitutes a 'reasonable' cause are numerous. All circumstances are taken into account. In some cases where the claim is very late the amount of benefit to be obtained by showing a good cause for the delay is substantial. It is well worth going into this matter very thoroughly.

Appeals. The time limits for different appeals vary

with the type of appeal. (You can find them in the regulations governing each type.) Be careful to make sure that you are within the time limit.

In a claim for disablement benefit the decision of the Medical Board will be implemented by the insurance officer almost immediately and you should receive benefit together with whatever allowance you are entitled to. If you dispute the *assessment* of the Medical Board the time limit for appeal to the Medical Appeal Tribunal is three months. If you dispute a decision on your *entitlement* to a particular allowance the time limit is 21 days and the appeal is to the Local Appeal Tribunal.

Usually when an appeal is late and there is a good reason, the authority to whom it is made has jurisdiction to allow it to be made out of time. A clear statement of all the reasons for delay should be sent with the appeal forms. When applying for leave to appeal out of time it helps if you can put the reasons for the appeal itself in full. If you have a good case, the authority will then know that if it refuses leave it will, in effect, be confirming a decision which is patently wrong.

Even if leave for a late appeal is refused you may still have grounds for a *review.*

Warning:
Fraud and Repayment of Benefit:

You should note that you can get into trouble with the criminal courts for making fraudulent claims.

There are provisions in the law for recovering money from you when you have been overpaid. Generally this power will not be used if you have acted in good faith.

13.

Organising

Organisation is the key to success in fighting for health and safety. The union movement cuts right across all the divisions of industry and law. It can reach down into the smallest slum workshops where no safety inspectors ever set foot. It is the only kind of organisation that can be committed solely to the interests of workers.

It has 10 million members, enormous power and the right to use it (a right which, in the case of health and safety, was not infringed by Phases 1 and 2 of the Tory 'freeze'). In the process of achieving this situation millions have died from injury, disease, malnutrition and the hangman's noose. Thousands more will die and millions will be maimed because this power is not being used in defence of its members' health and safety.

If the record of the employers is shameful, you can at least understand that they have a vested interest in getting safety on the cheap. How is the record of the trade union movement to be explained? There are plenty of excuses – there is work enough in fighting for good wages (and defending the right to fight for them), in protecting jobs and in handling all the mass of work generated by governments and employers who increasingly lay down *their* terms first. In a defensive situation, you don't open up another front.

It is said that there is no demand from the shop floor for action on hazards. It is true that workers in many industries have come to accept danger as part of the job, and have become dependent on special payments for danger, dust, dirt and, more recently, noise. Generations of workers have been conned into taking a pride in their ability to 'take' heat, cold, dust and overwork when it would be a lot 'tougher' to turn round and tell the employer to stuff his lousy conditions.

These excuses for lack of leadership have always been thin and they won't work much longer. There is a growing tide of awareness and concern about hazards among workers in all industries and occupations.

The time has come for an organised trade union offensive against hazards, to challenge the employers' right to set the levels of risk and to demand standards of health, safety and well-being acceptable to workers.

The needs are:

1. Leadership.

Action at shop floor level will develop naturally out of the present growing awareness, but it will be a lot easier to challenge employers if union leaders and the TUC make a declaration of war on hazards at national level. Each worker needs to get the message that 'You don't have to put up with it; it can be made safe and we will back you to the hilt'.

2. Information.

Workers in every trade need accurate information on the hazards of their work and the minimum standards of protection they should accept. The TUC should be producing information and developing standards which will give better protection than those adopted by the Government/industry partnership.

Each union should have a safety department distributing this information – plus its own material on any special risks faced by its members.

3. Training.

Workers need *union* training if they are to cut through management safety jargon and get at the real facts.

There is no point in pretending that the movement measures up to these needs. The higher you look in the trade union bureaucracy the less evidence you find for any serious **trade union** approach to safety, any willingness to recognise conflict or any leadership in the struggle for health.

The TUC :

The TUC, in its role as a 'responsible' establishment institution, seeks solutions through other institutions, such as Parliament and the CBI, rather than through the strength of its members.

Although experience should have shown that the law is at best a weak defender of workers' rights, including the right to safety, and at worst a threat to those rights, the TUC continues to make reform of the law one of the main planks of its policy. A strong comprehensive body of safety law would be valuable and it will always be a valid union objective. Unfortunately there is no reason to think that better law would be enforced any more than the strong parts of existing regulations are enforced. This cannot be the *main* plank of any realistic policy.

Other planks are equally worm-eaten. One of them is a joint statement on consultation on safety drawn up with the Confederation of British Industry. According to this authoritative document,

> o A clear written statement of a company's safety policy is the essential foundation stone for any effective safety organisation. The statement, we (the TUC and CBI) believe should include or be supported by a definition of the responsibilities of, and the functional relationship between, line management, a safety officer and other specialist advisers, employees and members of safety committees.

Notice that the initiative remains firmly with management: 'employees' are given no hand in laying this paper 'foundation stone'.

The joint TUC/CBI statement then refers to the importance of 'good communications' and the development of 'a genuine desire on the part of employees to improve the safety performance and health conditions, in their own *and the company's* interests.' (Our italics.)

This particular plank is not only worm-eaten but riddled with the particularly dangerous form of rot found between the covers of the Robens Report – that there is 'a greater natural identity of interest between the two sides of industry in relation to safety and health problems than in most other matters'.

Apart from its activities in the corridors of Parliament (where the unions have about 100 sponsored MPs) and the CBI, mentioned earlier, the TUC provides various services for its member unions:

The Medical Adviser:

Dr Robert Murray is the only doctor employed by the union movement. The TUC appears reluctant to employ a second doctor in spite of the fact that health problems faced by workers are getting more complicated and more enquiries are coming through all the time.

The TUC cannot expect one doctor to service the bulk of trade union enquiries *and* represent it at an ever-increasing number of conferences and meetings.

The TUC Centenary Institute of Occupational Health:

This body also handles inquiries from trade unions. Its information and advisory services work closely with the TUC medical adviser but the Institute is not part of the trade union movement. ○ One of its research publications in 1971 was entitled 'Skinfold Measurements of Obesity in British Businessmen'. The TUC contributed £125,000 in 1968 towards the cost of new premises for the existing occupational health department in London University. The name was changed to commemorate the gift and the centenary of the TUC, but the Institute remains part of the university system. Each year Congress contributes a further £25,000 towards the Institute's running costs. In return, unions have free, but not exclusive, access to the information service.

So far this huge investment by the trade union movement has brought small returns because the Institute's information role is passive: it waits for enquiries to come in rather than generating information for workers so that they can develop knowledge and skills of their own.

Some of the long-term research work on occupational health is undoubtedly valuable but so long as the results are buried in learned journals, the information may not reach even managements, let alone workers.

A series of leaflets setting out the hazards of different

materials would be more use to workers than a learned paper giving the exact percentage of say lung cancer among asbestos workers. **Many workers do not even know that asbestos causes asbestosis, let alone at least two types of cancer.**

This is not an attack on research into occupational health or on the TUC's sponsorship of it – providing the TUC does not think that the Institute can do its job for it.

TUC Training College:

Training in safety and health is only a small part of the college's work. You can take two courses: a one week course for stewards at the college in London and a postal course. The second is singularly lacking in trade union spirit. One of the questions asks you for suggestions on improving the accident prevention situation, and the model answer says you can 'draw attention to' dangerous conditions, make proposals to management for safer methods and help to discourage a careless attitude among workmates. Nothing about discouraging a careless attitude among employers.

The stewards' course in London gives you a lot of useful information but again lacks any coherent strategy for developing a safety campaign on the shop floor. Effective or not, its training is only scratching the surface of the problem: only about 200 stewards pass through each year. The T&GWU alone has 40,000 stewards.

Individual unions :

Most unions put the emphasis of their health and safety work on winning compensation for injuries rather than preventing them. In many cases, the legal department tackles safety enquiries as a sideline when not processing claims.

No-one is suggesting that the compensation effort can be cut back but the priority given to it has the unhealthy reek of the 19th century 'Coffin Club' unions.

Compensation 'winnings' are used as an index of how well the union is doing for its members. 'If you lads join the T&GWU', runs the recruitment patter to the long distance lorry drivers, 'you can get free legal assistance if you have an accident – surely that's worth 25p of anyone's wage?'

Given the risks that workers face in their jobs, it *is* quite a bargain. A free leaflet on toxic, corrosive and inflammable loads would also win members and might actually save life – not to mention future work for the legal department.

Unions which publicize hazards are accused by the employer of 'stirring' or agitation. Claims for compensation involve no such confrontation because the employer is insulated by his insurance company and lawyers. The insurance premium covers any damage that may be paid out as a result of his negligence.

Out of 130 trade unions only three have full-time safety officers, AUEW Engineering Section, EE/PTU and NUM. Only a handful are producing safety information for their members. None is producing enough to reach more than a few people on the shop floor. Some have some kind of training programme for stewards but their output is tiny. The AUEW Foundry Section has begun to develop a more specialist approach to training with the aid of the TUC Training College.

Shop-floor organisation :

All this is very depressing if you fall into the old trap of waiting for the word from London. But the offensive against hazards can only be fought and won on the shop floor. The flabbiness of the union leadership and the TUC in this field just means that the movement must put pressure not only on the employers but also on its own organisations.

Strong organisation at shop floor level is vital but present forms of organisation are just not designed for this kind of struggle. Traditional emphasis on wage bargaining, combined with the myth of 'identity of interest' on controlling hazards, produce a curious acceptance of **joint safety committees** as the answer to safety problems.

It may be that the resistance of employers at national and local level to joint committees has made them seem more desirable than they are.

Their weakness is that for all the appearance of balance between the two sides on the committee there is a manager in the chair: unless a less profit-orientated manager, like the safety officer, sides with the workers, the committee cannot reach decisions which are out of tune with management policy. If it does, management can still decide to ignore the committee.

This is not to say that safety committees are useless. Workers in a chemical plant found that when they insisted on appointing their own representatives to the committee, in place of yes-men who had been hand-picked by management, they were able to force improvements. Dangerously corroded chemical pipes were replaced and emergency showers installed throughout the plant.

o Post Office engineering workers have achieved advanced joint consultation procedures for approval of all new equipment before it is introduced.

Safety committees can be made to work better by demanding that they become more democratic, that workers have their turn in the chair, that decisions are binding on management and so on. If you don't have a joint safety committee it is a good idea to press for one, with such demands built in from the start.

But remember, the joint safety committee can only exist as a management institution. If you were to demand a truly democratic committee, on which workers' representatives would outnumber management's, 'identity of interest' would swiftly disappear.

In a situation of conflict, a management institution can never be a substitute for your own organisation. This can take many forms but the key figure is the safety steward or 'safety representative' elected by the shop floor.

In smaller places it may be that one steward will be responsible for both normal wage negotiations and grievance handling as well as safety. Where possible though it is better to separate the functions: identifying and trying to eradicate hazards is a full time job in itself. Also the two responsibilities tend to get in each other's way: when new processes are being introduced it is important to be able to bring as much skill to bear on safety and health implications as on wage questions. A safety steward can ensure that safety is not pushed into the background.

In larger workplaces there will have to be more safety stewards and experience will show how many are needed. It is impossible to lay down a blueprint for shopfloor safety organisation. You have to develop it to suit the situation but the important thing is to achieve close and frequent contact between safety representatives and all parts of the shop floor so that conditions can be constantly monitored and action quickly taken.

This may be easier to achieve if workers elect their own safety committee made up of safety stewards plus representatives who know the hazards of different operations. This would be really useful in the early stages of a safety campaign when you are building up a picture of all the hazards in the place and deciding on priorities for action (see Section 8).

Other suggestions:

Safety stewards should be members of the shop stewards' committee.

The safety steward, or senior safety steward in large establishments, should be in on any negotiations where safety could be involved – for example talks about productivity deals, manning or work measurement.

As safety, health and welfare problems come up they should be subject to normal procedure just like any other issue. Joint safety committees, some of which meet only once every three months, provide management with wonderful opportunities to delay these issues.

Effective shop floor safety organisation will put a heavy strain on the old 'identity of interest' line. If they are to function properly, safety stewards need clearly defined rights to:

○ **Move freely throughout the workplace at all times.**

○ **Carry out safety inspections, particularly after an accident. (Nothing should be disturbed, except for rescue and making safe, until the inspection has been made.)**

○ **Have free access to accident, first aid and sickness records.**

○ **Work from a special room where equipment – for**

example a camera or sound level meter – can be kept.

o Hold safety meetings during working hours.

o Call in outside advisers, eg, union safety officers, lawyers or people with equipment for measuring noise or contamination.

o Supervise and assist in training of young workers and new entrants.

o Take time off for training in safety and health, including courses run by unions or the TUC. (For other sources of training, see p328.)

Demands:

In the present state of most shop floor organisation management is effectively setting its own standards for health and safety. An aggressive shop floor safety organisation can investigate these standards and put forward its own demands based on conditions of health and safety acceptable to workers.

These demands will develop naturally out of the process of investigating hazards. There can be no hard and fast rules: sometimes simple compliance with the law would be a major breakthrough – for example the provision of proper eating, changing, washing and toilet facilities on pipeline construction sites.

In other cases, where the law is inadequate or non-existent, you can use the generally higher requirements of the International Labour Office's Model Code of *Safety Regulations for Industrial Establishments* (see publications list).

The important thing is to raise standards to levels you find acceptable and get them written into all contracts and agreements. Typical demands might include: better first aid and medical services, improved ventilation, reduction of noise to 85dBA or less, full sickness pay, better lighting.

The American Oil Chemical and Atomic Workers International Union (OCAW) made occupational health and safety a major point in the contracts they negotiated with oil companies in 1973. Their demands include the following:

1. Periodic surveys of refineries by industrial health consultants to uncover dangerous materials and conditions. Results of these surveys to be made known to workers.

2. Company-paid physical examinations and medical tests for all refinery workers.

3. Access to all company records of disease and death among workers.

4. Compensation for the time workers spend on plant inspections and health committee meetings.

All the major oil companies accepted these terms except Shell Oil Company. Five thousand OCAW members in Shell refineries all over the country went on strike in the last week of January 1973 and stayed out until the first week of June when most of their demands were met. The first national health and safety stoppage in America, this action also brought the first big tie up between unions and environmental groups – see page 119.

Summary:

1. Your need for health and safety is in direct conflict with the employers' drive for maximum profits.

2. Employers will expose you to danger if it makes production cheaper – and if they can get away with it.

3. They **can** get away with it because the law is soft and not intended to present any fundamental challenge to profits.

4. They can get away with it because the unions are soft and prepared to make criminal behaviour a subject for negotiation rather than the signal for a militant counteroffensive.

5. If you know the hazards of your job you can protect yourself to some extent by refusing to accept risks. But the scope for individual action is limited by the threat of victimisation and by the scale of the problems to be tackled. If you work in a steel mill there's not much you can do on your own to force management into spending tens of thousands on, say reducing noise to safe levels.

6. When you are organised to fight collectively for safety by answering any threat to health with a threat to profits you can begin to exert real control over hazards. But again there are limitations: suppose management says the

mill is already uneconomic and they'd close it rather than spend the money? With really strong combine organisation you might win that one too.

7. Some health problems go too deep for any shop-floor safety organisation, however strong. (What could you do about a new multi-million pound car plant where fast, automated lines are taking a heavy toll in stress and mental illness and the only solution for health would be a complete reconstruction to allow for more humane production methods?)

What can you do about the other hazards of a society which puts the profits of the few before the health of the majority – the hazards of unemployment, poverty, slums, overcrowded schools, polluted air, inadequate medical care?

Trade union organisations can bring improvements in some of these areas, some of the time, but the economic roots will live on, to plague another generation.

There can be no lasting solution until workers control society and can direct their skill and labour into meeting the needs of all people. In freeing them from the struggle for survival, they will free them for the boundless possibilities of human existence.

Organisations and publications:

Organisations or groups of organisations are given in alphabetical order.

British Society for Social Responsibility in Science (BSSRS):
70 Great Russell Street, London WC1. 01 – 242 8535
Wants to make its scientific knowledge and skills available to ordinary people. Has helped local groups fight problems like air pollution and wants to form links with workers. Is preparing leaflets on health hazards like lead.

Claimants Unions:
Local branches in most centres. Address in telephone book or in list of organisations at local library. Will help with claims for social security, injury benefits, etc. Useful leaflets for claimants, eg on social security for strikers.

Construction Industry Research and Information Association, 6 Storey's Gate, London SW1.
Publishes codes of practice listed on pages 92 and 93.

Consultants:

When management cannot give satisfactory answers to questions about the level of risk from hazards like noise or chemicals it may be necessary to force them to call in experts. **Industrial hygiene:** The Factory Inspectorate (see below) has its own industrial hygiene unit and a mobile laboratory for on-site investigation. Will investigate if District Inspector or management thinks there is a health risk. The TUC Centenary Institute (see below) offers an independent occupational hygiene service for industry. Other occupational hygiene laboratories are attached to universities at Newcastle, Manchester, Aston, and Dundee. **Noise and vibration:** The Institute of Sound and Vibration Research at Southampton University is among the best working in these fields. **Radiation:** The Radiological Protection Service at Harwell, Didcot, Berks. **Ergonomics:** Cranfield Institute of Technology; and departments at various universities.

International Labour Office:

40 Piccadilly, London W1. 01 – 734 6521.
International organisation with HQ in Geneva. Representatives from Governments, employers' and workers' organisations draw up standards for the protection of workers. Useful source of publications, many of them free. List of publications available from London office.

Industrial Health and Safety Centre:

97 Horseferry Road, Westminster, London SW1, 01 – 828 9255.
Permanent exhibition of safety equipment, much of it never seen in the average workplace. Open during hours when most people are at work. Book in advance if you want guided tour by a Factory Inspector.

Inspectorates and Employment Medical Advisers:

Inspectorates can be a source of information as well as agents of enforcement when safety laws are broken. Inspectors will only advise or enforce if your type of work comes within the scope of the law they enforce. Your local Employment Medical Adviser has a duty to advise you on any problem affecting your health at work – *whatever your occupation*. Addresses of local inspector and medical adviser should be given on the official abstract of the safety law (if any) covering your occupation. The abstract should be at the main entrance to your workplace. Otherwise look up in the telephone book. For agricultural inspectors look under 'Agriculture, Fisheries and Food, Ministry of'. Local authority inspectors, who enforce the Offices, Shops and Railway Premises Act, can be located by ringing main local authority number. See 'Local Government Authorities' heading in Yellow Pages. If Employment Medical Advisory Service is not in phone book, enquire at local office of Department of Employment. Labour Exchange should know.

Noise Abatement Society:
6 Old Bond Street, London W1. 01 – 493 5877.
Takes an aggressive attitude about noise at work; suggests stewards should have noise meters (it sells 'noise torches' for about £10).

Poisons Information Service:
24-hour service for doctors and nurses needing information on treatments for poisoning. Not supposed to be a service for the public but if you know what substance has caused poisoning and know that it will be some time before victim can get expert medical attention, the service will advise you on first aid treatment. Use only in an emergency **after** sending for doctor or ambulance. The main unit is at Guy's Hospital, London (Tel. 01 – 407 7600); hospitals at Edinburgh, Cardiff, Belfast and Dublin will give the same service.

Publicity:

Can be a powerful pressure on stubborn managements when conditions are bad. Publicity about Rio Tinto Zinc's leaky lead smelter at Avonmouth helped expose scandalous conditions throughout the lead industry. The Factory Inspectorate had to take on more staff to deal with extra investigations needed to satisfy demands from workers. External pollution is still more fashionable than internal. Because the two are often linked it may be best to emphasise this aspect first and hope that you can interest them in shopfloor hazards later. Remember the media like their problems packaged in terms of actions and events; ideally there should be something they can take a picture of, even if quite irrelevant. Newsmen like to think they are onto something nobody else knows about.

If the problem is a strictly local one, especially if it involves the main employer in a small town, a report in the local paper can be effective. If it involves a national company or current 'cause for concern' try one of the heavier national papers; probably *Guardian* or *Sunday Times*. Among the nationally networked TV programmes, *World in Action* (Granada, Manchester) and *This Week* (Thames, London) have both investigated work hazards. They are unlikely to be interested unless your particular situation has significant implications for all workers or is part of an emerging pattern.

Safety Organisations:

Royal Society for the Prevention of Accidents (RoSPA)
Head office: Royal Oak Centre, Brighton Road, Purley, Surrey, CR2 2UR. 01 – 668 4272.
Industrial Safety – Training Dept: Fanhams Hall, Ware, Herts. Ware 5929. Information Division: 6 Buckingham Place, London SW1. 01– 828 7444. Genteel safety organ-isation. Not the place for workers to get help in an emer-gency but useful source of information on hazards (keeps

one of few sets of CIS cards – abstracts of latest international research on occupational health). Runs various training schemes, eg for power press operators at its Birmingham training centre.

British Safety Council.
62 Chancellors Road, London W6. 01 – 741 1231.
'Aggressive' safety organisation. Uses American methods to 'sell' safety to managements. Has been known to help workers, unofficially, though this is not likely to happen if employer subscribes to the BSC service.

Sampling instruments:

If you are forced to make your own investigation of air-borne contaminants, as outlined in Section 6, these two firms supply hand-pump air samplers and detector tubes:
Draeger Normalair Ltd, Blyth, Northumberland NE24 4RH. Blyth 2891.
D.A.Pitman Ltd, Mill Works, Jessamy Road, Weybridge, Surrey. Weybridge 44405.

Socialist Medical Association.
14-16 Bristol Street, Birmingham. 021 – 622 2020.
Association of socialist doctors campaigning for a health service that will meet the needs of all people. An occupational health service is one of its main objectives. Has a trade union liaison committee and publishes some good pamphlets on health at work.

Training:

TUC Training College at Congress House (see below) runs postal and residential courses in health and safety on a totally inadequate scale.

TUC Regional Education Officers will organise day-release courses in safety for shop stewards. You can use the service direct – without going through your own union bureaucracy. Officers are based at Newcastle, Nottingham, Sheffield, Liverpool, Pontypridd, Birmingham, Bristol, Belfast, Glasgow and London. Listed in telephone book under 'TUC Regional Education Service'.

Individual unions run weekend schools.

Industrial Training Boards have been set up for major industries or groups of industries to train workers in the skills of their trades; safety is usually an integral part of the teaching.

Safety organisations (see above) run various courses, mainly emphasising accident prevention.

Red Cross and St John Ambulance (addresses in phone book) give training in first aid.

University of Aston at Birmingham is developing courses for stewards in accident prevention, noise and other subjects.

Trade Union Services :

TUC Medical Adviser: Congress House, Great Russell Street, London WC1B 3LS. 01 – 636 4030.

Handles enquiries on health and safety problems from unions; passes some on to the TUC Centenary Institute.

TUC Centenary Institute of Occupational Health: Keppel Street, Gower Street, London WC1. 01 – 580 2386.

Handles inquiries passed on by the Medical Adviser and also those coming direct from unions, workers, management, doctors and general public. Only unions and their members get the service free, thanks to a hefty annual grant from the TUC. See also entry under 'Consultants', above.

Individual unions: Only a handful have safety officers and can give quick answers to straightforward questions. Others pass almost all problems straight to one of the above. Whatever the arrangement, the more you demand of it, the more useful it will become. All unions should have health and safety departments.

All have some kind of legal service and injury benefit scheme.

Publications:
Introduction:

No single book can cover the full range of occupational health and safety subjects and it is important to collect as much additional information as you can, particularly where your job involves special risks. Fortunately you can build up a useful library on hazards at little cost. Many publications can be obtained free from union and government sources. It is a good idea to get lists of publications from organisations working in this field.

One of the best sources of technical information on a wide range of hazards is the collection of **Technical Data Notes** published by the Factory Inspectorate. They are written for management but stewards should be able to obtain a complete set, free, from the District Inspector of Factories. There is no rule that workers can't have them.

Many cheap booklets on hazards and their control are available from Her Majesty's Stationery Office. These are listed in:

Department of Employment Sectional List No.21, obtainable free from HMSO.

Other useful sectional lists are:
Department of Health and Social Security No.11, and
Department of Employment No.18.

HMSO publications can be ordered by post from the following offices:

PO Box No.569, **London** SE1
Brazenose Street, **Manchester** M60 8AS
109 St.Mary Street, **Cardiff** CF1 1JW
13a Castle Street, **Edinburgh** EH2 3AR
258-259 Broad Street, **Birmingham** 1
50 Fairfax Street, **Bristol** BS1 3DE
7-11 Linehall Street, **Belfast** BT2 8AY

They like you to order from the nearest one.

Libraries:

Public libraries will stock more books on occupational health if enough people ask for them. Smaller libraries can tell you which is the nearest library with a reference section specialising in any subject you want to read up. Or they can borrow obscure titles for you.

Books and booklets:

Encyclopaedia of Occupational Health and Safety, International Labour Office. Should be in reference section of all but the smallest public libraries and on all union bookshelves.

Dangerous Properties of Industrial Materials by N.I.Sax, Reinhold, New York.
The standard work on toxic chemicals, this massive and

expensive book should be in the reference section of larger libraries. Union safety departments should have one and it would be a valuable investment for safety stewards handling a lot of problems to do with chemicals.

Industrial Hygiene and Toxicology by F.A.Patty, editor, Volume II, Interscience Publishers, New York. Useful addition to the above.

Health in Industry by Donald Hunter, Penguin Books. Out of print but should be available through local library. Useful general introduction to occupational health and safety by one of the greatest experts on industrial disease, whose book **The Diseases of Occupations** (English Universities Press) is a standard work.

Work is Dangerous to Your Health by A.Jeanne M. Stellman and Susan M.Daum, Random House, New York. American book for workers. Sequel to the manual for oil and chemical workers which inspired this handbook.

The Toxic Metals by Anthony Tucker, Pan/Ballantine. Worthwhile background reading for a highly critical round-up of current abuses of toxic metals and the way they threaten to erode the health of millions.

Chemistry and Industry – annual Buyers Guide. By post from Publications Sales Officer, Chemical Society, Blackhorse Road, Letchworth, Herts SG6 1HN. Useful in tracking down branded chemicals.

Approved Products for Farmers and Growers, 1973, Ministry of Agriculture, Fisheries and Food. Available free from Publications Dept., Ministry of Agriculture, Tolcarne Drive, Pinner, Middlesex. Lists chemicals approved for agricultural use, their hazards and precautions for use.

Overtime and Shift Working – a guide for negotiators, TUC. Contains good material on the nuts and bolts of shift systems, plus a load of statistics.

Computer Aided Design – its nature and implications by M.J.E.Cooley, an AUEW (TASS) publication. Free. Automation and speed-up in the drawing-office and how it can threaten shop floor as well as white collar workers.

The Power Game by Colin Barker, Pluto Press. Describes the sell-out to productivity and work intensifica-

M

tion methods in the electricity supply industry and how workers can resist further attacks on working conditions.

Danger and Disease at Work, Socialist Medical Association pamphlet.

An Occupational Health Service Now, SMA pamphlet.

Bronchitis – the slaughter can be stopped, SMA pamphlet.

Accident Prevention, International Labour Office. A 'workers' education manual' with a flavour of RoSPA about it. Probably worth getting.

Factory Accidents – their causes and prevention, RoSPA.
Very good by RoSPA standards – clear and factual, without the 'careless worker' bit.

Common Causes of Factory Accidents, British Safety Council.
Apparently they are mostly the workers' fault but this contains some worthwhile additional material on the agents of injury.

Safety Code for the Use of Electricity in Industry, British Safety Council.
Good factual account of electrical hazards and prevention.

2,000 Accidents – A shop floor study of their causes, National Institute of Industrial Psychology. Most revealing (and readable) book shows that accidents are built into dangerous work systems. A breath of fresh air, well worth inhaling as an antidote to the 'careless worker' poison.

Accidents and Ill-health at Work, John L. Williams, Staples Press. A comprehensive review of official and other machinery for preserving workers' health, and the reasons for its failure.

The Factories Act 1961 – A Short Guide, HMSO

The Offices Shops and Railway Premises Act 1963 – A General Guide, HMSO

The Offices Shops and Railway Premises Act 1963. Abstract in Booklet Form for Issue to Employees, HMSO
The above are useful introductions to the law, though stewards will need to consult **Redgrave's Factories Acts** and

Redgrave's Offices and Shops, Butterworth, for more
detailed provisions.

**What to Do if you Have an Accident at Work or on
the Road** by Frank Clifford, Charles Mitchell Ltd, Cherry
Street, Woking, Surrey.
Cheap (15p) guide to legal first aid by an aggressive compensation lawyer.

Guide to the Mines and Quarries Act 1954

**Guide to Accident Site Observers (Mines and Quarries
Act 1954),** National Union of Mineworkers. Clear accounts
of the law and how it should be interpreted.

Health, Safety and Welfare in Foundries, AUEW
Foundry Workers Section
The law reprinted, unfortunately without trade union
interpretation.

Safety and Health at Work, Report of the Robens
Committee, HMSO
For background information, and guide to the shape of
legislation based on 'self-regulation by industry' that Robens
would like to see.

HM Chief Inspector of Factories Annual Report,
HMSO
Statistics, details of investigations of health risks, facts on
new hazards.

**HM Chief Inspector of Mines and Quarries Annual
Report,** HMSO. Statistics, etc.

**The Offices, Shops and Railway Premises Act 1963,
Annual Report by the Secretary of State for Employment,**
HMSO. Statistics, etc.

**Report on Safety, Health, Welfare and Wages in
Agriculture,** HMSO. Statistics, etc.

**Shipping Casualties and Deaths, Vessels Registered in
the United Kingdom, Annual Return by the Department of
Trade and Industry,** HMSO. Statistics.

**Department of Health and Social Security Annual
Report,** HMSO. The most comprehensive (though still
inadequate) source of statistics on occupational injury,
disease and death. Also has useful data on the Health
Service, staffing, etc.

Codes of practice:

Model Code of Safety Regulations for Industrial Establishments, International Labour Office. Comprehensive regulations, fully indexed and easy to understand, set higher standards than many UK safety statutes. Could be used as basis for better minimum standards of safety in drawing up plant safety agreements.

Department of Employment Code of Practice for reducing the exposure of employed persons to noise, HMSO. Not a code for true safety but a bargaining point in the absence of any statutory standard.

Department of Employment Code of Practice for the protection of persons exposed to Ionising Radiations in Research and Teaching, HMSO. Important to see that this code is enforced because these areas are mostly outside any safety legislation.

Code of Practice for protection of persons against Ionising Radiations arising from Medical and Dental Use, HMSO. See note above.

Guide on the protection of persons against hazards from laser radiation. BS4803:1972, British Standards Institution.

Directory of
Toxic Substances

Prepared by Dr Bob Hider and Mr Dick Ranson, of the Department of Chemistry at Essex University.

About this section:
Although the list is extensive it is far from comprehensive; it deals with the more commonly used toxic chemicals. Some, less common but equally toxic, may have been omitted. **Because a chemical is not mentioned, don't take it to be harmless.**

Many substances are dealt with more fully in other sections of the book, particularly Section 5, Disease. You will find references in the Index. The directory itself is not indexed.

Books listed earlier under 'Publications' should be consulted whenever possible, particularly **'Dangerous Properties of Industrial Materials'**.

One of the main uses for the directory will be in building up a list of substances used in your workplace. This is an essential part of any campaign to identify and control hazards. See Section 8, Action.

Any that are likely to produce acute poisoning needing quick first aid should be listed, with treatment required, and posted on the wall where people can see it easily.

**Information on each chemical is given
in the following order:**
**Physical state: Gas, liquid, solid, solution or
suspension.**
**Inflammability: (this is a rough guide only and
does not conform to any approved grading system.)**
Toxicology (see below).
First aid (see below).
**Occupations or processes: where the substance
is most likely to be met.**

If any of the chemicals you use require treatments given in the list below, it is important to remove all contaminated clothing quickly. Emergency showers or baths, eyewash bottles, washbasins and drinking water taps should be close at hand. Taps should be mounted so that you can get your head under to wash out mouth and nose. Check that all equipment works.

- **Irrigate thoroughly with water**
- **Drench with water and then wash with soap and water**
- **Drench with water and apply magnesia/glycerol paste**
- **Bath in dilute sodium thiosulphate solution**
- **Wash with water for at least 15 minutes**

Contaminated clothing must be washed well before it is worn again.

Check that special first aid preparations such as magnesia/glycerol paste are available.

The best treatment for chemical hazards is prevention. Insist on good control of toxic substances; the best possible handling methods; and full time medical and first aid services to watch over health and tackle emergencies.

Toxicology:

There is only a superficial knowledge of the toxicology of many substances. Often what is known is based *only* on animal experiments. Many substances are cumulative – they collect in the body over a period of years and it cannot get rid of them. In many cases, scientists can only guess at the damage they do.

For this reason the Threshold Limit Values (TLV) which appear at the end of many entries should not be taken as a guide to the level of risk. TLVs certainly cannot be treated as *safe* limits, as explained in Section 4, Chemical Hazards.

Don't be lulled into a false sense of security by high threshold values. Treat all chemicals with respect. All contact should be avoided – not just when it is convenient.

First aid:

Treatments are suggested for exposure by inhalation and contact with skin or eyes.

No treatment for swallowed chemicals is given because this is a rare occurrence in industry. But most are poisonous if you swallow them.

Induced vomiting used to be a standard treatment for swallowed poisons but death caused by choking on vomit and by overdoses of salt have made it controversial. It should be used only in severe cases where the acute effects of the poison could be fatal and expert medical help cannot be expected for some time. Make the victim drink the following mixture:

o One tablespoon only of ordinary household salt mixed into two glasses of water. The proportions are important: more salt can cause poisoning; more water and the mixture may be too dilute to cause vomiting. The patient's body will then start to absorb the salt.

Vomiting can also be induced by tickling the back of the victim's throat with a *clean* finger.

Vomiting should not be induced when any of the following has been swallowed:

Petrol, paraffin, turpentine, methyl alcohol, ethyl alcohol, other organic solvents; ether; corrosive or caustic substances.

Abavit. See mercury toxic compounds.
TLV 0.01mg/cu.m

Acetates (eg propyl acetate, amyl-acetate). Liquids; high inflammability; irritant to eyes, nose and throat; narcotic; skin sensitizer, dermatitis on prolonged exposure; vapour may cause dizziness, nausea and headache.

o Treatment after inhalation: remove from exposure, rest, keep warm; o after exposure to eyes: irrigate thoroughly with water, seek medical attention in severe cases; o after exposure to skin: drench with water and then wash with soap and water.

Solvents found throughout industry; used in lacquers, varnishes and adhesives.

Acetic anhydride. Liquid; high inflammability; irritant to eyes, nose and throat; skin sensitizer, dermatitis on prolonged exposure; irritates or burns skin.

o Treatment after inhalation: remove from exposure, rest, keep warm; give drinks to relieve throat irritation; o after exposure to eyes: irrigate thoroughly with water, seek medical attention in severe cases; o after exposure to skin: drench with water and then wash with soap and water.

Used in chemical industry. TLV 5ppm.

Acetone cyanohydrin. See cyanopropanol.

Acetonitrile. Liquid; high inflammability; vapour may cause dizziness, nausea and headache; vomiting and stomach pains, paralysis: o Treatment after inhalation: remove from exposure, rest, keep warm; seek medical attention in severe cases; o after exposure to eyes: irrigate thoroughly with water; seek medical attention in severe cases; o exposure to skin: drench with water, then wash with soap and water.

Used in chemical industry. TLV 40ppm.

Acetylacetone. Liquid; high inflammability; irritant to eyes, nose and throat; irritates or burns skin.

o Treatment after inhalation: remove from exposure, rest, keep warm; o after exposure to eyes: irrigate thoroughly with water, seek medical attention in severe cases; o after exposure to skin: drench with water and then wash with soap and water.

Used in chemical industry.

2-acetyl-amino-fluorene. Powerful bladder carcinogen. Don't have anything to do with it unless plant is completely sealed and every precaution taken.

Acetylbromide. Liquid; high inflammability; irritant to eyes, nose and throat; irritates or burns skin.

o Treatment after inhalation: remove from exposure, rest, keep warm; seek medical attention in severe cases; o after exposure to eyes: irrigate thoroughly with water; seek medical attention in severe cases; o after exposure to skin: drench with water, then wash with soap and water.

Used in chemical industry.

Acetylchloride. Liquid; high inflammability; irritant to eyes, nose and throat; irritates or burns skin. o Treatment after inhalation: remove from exposure, rest, keep warm; seek medical attention in severe cases; o after exposure to eyes: irrigate thoroughly with water; seek medical attention in severe cases; o after exposure to skin: drench with water, then wash with soap and water.

Used in chemical industry.

Acetylene dichloride. See 1,2-dichloro ethylene.

Acetylene tetrachloride. See tetrachloroethane.

Acids. Solid/liquid/solution or suspension; generally low inflammability; irritant to eyes, nose and throat; irritate or burn skin. o Treatment after inhalation: remove from exposure, rest, keep warm; o after exposure to eyes: irrigate thoroughly with water, seek medical attention; o after exposure to skin: drench with water and apply magnesia/glycerol paste; burns require medical attention. Found extensively throughout industry. See Section 5, Disease.

Acroleic acid. See acrylic acid.

Acrolein. Liquid (smells like burning fat); high inflammability; irritant to eyes, nose and throat; asthmatic reaction. o Treatment after inhalation: remove from exposure, rest, keep warm; seek medical attention in severe cases; o after exposure to eyes: irrigate thoroughly with water; seek medical attention in severe cases; o after exposure to skin: irrigate thoroughly with water.

Used in chemical industry; plastics, rubbers and resins; greases and lubricants. TLV 0.1ppm.

Acrylaldehyde, See acrolein.

Acrylates. Liquids; high inflammability; irritant to eyes, nose and throat; irritates or burns skin. o Treatment after inhalation: remove from exposure, rest, keep warm; o after exposure to eyes: irrigate thoroughly with water; seek medical attention in severe cases; o after exposure to skin: irrigate thoroughly with water.

Plastics, rubbers and resins.

Acrylic acid. Liquid; high inflammability; irritant to eyes, nose and throat; irritates or burns skin; o after inhalation: remove, rest, keep warm; o after exposure to eyes: irrigate thoroughly with water; seek medical attention in severe cases; o after exposure to skin: drench with water and apply magnesia/glycerol paste; burns require medical attention.

Plastics, rubbers and resins.

Acrylic aldehyde. See acrolein.

Acrylonitrile. Liquid; high inflammability; skin sensitizer; dermatitis on prolonged exposure; vapour may cause dizziness, nausea and headache; prolonged exposure may lead to liver and/or kidney damage; unconsciousness. o Treatment after inhalation: remove from exposure, rest, keep warm; break amyl nitrite capsule for inhalation; seek medical attention with-

out delay; o after exposure to eyes: irrigate thoroughly with water, seek medical attention without delay; o after exposure to skin: irrigate thoroughly with water; seek medical attention without delay. Plastics, rubbers and resins. TLV 20ppm.

Agrosan. See mercury compounds.

Agrosol. See mercury compounds.

Aldrin. Solid/solution or suspension; low inflammability; prolonged exposure may lead to liver and/or kidney damage; interferes with nervous system. o Treatment after inhalation: remove from exposure, rest, keep warm; seek medical attention in severe cases; o after exposure to eyes: irrigate thoroughly with water; o after exposure to skin: drench with water, then wash with soap and water. Pesticides. TLV 0.25mg/cu m.

Alkalis. Solid/solution or suspension; generally low inflammability; burn skin and eyes; skin sensitizers; dermatitis on prolonged exposure. o Treatment after exposure to eyes: irrigate thoroughly with water; seek medical attention in severe cases; o after exposure to skin: irrigate thoroughly with water. Found extensively throughout industry.

"Alkron". Liquid; high inflammability; see parathion. TLV 0.1mg/cu.m.

Allyl alcohol. Liquid (alcoholic smell, not unpleasant); high inflammability; irritant to eyes, nose and throat; skin sensitizer; dermatitis on prolonged exposure. o Treatment after inhalation: remove from exposure, rest, keep warm; seek medical attention in severe cases; o after exposure to eyes: irrigate thoroughly with water; seek medical attention in severe cases; o after exposure to skin: drench with water, then wash with soap and water. Used in chemical industry. TLV 2ppm.

Allyl bromide. Liquid; high inflammability; irritant to eyes, nose and throat; vapour may cause dizziness, nausea and headache. o Treatment after inhalation: remove from exposure, rest, keep warm; o after exposure to eyes: irrigate thoroughly with water; seek medical attention in severe cases; o after exposure to skin: drench with water, then wash with soap and water. Used in chemical industry.

Allyl chloride. Liquid; high inflammability; irritant to eyes, nose and throat; vapour may cause dizziness, nausea and headache. o Treatment after inhalation: remove from exposure, rest, keep warm; o after exposure to eyes: irrigate thoroughly with water; seek medical attention in severe cases; o after exposure to skin: drench with water, then wash with soap and water. Used in chemical industry. TLV 1ppm.

Aluminium chloride (anhydrous). Solid; nonflammable; irritant to eyes, nose and throat; irritates or burns skin. o Treatment after inhalation: remove from exposure, rest, keep warm; o after exposure to eyes: irrigate thoroughly with water; seek medical attention in severe cases; o after exposure to skin: irrigate thoroughly with water. Used in chemical industry. Petroleum and oil.

Amines. Generally liquid; generally high inflammability;

irritant to eyes, nose and throat; irritates or burns skin; interferes with nervous system. o Treatment after inhalation: remove from exposure, rest, keep warm; seek medical attention in severe cases; o after exposure to eyes: irrigate thoroughly with water; seek medical attention in severe cases; o after exposure to skin: irrigate thoroughly with water. Used in chemical industry, and throughout industry; pharmaceuticals and medicinals; plastics, rubbers and resins; printing and dyestuffs.

Aminobenzene. See aniline.

Aminodiphenyl. Solid; low inflammability; prolonged exposure may lead to liver and/or kidney damage; carcinogen (causes bladder cancer). The use of this substance is prohibited in the U.K. under the Carcinogenic Substances Regulations 1967.

2-aminoethanol. Liquid; high inflammability; see amines. TLV 3ppm.

Aminonitrobenzenes. See nitroanilines.

Ammonia. Gas; low inflammability; irritant to eyes, nose and throat. o Treatment after inhalation: remove from exposure, rest, keep warm; seek medical attention in severe cases; o after exposure to eyes: irrigate thoroughly with water; seek medical attention in severe cases; o after exposure to skin: irrigate thoroughly with water. Used in chemical industry; fertilizers; printing and dyestuffs. TLV 25ppm.

Ammonia solution. Liquid; nonflammable; see alkalis. Used in chemical industry; printing and dyestuffs; refrigeration; metal industry and metal plating.

Ammonium dichromate. Solid; low inflammability; see chromates.
Used in chemical industry.

Ammonium fluoride. Solid; nonflammable; see fluorides; Used in glass industry.

Amyl acetates. Liquid (smell of bananas); high inflammability; irritant to eyes, nose and throat; vapour may cause dizziness, nausea and headache. o Treatment after inhalation: remove from exposure, rest, keep warm; o after exposure to eyes: irrigate thoroughly with water; seek medical attention in severe cases; o after exposure to skin: drench with water, then wash with soap and water.
Used in cosmetics industry; food additive; paints. TLVs: n-amyl acetate 100ppm; sec-amyl acetate 125ppm.

Amyl alcohols. Liquid; high inflammability; irritant to eyes, nose and throat; narcotic. o Treatment after inhalation: remove from exposure, rest, keep warm; o after exposure to eyes: irrigate thoroughly with water; seek medical attention in severe cases; o after exposure to skin: drench with water, then wash with soap and water.
Used in chemical industry; lacquers, varnishes and adhesives; paints.

Amyl formate. Liquid; high inflammability; irritant to eyes, nose and throat; interferes with nervous system. o Treatment after inhalation: remove from exposure, rest, keep warm; seek medical attention in severe cases; o after exposure to eyes: irrigate thoroughly with water; seek medical attention in severe cases; o after exposure to skin: drench with water, then wash with soap and water.

Lacquers, varnishes and adhesives.

Amyl lactate. Liquid; high inflammability; vapour may cause dizziness, nausea and headache; narcotic. o Treatment after inhalation: remove from exposure, rest, keep warm; seek medical attention in severe cases; o after exposure to eyes: irrigate thoroughly with water; seek medical attention in severe cases; o after exposure to skin: drench with water, then wash with soap and water.
Lacquers, varnishes and adhesives.

Amyl propionate. Liquid; high inflammability; irritant to eyes, nose and throat; vapour may cause dizziness, nausea and headache. o Treatment after inhalation: remove from exposure, rest, keep warm; seek medical attention in severe cases; o after exposure to eyes: irrigate thoroughly with water; seek medical attention in severe cases; o after exposure to skin: drench with water, then wash with soap and water.
Lacquers, varnishes and adhesives.

Aniline. Liquid; easily penetrates clothing, rubber and skin; high inflammability; irritant to eyes, nose and throat; vapour may cause dizziness, nausea and headache; interferes with nervous system; long exposure may cause liver damage, anaemia, heart disease. Blood poison (methaemoglobin formed). o Treatment after inhalation: remove from exposure, rest, keep warm; seek medical attention in severe cases; o after exposure to eyes: irrigate thoroughly with water; seek medical attention in severe cases; o after exposure to

skin: get any contaminated clothing off immediately; drench with water, then wash with soap and water.
Pharmaceuticals and medicinals; paints, plastics, rubbers and resins; printing and dyestuffs.
TLV 5ppm.

Anisidines. Liquid, solid, high inflammability; see aniline.
Used in chemical industry; printing and dyestuffs.
TLV 0.5mg/cu.m.

Anthracene. Solid; low inflammability; possible carcinogen.
o Treatment after exposure to skin: drench with water, then wash with soap and water.
Used in chemical industry.

Anthraquinone. Solid; low inflammability; skin sensitizer; dermatitis on prolonged exposure. o Treatment after exposure to skin: drench with water, then wash with soap and water.
Printing and dyestuffs.

Antimony and compounds. Gas (stibine), liquid, solid; generally low inflammability; irritant to eyes, nose and throat. Chronic effects: heart disease; dermatitis on prolonged exposure. o Treatment (stibine only); after inhalation: remove from exposure, rest, keep warm; seek medical attention in severe cases; o after exposure to eyes: irrigate thoroughly with water; seek medical attention in severe cases; o after exposure to skin: drench with water, then wash with soap and water.
Printing (metal) and dyestuffs; lead-acid batteries.
TLV 0.5 mg/cu.m.

Aqua fortis. See nitric acid.

Aretan. See mercury compounds.
Pesticides.

Arlothane. See hexachloroethane.

Armeen. See amines.
Used in chemical industry.

Aroclor. Liquid, solution or suspension; low inflammability; see chlorinated biphenyls.
Pesticides and herbicides.

Arsenic and compounds. Highly poisonous substances. Gas, liquid, solid; generally low inflammability; irritant to eyes, nose and throat; skin sensitizers; dermatitis on prolonged exposure; prolonged exposure may also lead to liver and/or kidney damage; possible carcinogen (may cause cancer). o Treatment after inhalation: remove from exposure, rest, keep warm; seek medical attention in severe cases; o after exposure to eyes: irrigate thoroughly with water; seek medical attention in severe cases; o after exposure to skin: drench with water, then wash with soap and water.
Pesticides.
TLV 0.5 mg/cu.m.

Arsenic hydride (Arsine). Gas; low inflammability; affects blood. See arsenic compounds.
Metal pickling.
TLV 0.05ppm.

Arsine. See arsenic hydride.

Asbestos. Very dangerous material; solid; nonflammable; no short-term effects but small exposures can cause fibrosis of lungs (asbestosis) and various cancers. Blue asbestos (rich lavender blue colour) particularly deadly. Increasing use (except blue) in industry, for thermal and acoustic insulation, fireproofing, fibre reinforcing; construction, shipbuilding, demolition, auto industry (friction materials, gaskets).
See full description, including TLV, in text.

Asphalt. Solid/liquid; inflammable; no short term effects (except burns from hot material); may cause skin cancer on prolonged exposure. Construction.
TLV asphalt (petroleum fumes) 5mg/cu.m.

Auramine. Causes bladder cancer. Controlled substance under Carcinogenic Substances Regulations 1967.

Barium compounds. eg barium chloride. Solid; nonflammable; dermatitis on prolonged exposure (chloride-sulphide is not irritant).
o Treatment after exposure to skin: drench with water, then wash with soap and water. Paints, lacquers, varnishes and adhesives; plastics, rubbers and resins; printing and dyestuffs.
TLV (soluble compounds) 0.5 mg/cu.m.

Becspray. See tar and pitch.

Bectaphatt. See tar and pitch.

Bentalol. See benzyl alcohol.

Benzene. Liquid; high inflammability; narcotic; vapour may cause dizziness, nausea and headache; unconsciousness; carcinogen (may cause cancer); blood cell damage (employer should carry out regular blood tests). o Treatment after inhalation: remove from exposure, rest, keep warm; seek medical attention in severe cases; o after exposure to eyes: irrigate thoroughly with water; seek medical attention in severe cases; o after exposure to skin drench with water, then wash with soap and water.
Solvent found extensively throughout industry; chemical industry, particularly in making styrene; lacquers, varnishes, adhesives; paints; is con-

tained in petrol, may be in toluene.
TLV 25ppm (if you can smell it, it's over the TLV. But nose loses sensitivity to it.)

BHC, benzene hexachloride. Solid, solution or suspension; low inflammability; irritant to eyes, nose and throat; skin sensitizer; dermatitis on prolonged exposure; vapour may cause dizziness, nausea and headache; interferes with nervous system. o Treatment after inhalation: remove from exposure, rest, keep warm; seek medical attention in severe cases; o after exposure to eyes: irrigate thoroughly with water; seek medical attention in severe cases; o after exposure to skin: drench with water, then wash with soap and water.
Used in chemical industry; pesticides and herbicides.

Benzene sulphonic acid. Solid; low inflammability; see acids. Used in chemical industry.

Benzidine. Powerful bladder carcinogen; the use of this compound is prohibited in the U.K. under the Carcinogenic Substances Regulations, 1967.

Benzol. See benzene.

Benzoquinone. Solid; low inflammability; irritant to eyes, nose and throat; irritates or burns skin. o Treatment after inhalation: remove from exposure, rest, keep warm; seek medical attention in severe cases; o after exposure to eyes: irrigate thoroughly with water; seek medical attention in severe cases; o after exposure to skin: drench with water, then wash with soap and water.
Used in chemical industry; cosmetics industry; printing and dyestuffs; textiles and paper.

Benzoyl chloride. Liquid; high inflammability; irritant to eyes, nose and throat; irritates or burns skin. o Treatment after inhalation: remove from exposure, rest, keep warm; seek medical attention in severe cases; o after exposure to eyes: irrigate thoroughly with water; seek medical attention in severe cases; o after exposure to skin: drench with water, then wash with soap and water.
Used in chemical industry.

Benzyl alcohol. Liquid; high inflammability; irritant to eyes, nose and throat; vapour may cause dizziness, nausea and headache. o Treatment after inhalation: remove from exposure, rest, keep warm; o after exposure to eyes: irrigate thoroughly with water; seek medical attention in severe cases; o after exposure to skin: drench with water, then wash with soap and water.
Used in cosmetics industry; lacquers, varnishes and adhesives.

Benzyl amine. Liquid; high inflammability; see amines.

Benzyl bromide. Liquid; high inflammability; irritant to eyes, nose and throat; irritates or burns skin. o Treatment after inhalation: remove from exposure, rest, keep warm; o after exposure to eyes: irrigate thoroughly with water; seek medical attention in severe cases; o after exposure to skin: drench with water, then wash with soap and water.
Used in chemical industry.

Benzyl chloride. Liquid; high inflammability; irritant to eyes (makes you cry), nose and throat; irritates or burns skin. o Treatment after inhalation: remove from exposure, rest, keep warm; o after

exposure to eyes: irrigate thoroughly with water; seek medical attention in severe cases; o after exposure to skin: drench with water, then wash with soap and water.
Used in cosmetics industry; pharmaceuticals and medicinals; plastics, rubbers and resins, printing and dyestuffs. TLV 1ppm.

Beryllium and compounds. eg beryllium chloride. Solid; nonflammable; causes acute lung inflammation and whole body sensitization; may cause lung cancer. o Treatment after inhalation: remove from exposure, rest, keep warm; seek medical attention in all cases; o after exposure to eyes: irrigate thoroughly with water; seek medical attention in severe cases; o after exposure to skin: irrigate thoroughly with water.
Metal industry and metal plating; particularly processing copper-beryllium alloys; electronic valves and components.
See full description in text. TLV 0.002mg/cu.m.

Bichromates. See chromates.

Biphenylamine. See aminodiphenyl.

Bleaching powder. See chloride of lime.

Bone meal. Solid; nonflammable; may carry anthrax (see Section 5, Disease). Agriculture, horticulture.

Boron hydrides. Gas, liquid; high inflammability; irritant to eyes, nose and throat; prolonged exposure may lead to liver and/or kidney damage; interferes with nervous system. o Treatment after inhalation: remove from exposure, rest, keep warm; seek medical attention in severe cases; o after exposure to eyes: irrigate thoroughly with

water; seek medical attention in severe cases; o after exposure to skin: drench with water, then wash with soap and water.
Fuels and propellants.

Bromine. Liquid; nonflammable; irritant to eyes, nose and throat; irritates or burns skin. o Treatment after inhalation: remove from exposure, rest, keep warm; seek medical attention in severe cases; o after exposure to eyes: irrigate thoroughly with water; seek medical attention in severe cases; o after exposure to skin: irrigate thoroughly with water; bathe in dilute sodium thiosulphate solution; seek medical attention in severe cases.
Used in chemical industry.
TLV 0.1ppm.

Bromoacetic acid. Solid; low inflammability; see acids.
Used in chemical industry.

Bromoethane. Liquid; high inflammability; see ethyl bromide.

Bromomethane. Liquid; high inflammability; see methyl bromide.

3-bromopropene. Liquid; high inflammability; see allyl bromide.

3-bromopropyne. Liquid; high inflammability; irritant to eyes, nose and throat; irritates or burns skin. o Treatment after inhalation: remove from exposure, rest, keep warm; o after exposure to eyes: irrigate thoroughly with water; seek medical attention in severe cases; o after exposure to skin: drench with water, then wash with soap and water.
Used in chemical industry.

α-bromotoluene. See benzyl bromide.

Buck. See alkalis.

Butadiene (1,3-butadiene). Gas; high inflammability;

narcotic; irritates or burns skin; unconsciousness.
o Treatment after inhalation: remove from exposure, rest, keep warm.
Plastics, rubbers and resins.
TLV 1,000ppm.

Butanols. See butyl alcohols.

Butyl acetate. Liquid; high inflammability; see acetates.
Solvent – found throughout industry; used in chemical industry; lacquers, varnishes and adhesives; plastics, rubbers and resins.
TLV 150ppm.

Butyl acrylate. Liquid; high inflammability; see acrylates.

Butyl alcohols. Liquid, solid; high inflammability; irritant to eyes, nose and throat; skin sensitizer; dermatitis on prolonged exposure; irritates or burns skin; vapour may cause dizziness, nausea and headache. o Treatment after inhalation: remove from exposure, rest, keep warm; o after exposure to eyes: irrigate thoroughly with water; seek medical attention in severe cases; o after exposure to skin: drench with water, then wash with soap and water.
Plastics, rubbers and resins; printing and dyestuffs.
TLV 100ppm.

Butyl amines. Liquid; high inflammability; see amines.

Butyl carbitol. Liquid, high inflammability; narcotic; prolonged exposure may lead to liver and/or kidney damage.
o Treatment after inhalation: remove from exposure, rest, keep warm; o after exposure to eyes; irrigate thoroughly with water; seek medical attention in severe cases; o after exposure to skin: drench with water, then wash with soap and water.
Lacquers, varnishes and adhesives; printing and dyestuffs.

Butyl cellosolve. Liquid; high inflammability; narcotic; prolonged exposure may lead to liver and/or kidney damage. o Treatment after inhalation: remove from exposure, rest, keep warm; o after exposure to eyes: irrigate thoroughly with water; seek medical attention in severe cases; o after exposure to skin: drench with water, then wash with soap and water.
Lacquers, varnishes and adhesives; detergents and soaps; cleaning agents.

Butyl formate. Liquid; high inflammability; irritant to eyes, nose and throat; irritates or burns skin; vapour may cause dizziness, nausea, headache. o Treatment after inhalation: remove from exposure, rest, keep warm; seek medical attention in severe cases; o after exposure to eyes: irrigate thoroughly with water; seek medical attention in severe cases; o after exposure to skin: drench with water, then wash with soap and water.
Solvent – found throughout industry; used in cosmetics industry; lacquers, varnishes and adhesives.

Butyric acid. Liquid; high inflammability; see acids.
Food additive.

Butyronitrile. Liquid; high inflammability; see acetonitrile.

p-tertiary butyl toluene. Liquid; high inflammability; irritant to eyes, nose and throat; prolonged exposure may lead to liver and/or kidney damage; interferes with nervous system; blood poison. o Treatment after inhalation: remove from exposure, rest, keep warm; seek medical attention in severe cases; o after exposure to eyes: irrigate thoroughly with water; seek medical attention in severe cases; o after exposure to skin: drench with water, then wash with soap and water. Used in chemical industry; petroleum and oil. TLV 10ppm.

Cadmium and cadmium compounds. Solid; nonflammable; vapour may cause dizziness, nausea and headache; prolonged exposure may lead to liver and/or kidney damage; inflammation of lungs. o Treatment after inhalation: remove from exposure, rest, keep warm; seek medical attention in severe cases; o after exposure to skin: drench with water, then wash with soap and water.
Paints (pigments); fruit tree sprays; metal plating; silver soldering; flame cutting of plated parts.
TLV 0.1mg/cu.m.

Calcium carbimide. See calcium cyanamide.

Calcium cyanamide. Solid; nonflammable; irritant to eyes, nose and throat; skin sensitizer; dermatitis on prolonged exposure; irritates or burns skin. o Treatment after inhalation: remove from exposure, rest, keep warm; o after exposure to eyes: irrigate thoroughly with water; seek medical attention in severe cases; o after exposure to skin: irrigate thoroughly with water.
Used in chemical industry; fertilisers.

Calcium hypochlorite. See chloride of lime.

Caradate. See isocyanates.
Plastics, rubbers and resins.

Carbergan. See carbon tetrachloride.

Carbitol. Liquid; high inflammability; narcotic; prolonged exposure may lead to liver and/or kidney damage. o

Treatment after inhalation: remove from exposure, rest, keep warm; o after exposure to eyes: irrigate thoroughly with water; seek medical attention in severe cases; o after exposure to skin: drench with water, then wash with soap and water.
Lacquers, varnishes and adhesives; cleaning agents.

Carbolic acid. See phenol.

Carbon bisulphide. Liquid (aromatic smell, slightly pungent); high inflammability; irritant to eyes, nose and throat; narcotic; vapour may cause dizziness, nausea, headache; interferes with nervous system; unconsciousness; paralysis; more than doubles your chance of heart disease. o Treatment after inhalation: remove from exposure, rest, keep warm, seek medical attention; o after exposure to eyes: irrigate thoroughly with water; seek medical attention in severe cases; o after exposure to skin: drench with water, then wash with soap and water.
Used in chemical industry; lacquers, varnishes and adhesives; plastics, rubbers and resins; viscose rayon manufacture; cellulose filaments and films.
TLV 20ppm.

Carbon disulphide. See carbon bisulphide.

Carbon monoxide. Gas; low inflammability; may cause dizziness, headache, nausea; unconsciousness. o Treatment after inhalation: remove from exposure, rest, keep warm; seek medical attention in severe cases.
Fumes from vehicles, welding, pre-heating; in steel works, town gas, coke works.
TLV 50ppm.

Carbon tetrachloride. Liquid; nonflammable; irritant to eyes, nose and throat; narcotic; skin sensitizer; dermatitis on prolonged exposure, vapour may cause dizziness, nausea and headache, prolonged exposure may lead to liver and/or kidney damage; vomiting and stomach pains; unconsciousness; inflammation of lungs; induces bronchitis. o Treatment after inhalation: remove from exposure, rest, keep warm; seek medical attention in severe cases; o after exposure to eyes: irrigate thoroughly with water; seek medical attention in severe cases; o after exposure to skin: drench with water, then wash with soap and water.
Solvent – found throughout industry; lacquers, varnishes and adhesives; paints; cleaning agents. In some fire extinguishers; this type should not be kept or used indoors.
TLV 10ppm.

Carbonyl chloride. See phosgene.

Cassel. See cyanides.

Catechol. Solid; low inflammability. See phenol.
Used in chemical industry; disinfectants and fumigants.

Caustic potash. See potassium hydroxide.

Caustic soda. See sodium hydroxide.

Cellosolve. Liquid; high inflammability; narcotic; prolonged exposure may lead to liver and/or kidney damage. o Treatment after inhalation remove from exposure, rest, keep warm; seek medical attention in severe cases; o after exposure to eyes: irrigate thoroughly with water; seek medical attention in severe cases; o after exposure to skin: drench with water, then wash with soap and water. Solvent – used throughout industry; lacquers, inks, varnishes and adhesives; paints. TLV 25ppm.

Cellosolve acetate. Liquid; high inflammability; narcotic; irritates or burns skin. o Treatment after inhalation: remove from exposure, rest, keep warm; seek medical attention in severe cases; o after exposure to eyes: irrigate thoroughly with water; seek medical attention in severe cases; o after exposure to skin: drench with water, then wash with soap and water. Solvent – used throughout industry; lacquers, varnishes and adhesives; paints.

Chlordane. Liquid; low inflammability; prolonged exposure may lead to liver and/or kidney damage; interferes with nervous system. o Treatment after inhalation: remove from exposure, rest, keep warm; seek medical attention in severe cases; o after exposure to eyes: irrigate thoroughly with water; seek medical attention in severe cases; o after exposure to skin: drench with water, then wash with soap and water. Pesticides and herbicides. TLV 0.5 mg/cu.m.

Chlorex. See dichloroethyl ether.

Chloride of lime. Solid; non-flammable; irritant to eyes, nose and throat; skin sensitizer; dermatitis on prolonged exposure; irritates or burns skin. o Treatment after inhalation: remove from exposure, rest, keep warm; seek medical attention in severe cases; o after exposure to eyes; irrigate thoroughly with water; seek medical attention in severe cases; o after exposure to skin: drench with

water, then wash with soap and water. Used in cosmetics industry; disinfectants and fumigants; printing and dyestuffs; textiles and paper.

Chlorinated camphene. See toxaphene. TLV 0.5 mg/cu.m.

Chlorinated hydrocarbons. Gas, liquid, solid; nonflammable to high inflammability; narcotic; skin sensitizer, dermatitis on prolonged exposure; vapour may cause dizziness, nausea and headache; prolonged exposure may lead to liver and/or kidney damage. o Treatment after inhalation: remove from exposure, rest, keep warm; seek medical attention in severe cases; o after exposure to eyes: irrigate thoroughly with water; seek medical attention in severe cases; o after exposure to skin: drench with water, then wash with soap and water. Found extensively throughout industry – solvents, pesticides.

Chlorinated biphenyls. Liquid, solid; low inflammability; skin sensitizers; dermatitis on prolonged exposure; vapour may cause dizziness, nausea and headache; prolonged exposure may lead to liver and/or kidney damage. o Treatment after inhalation: remove from exposure, rest, keep warm; seek medical attention in severe cases; o after exposure to eyes: irrigate thoroughly with water; seek medical attention in severe cases; o after exposure to skin: drench with water, then wash with soap and water. Lacquers, varnishes and adhesives; paints; plastics, rubbers and resins. TLV (chlorinated diphenyl-oxide) 0.5 mg/cu.m.

Chlorinated naphthalenes.
Solid; low inflammability; see chlorinated biphenyls.
Used in chemical industry; thermal and/or electrical insulation; greases and lubricants; lacquers, varnishes and adhesives; paints; cleaning agents.

Chlorine. Gas; low inflammability and strong oxidizing agent – spontaneous ignition is possible on contact with other substances; irritant to eyes, nose and throat; irritates or burns skin; inflammation of lungs. o Treatment after inhalation: remove from exposure, rest and keep warm, seek medical attention; o after exposure to eyes: irrigate thoroughly with water; seek medical attention; o after exposure to skin: irrigate thoroughly with water.
Used in chemical industry; disinfectants and fumigants; textiles and paper; refrigeration systems.
TLV 1ppm. (If you can smell it, it's above the safe limit.)

Chlorine trifluoride. Gas; non-flammable; irritant to eyes, nose and throat; irritates or burns skin. o Treatment after inhalation: remove from exposure, rest, keep warm; seek medical attention in severe cases; o after exposure to eyes: wash with water for at least 15 minutes; seek medical attention in severe cases; o after exposure to skin: drench with water and apply magnesia/glycerol paste; get medical attention; burns must have medical attention; wash with water for at least 15 minutes.
Fuels and propellants.
TLV 0.1ppm.

Chloroacetic acid. Solid; low inflammability; see acids.
Used in chemical industry.

Chloroacetyl chloride. Liquid; low inflammability; see acetyl chloride.
Used in chemical industry.

Chloroanilines. Liquid; high inflammability; see aniline.
Used in chemical industry.

Chlorobenzene. Liquid; high inflammability; see chlorinated hydrocarbons.
Solvent – found throughout industry; plastics, rubbers and resins.

Chlorobiphenyls. See chlorinated biphenyls.

2-chloro-1, 3-butadiene. See chloroprene.

Chloroethane. See ethyl chloride.

2-chloroethanol. Liquid; high inflammability; irritant to eyes, nose and throat; narcotic, vapour may cause dizziness, nausea and headache; prolonged exposure may lead to liver and/or kidney damage; inflammation of lungs; vomiting and stomach pains. o Treatment after inhalation: remove from exposure, rest, keep warm; seek medical attention in severe cases; o after exposure to eyes: irrigate thoroughly with water; seek medical attention in severe cases; o after exposure to skin: drench with water, then wash with soap and water; seek medical attention in severe cases.
Solvent – found throughout industry; plastics, rubbers and resins.
TLV 5ppm.

Chloroethylene. See vinyl chloride.

Chloroform. Liquid; low inflammability; irritant to eyes, nose and throat; vapour may cause dizziness, nausea and headache; prolonged exposure may lead to liver and/or kidney damage; unconsciousness; vomiting and stomach pains; paralysis. o Treatment after inhalation: remove from exposure, rest, keep warm; seek medical attention in severe cases; o after exposure to eyes: irrigate thoroughly with water; seek medical attention in severe cases.

Solvent – used throughout industry; plastics, rubbers and resins.

Chloromethane. See methyl chloride.

Chloronitroanilines. Solid; low inflammability; skin sensitizer; dermatitis on prolonged exposure; prolonged exposure may also lead to liver and/or kidney damage. o Treatment after exposure to eyes: irrigate thoroughly with water; seek medical attention in severe cases; o after exposure to skin: irrigate thoroughly with water.

Used in chemical industry.

Chloronitrobenzenes. Solid; low inflammability; irritant to eyes, nose and throat; skin sensitizer; dermatitis on prolonged exposure; prolonged exposure may also lead to liver and/or kidney damage. o Treatment after inhalation: remove from exposure, rest, keep warm; seek medical attention in severe cases; o after exposure to eyes: irrigate thoroughly with water; seek medical attention in severe cases; o after exposure to skin: irrigate thoroughly with water.

Used in chemical industry.

1-chloro-1-nitropropane. Liquid; high inflammability; irritates or burns skin; prolonged exposure may lead to liver and/or kidney damage. o Treatment after exposure to eyes: irrigate thoroughly with water; seek medical attention in severe cases; o after exposure to skin: drench with

water, then wash with soap and water.

Plastics, rubbers and resins. TLV 20ppm.

Chlorophenols. Liquid; solid (medicinal smell); low inflammability – high inflammability; see phenol. Disinfectants and fumigants; pharmaceuticals and medicinals.

Chloroprene. Liquid; high inflammability; irritant to eyes, nose and throat; narcotic, skin sensitizer; dermatitis on prolonged exposure; irritates or burns skin; prolonged exposure may lead to liver and/or kidney damage; inflammation of lungs; blood poison. o Treatment after inhalation: remove from exposure, rest, keep warm; seek medical attention in severe cases; o after exposure to eyes: irrigate thoroughly with water; seek medical attention in severe cases; o after exposure to skin: drench with water, then wash with soap and water.

Plastics, rubbers and resins. TLV 25ppm.

3-chloropropene. See allyl chloride.

Chlorosulphonic acid. Liquid; low inflammability; see acids. Used in chemical industry.

Chlorotoluene. Liquid; high inflammability; see chlorohydrocarbons.

α-chlorotoluene. See benzyl chloride.

Chromates. Solid; nonflammable; strong oxidity agent – spontaneous ignition is possible on contact with other substances; irritant to eyes, nose, throat; skin sensitizer, dermatitis and skin 'holes' on prolonged exposure; prolonged exposure may also damage liver and/or kidney and nose; carcinogens (may cause cancer). o Treatment after inhalation: remove from exposure,

rest, keep warm; o after exposure to eyes: irrigate thoroughly with water; seek medical attention in severe cases; o skin: see page 136.
Printing and dyestuffs; metal industry and metal plating; welding.
TLV 0.1mg/cu.m.

Chromic acid. Solid or solution; nonflammable; strong oxidizing agent – spontaneous ignition is possible on contact with other substances; see acids; dermatitis, chrome ulcers and nose damage. See page 136.
Found extensively throughout industry; metal industry, chrome plating; cleaning agents.
TLV 0.1mg/cu.m.

Chromium trioxide. Solid; nonflammable; strong oxidizing agent – spontaneous ignition is possible on contact with other substances; see chromic acid.

Coal dust. Solid; explosive; causes pneumoconiosis (see Section 5, Disease).
TLV 2mg/cu.m.

Coal tar. See naphtha; can cause skin cancer.
TLV (pitch volatiles, 0.2mg/cu.m.

Cotton dust. Can cause byssinosis (see Section 5, Disease).
TLV 0.5mg/cu.m.

Cresols. Liquid, solid; low flammability – high inflammability; see phenol.
Disinfectants and fumigants; plastics, rubbers and resins; oil refining.
TLV 5ppm.

Cresylic acid. See cresols.

Crotonaldehyde. Liquid; high inflammability; irritant to eyes, nose and throat; irritates or burns skin. o Treatment after inhalation: remove from exposure, rest, keep warm; seek medical attention in

severe cases; o after exposure to eyes: irrigate thoroughly with water; seek medical attention in severe cases; o after exposure to skin: irrigate thoroughly with water.
Solvent – used throughout industry; plastics, rubbers and resins.
TLV 2ppm.

Cumene. Liquid; high inflammability; irritant to eyes, nose and throat; narcotic; irritates or burns skin; possible carcinogen (may cause cancer).
o Treatment after inhalation: remove from exposure, rest, keep warm; o after exposure to eyes: irrigate thoroughly with water; seek medical attention in severe cases; o after exposure to skin: drench with water, then wash with soap and water.
Solvent– used throughout industry; paints; petroleum and oil.
TLV 50ppm.

Cyanides. Highly toxic. Gas, liquid, solid; nonflammable – high inflammability; vapour may cause dizziness, nausea and headache; vomiting and stomach pains; unconsciousness. o Treatment after inhalation: remove from exposure, rest, keep warm; break amyl nitrite capsule for inhalation; seek medical attention without delay; o after exposure to eyes: irrigate thoroughly with water; seek medical attention in severe cases; o after exposure to skin: drench with water, then wash with soap and water; seek medical attention in severe cases.
Used in chemical industry; disinfectants and fumigants; pesticides and herbicides; metal industry and metal plating; found in road salt.
TLV 5mg/cu.m.

Cyanogen. Highly toxic. Gas; high inflammability; irritant to eyes, nose and throat; vapour may cause dizziness, nausea and headache; unconsciousness; vomiting and stomach pains. o Treatment after inhalation: remove from exposure, rest, keep warm; break amyl nitrite capsule for inhalation; seek medical attention without delay; o after exposure to eyes: irrigate thoroughly with water; seek medical attention in severe cases; o after exposure to skin: irrigate thoroughly with water; seek medical attention in severe cases.
Used in chemical industry; printing and dyestuffs; metal industry and metal plating. TLV 10ppm.

Cyanoids. See cyanides.

Cyanoline. See cyanides.

Cyanopropanol. Liquid; high inflammability; vapour may cause dizziness, nausea and headache; unconsciousness. o Treatment after inhalation: remove from exposure, rest, keep warm; break amyl nitrite capsule for inhalation; seek medical attention without delay; o after exposure to eyes: irrigate thoroughly with water; seek medical attention in severe cases; o after exposure to skin: irrigate thoroughly with water; seek medical attention in severe cases.
Used in chemical industry.

Cyclohexanol. Liquid; high inflammability; irritant to eyes, nose and throat; narcotic; irritates or burns skin; prolonged exposure may lead to liver and/or kidney damage. o Treatment after inhalation: remove from exposure, rest, keep warm; o after exposure to eyes: irrigate thoroughly with water; seek medical attention in severe cases; o after

exposure to skin: drench with water, then wash with soap and water.
Solvent – found throughout industry; plastics, rubbers and resins; textiles and paper. TLV 50ppm.

Cyclohexanone. Liquid; high inflammability; irritant to eyes, nose and throat; narcotic; irritates or burns skin. o Treatment after inhalation; remove from exposure, rest, keep warm; o after exposure to eyes: irrigate thoroughly with water; seek medical attention in severe cases; o after exposure to skin: drench with water, then wash with soap and water.
Solvent – found throughout industry; plastics, rubbers and resins.
TLV 50ppm.

Cyclopentadiene. Liquid; high inflammability; vapour may cause dizziness, nausea and headache; prolonged exposure may lead to liver and/or kidney damage; interferes with nervous system; blood poison. o Treatment after inhalation: remove from exposure, rest, keep warm; seek medical attention in severe cases; o after exposure to eyes: irrigate thoroughly with water; seek medical attention in severe cases; o after exposure to skin: drench with water, then wash with soap and water.
Plastics, rubbers and resins. TLV 75ppm.

2,4-D. See 2,4-dichlorophenoxy acetic acid. TLV 10mg/cu.m.

DDT. See dichlorodiphenyltrichloroethane.
TLV 1mg/cu.m.

Diacetone alcohol. Liquid; high inflammability; narcotic; irritates or burns skin; prolonged exposure may lead to liver and/or kidney damage;

blood poison. o Treatment after inhalation: remove from exposure, rest, keep warm; o after exposure to eyes: irrigate thoroughly with water; seek medical attention in severe cases; o after exposure to skin: irrigate thoroughly with water.
Solvent – found throughout industry; lacquers, varnishes and adhesives; plastics, rubbers and resins; printing and dyestuffs; cleaning agents. TLV 50ppm.

p-diaminodiphenyl. See benzidine.

Diaminoethane. See ethylene diamine.

Dianisidine. Liquid; high inflammability; possible carcinogen (may cause bladder cancer); Controlled substance under Carcinogenic Substances Regulations 1967.
o Treatment after inhalation: wash out nose and mouth with water; o after exposure to eyes: irrigate thoroughly with water; seek medical attention in severe cases; o after exposure to skin: drench with water, then wash with soap and water.
Analytical work.

Diazomethane. Gas or solution; high inflammability, irritant to eyes, nose and throat; irritates or burns skin; dermatitis; asthmatic reaction; vapour may cause dizziness, nausea and headache, unconsciousness; inflammation of lungs. o Treatment after inhalation: remove from exposure, rest, keep warm; seek medical attention without delay; o after exposure to eyes: irrigate thoroughly with water; seek medical attention in severe cases; o after exposure to skin: drench with water, then wash with soap and water.

Used in chemical industry. TLV 0.2ppm.

Dibenzylamine. Liquid; high inflammability; see amines.

Diborane. Gas; high inflammability; see boron hydrides. TLV 0.1ppm.

1-2 dibromoethane. See ethylene dibromide.

Dicestal. See chlorinated hydrocarbons.

0-dichlorbenzene. Liquid; high inflammability. See chlorinated biphenyls.

Dichlorobenzidine. Powerful bladder carcinogen. Controlled Substance under Carcinogenic Substances Regulations 1967.

Dichlorodiphenyltrichloroethane (DDT). Solid/solution or suspension; low inflammability; prolonged exposure may lead to liver and/or kidney damage; interferes with nervous system; blood poison. o Treatment after inhalation: remove from exposure, rest, keep warm; seek medical attention in severe cases; o after exposure to eyes: irrigate thoroughly with water; seek medical attention in severe cases; o after exposure to skin: drench with water, then wash with soap and water. Pesticide.
TLV 1mg/cu.m.

1-2-dichloroethane. Liquid; high inflammability; one of the most toxic chlorohydrocarbons; irritant to eyes, nose and throat; skin sensitizer; dermatitis on prolonged exposure; irritates or burns skin; vapour may cause dizziness, nausea and headache; prolonged exposure may lead to liver and/or kidney damage; vomiting and stomach pains. o Treatment after inhalation: remove from exposure, rest, keep warm; seek medical attention in severe cases; o after exposure to eyes: irrigate thoroughly with water; seek medical attention in severe cases; o after exposure to skin; drench with water, then wash with soap and water.

Solvent – found throughout industry; used in chemical industry; lacquers, varnishes and adhesives; paints; cleaning agents.

TLV 50ppm.

1,2-dichloroethylene. Liquid; high inflammability; irritant to eyes, nose and throat; skin sensitizer; dermatitis on prolonged exposure; prolonged exposure may also lead to liver and/or kidney damage; unconsciousness. o Treatment after inhalation: remove from exposure, rest, keep warm; o after exposure to eyes: irrigate thoroughly with water; seek medical attention in severe cases; o after exposure to skin: drench with water, then wash with soap and water.

Used in cosmetics industry; lacquers, varnishes and adhesives; plastics, rubbers and resins; printing and dyestuffs; pesticides and herbicides; cleaning agents.

TLV 200ppm.

Dichloroethyl ether. Liquid; high inflammability; irritant to skin, eyes, nose and throat; narcotic; prolonged exposure may lead to liver and/or kidney damage; inflammation of lungs. o Treatment after inhalation: remove from exposure, rest, keep warm; seek medical attention in severe cases; o after exposure to eyes: irrigate thoroughly with water; seek medical attention in severe cases; o after exposure to skin: drench with water, then wash with soap and water.

Used in chemical industry;

greases and lubricants.

TLV 5ppm.

Dichloromethane. Liquid; low inflammability; irritant to eyes, nose and throat; narcotic; vapour may cause dizziness, nausea and headache; unconsciousness. o Treatment after inhalation: remove from exposure, rest, keep warm; seek medical attention in severe cases; o after exposure to eyes: irrigate thoroughly with water; seek medical attention in severe cases; o after exposure to skin: drench with water, then wash with soap and water.

Paints; plastics, rubbers and resins; cleaning agents.

TLV 500ppm.

Dichloromethyl ether. Liquid; high inflammability; see dichloroethyl ether.

Dichloronitroethane. Liquid; high inflammability; irritates or burns skin; prolonged exposure may lead to liver and/or kidney damage; inflammation of lungs. o Treatment after inhalation: remove from exposure, rest, keep warm; o after exposure to eyes: irrigate thoroughly with water; seek medical attention in severe cases; o after exposure to skin: drench with water, then wash with soap and water.

Disinfectants and fumigants.

2,4-dichlorophenoxy acetic acid. Solid; low inflammability; vapour may cause dizziness, nausea and headache; prolonged exposure may lead to liver and/or kidney damage; interferes with nervous system. o Treatment after inhalation: remove from exposure, rest, keep warm; seek medical attention in severe cases; o after exposure to eyes: irrigate thoroughly with water; seek medical attention in severe cases; o after exposure to skin: drench with water, then wash with soap and water.

Used in chemical industry.

1,2-dichloro-propane. See propylene dichloride.

Dichromates. See chromates.

Didi-col. See DDT.

Didimac. See DDT.

Dieldrin. Solid, solution or suspension; low inflammability; vapour may cause dizziness, nausea and headache; prolonged exposure may lead to liver and/or kidney damage; interferes with nervous system; vomiting and stomach pains. o Treatment after inhalation: remove from exposure, rest, keep warm; seek medical attention in severe cases; o after exposure to eyes: irrigate thoroughly with water; seek medical attention in severe cases. o after exposure to skin: drench with water, then wash with soap and water.

Pesticides.

TLV 0.25 mg/cu.m.

Diethylamine. Liquid; high inflammability; see amines.

TLV 25ppm.

Diethylene dioxide. See dioxan.

Diethylene glycol monobutyl ether. See butyl carbitol.

Diethylene glycol monoethyl ether. See carbitol.

Diethyl sulphate. See dimethylsulphate.

Di-isocyanates. See tolylene di-isocyanate.

Di-(isocyanatophenyl)-methane. Solid; low inflammability; irritant to eyes, nose and throat; irritates or burns skin. o Treatment after inhalation: remove from exposure, rest, keep warm; seek medical attention in severe cases; o after exposure to eyes: irrigate thoroughly with water; seek medical attention

in severe cases; o after exposure to skin: drench with water, then wash with soap and water.

Plastics, rubbers and resins.

Di(isocyanatotoluene). See tolylene di-isocyanate.

Di-isopropyl ether. See isopropyl ether.

Dimethylamine. Gas, solution or suspension; high inflammability; see amines.

TLV 10ppm.

4-dimethylaminoazobenzene. Powerful carcinogen. Don't work in same place as it unless it is in a completely sealed system with every possible safeguard.

N,N-dimethyl aniline. Liquid; high inflammability; irritant to eyes, nose and throat; vapour may cause dizziness, nausea and headache; interferes with nervous system. o Treatment after inhalation: remove from exposure, rest, keep warm, seek medical attention in severe cases; o after exposure to eyes: irrigate thoroughly with water; seek medical attention in severe cases; o after exposure to skin: drench with water, then wash with soap and water.

Solvent – used throughout industry; printing and dyestuffs.

TLV 5ppm.

Dimethyl sulphate. Liquid; low inflammability; irritant to eyes, nose and throat; irritates or burns skin; prolonged exposure may lead to liver and/or kidney damage; inflammation of lungs; often delayed action. o Treatment after inhalation: remove from exposure, rest, keep warm; seek medical attention in severe cases; after exposure to eyes: wash with water for at least 15 minutes; seek medical attention in severe cases; o after exposure to skin: irrigate thoroughly with water; seek medical attention in severe cases.

Used in chemical industry; cosmetics industry.

TLV 1ppm.

"Dinitro". See 2,4-dinitro-O-cresol.

Dinitrobenzene. Solid; low inflammability; irritant to eyes, nose and throat; vapour may cause dizziness, nausea and headache; interferes with nervous system; unconsciousness; easily penetrates skin and affects blood (it can't carry oxygen and you may go blue); prolonged exposure may lead to liver and/or kidney damage. o Treatment after inhalation: remove from exposure, rest, keep warm; o after exposure to eyes: irrigate thoroughly with water; seek medical attention in severe cases; o after exposure to skin: drench with water, then wash with soap and water.

Used in cosmetics industry; printing and dyestuffs.

TLV 1mg/cu.m.

Dinitrobenzol. See dinitrobenzene.

2,4-dinitro-O-cresol. Solid; low inflammability; skin sensitizer; dermatitis on prolonged exposure; asthmatic reaction; sweating. o Treatment after inhalation: remove from exposure, rest, keep warm; seek medical attention in severe cases; o after exposure to eyes: irrigate thoroughly with water; seek medical attention in severe cases; o after exposure to skin: irrigate thoroughly with water; swab with glycerol for 10 minutes; seek medical attention in severe cases.

Pesticides and herbicides.

Dinitro-phenols. Solid; low inflammability; skin sensitizer; dermatitis on prolonged expo-

sure; asthmatic reaction; prolonged exposure may lead to liver and/or kidney damage; sweating. o Treatment after inhalation: remove from exposure, rest, keep warm; seek medical attention in severe cases; o after exposure to eyes; irrigate thoroughly with water; seek medical attention in severe cases; o after exposure to skin: irrigate thoroughly with water; swab with glycerol for 10 minutes; seek medical attention in severe cases.

Printing and dyestuffs; explosives.

2,4-dinitrotoluene. Solid; low inflammability; irritant to eyes, nose and throat; irritates or burns skin; prolonged exposure may lead to liver and/or kidney damage; blood poison. o Treatment after exposure to eyes: irrigate thoroughly with water; seek medical attention in severe cases; o after exposure to skin: drench with water, then wash with soap and water.

Explosives.

2,4-dinitrotoluol. See 2,4-dinitrotoluene.

Dioxan. Liquid; high inflammability; irritant to eyes, nose and throat; narcotic; vapour may cause dizziness, nausea and headache; prolonged exposure may lead to liver and/or kidney damage; inflammation of lungs; vomiting and stomach pains. o Treatment after inhalation: remove from exposure, rest, keep warm; seek medical attention in severe cases; o after exposure to eyes: irrigate thoroughly with water; seek medical attention in severe cases; o after exposure to skin: irrigate thoroughly with water.

Solvent – found throughout industry; lacquers, varnishes

and adhesives; plastics, rubbers and resins; printing and dyestuffs. TLV 100ppm.

Diphenylamine. Solid; low inflammability; see aniline and amines.
TLV 10mg/cu.m.

Diphenylmethane di-isocyanate. See di-(isocyanatophenyl)methane.

Dipping acid. See sulphuric acid.

Duomeen. See amines.

Embafume. See methyl bromide.

Enzymes. Dust; sensitizers; asthmatic reaction.
Detergent manufacture. Proteolytic enzymes (as 100 per cent pure crystalline enzyme) have been given a
TLV of 0.003 mg/cu.m.

Epoxy resins. Powders/liquids; skin sensitizers – dermatitis risk; remove from skin immediately; may cause cancer. Plastics; construction; glass fibre moulding; adhesives.

1,2-epoxyethane. See ethylene oxide.

Erythrene. See butadiene.

Ethide. See dichloronitroethane.

Ethyl acetate. Liquid; high inflammability; irritant to eyes, nose and throat; narcotic; skin sensitizer; dermatitis on prolonged exposure. o Treatment after inhalation: remove from exposure, rest, keep warm; o after exposure to eyes: irrigate thoroughly with water; seek medical attention in severe cases; o after exposure to skin: drench with water, then wash with soap and water.
Solvent – found throughout industry; food additive; lacquers, varnishes and adhesives; pharmaceuticals and medicinals; explosives.
TLV 400ppm.

Ethyl acrylate. Liquid; high inflammability; see acrylates.
TLV 25ppm.

Ethyl amine. Liquid, solution or suspension; high inflammability; see amines.
TLV 10ppm.

Ethyl benzene. Liquid; high inflammability. See benzene (does not have the same action on bone marrow as benzene.)
TLV 100ppm.

Ethyl benzol. See ethyl benzene.

Ethyl bromide. Liquid; high inflammability; irritant to eyes, nose and throat; narcotic, prolonged exposure may lead to liver and/or kidney damage; unconsciousness. o Treatment after inhalation: remove from exposure, rest, keep warm; o after exposure to eyes: irrigate thoroughly with water; seek medical attention in severe cases; o after exposure to skin: drench with water, then wash with soap and water.
Refrigeration systems.
TLV 200ppm.

Ethyl carbamate. Solid; low inflammability; vapour may cause dizziness, nausea and headache; interferes with nervous system; possible carcinogen. o Treatment after inhalation: wash out nose and mouth with water; seek medical attention in severe cases; o after exposure to skin: drench with water, then wash with soap and water.
Used in chemical industry; pharmaceuticals and medicinals.

Ethyl chloride. Gas/liquid; high inflammability; irritant to eyes, nose and throat; narcotic. o Treatment after inhalation: remove from exposure, rest, keep warm; o after exposure to eyes: irrigate thoroughly with water; seek medical attention in severe cases; o after exposure to skin: drench with water, then wash with soap and water. Used in cosmetics industry; pharmaceuticals and medicinals; refrigerator systems. TLV 1,000ppm.

Ethyl silicate. Liquid; low inflammability; irritant to eyes, nose and throat; narcotic; irritates or burns skin; prolonged exposure may lead to liver and/or kidney damage. o Treatment after inhalation: remove from exposure, rest, keep warm; seek medical attention in severe cases; o after exposure to eyes: irrigate thoroughly with water; seek medical attention in severe cases; o after exposure to skin: drench with water, then wash with soap and water. Glass industry. TLV 100ppm.

Ethylene chlorhydrin. See chloroethanol. TLV 5ppm.

Ethylene diamine. Liquid; high inflammability; irritant to eyes, nose and throat; skin sensitizer; dermatitis on prolonged exposure; irritates or burns skin; asthmatic reaction. o Treatment after inhalation: remove from exposure, rest, keep warm; o after exposure to eyes; irrigate thoroughly with water; seek medical attention in severe cases; o after exposure to skin: irrigate thoroughly with water. Used in cosmetics industry; lacquers, varnishes and adhesives; plastics, rubbers and resins; cleaning agents; analytical work. TLV 10ppm.

Ethylene dibromide. Liquid; low inflammability; irritant to eyes, nose and throat; narcotic; skin sensitizer; derma-

titis on prolonged exposure; irritates or burns skin; prolonged exposure may lead to liver and/or kidney damage; inflammation of lungs. o Treatment after inhalation: remove from exposure, rest, keep warm; o after exposure to eyes: irrigate thoroughly with water; seek medical attention in severe cases; o after exposure to skin: drench with water, then wash with soap and water. Petroleum and oil, plastics, rubbers and resins.

Ethylene dichloride. See 1,2-dichloroethane. TLV 20ppm.

Ethylene glycol monoethyl ether. See cellosolve.

Ethylene glycol monoethyl ether acetate. See cellosolve acetate. TVL 25ppm.

Ethylene glycol monomethyl ether. See methyl cellosolve.

Ethylene imine. Liquid; high inflammability; irritant to eyes, nose and throat; irritates or burns skin; prolonged exposure may lead to liver and/or kidney damage. o Treatment after inhalation: remove from exposure, rest, keep warm; o after exposure to eyes: irrigate thoroughly with water; seek medical attention in severe cases; o after exposure to skin: drench with water, then wash with soap and water. Used in chemical industry. TLV 0.5ppm.

Ethylene oxide. Very dangerous. Liquid/gas; high inflammability; irritant to eyes, nose and throat; irritates or burns skin; vapour may cause dizziness, nausea and headache; inflammation of lungs, vomiting and stomach pains; often delayed action. o Treatment after inhalation: remove from

exposure, rest, keep warm; seek medical attention in severe cases; o after exposure to eyes: irrigate thoroughly with water; seek medical attention in severe cases; o after exposure to skin: irrigate thoroughly with water.
Used in chemical industry; pesticides and herbicides; sterilizing.
TLV 50ppm.

Ethylene trichloride. See trichloroethylene.

Ethyl methyl ketone. See methyl ethyl ketone.

Flint dust. Solid; nonflammable; can cause silicosis. See section on industrial diseases.
Used in potteries.

Fluorides. Gas, liquid, solid; nonflammable – high inflammability; irritant to eyes, nose and throat; irritates or burns skin; vapour may cause dizziness, nausea, headache; vomiting and stomach pains. o Treatment after inhalation: remove from exposure, rest, keep warm; seek medical attention in severe cases; o after exposure to eyes: irrigate thoroughly with water; seek medical attention in severe cases; o after exposure to skin: irrigate thoroughly with water.
Found extensively throughout industry: disinfectants and fumigants; food additive; pharmaceuticals and medicinals; pesticides and herbicides; analytical work.
TLV 2.5mg/cu.m.

Fluorine. Gas; nonflammable; irritant to eyes, nose and throat; irritates or burns skin. o Treatment after inhalation: remove from exposure, rest, keep warm; seek medical attention in severe cases; o after exposure to eyes: wash with water for at least 15 minutes;

seek medical attention without delay; o after exposure to skin: irrigate thoroughly with water; burns and blisters must receive medical attention quickly.
Used in chemical industry; glass industry.
TLV 1ppm.

Fluoroboric acid. Liquid; nonflammable; irritant to eyes, nose and throat; irritates or burns skin. o Treatment after inhalation: remove from exposure, rest, keep warm; o after exposure to eyes: irrigate thoroughly with water; seek medical attention in severe cases; o after exposure to skin: drench with water and apply magnesia/glycerol paste; burns require medical attention.
Used in chemical industry.

Fluorosilicic acid. Liquid; nonflammable; irritant to eyes, nose and throat; irritates or burns skin. o Treatment after inhalation: remove from exposure, rest, keep warm; seek medical attention in severe cases; o after exposure to eyes: irrigate thoroughly with water; seek medical attention in severe cases; o after exposure to skin: drench with water, and apply magnesia/glycerol paste; burns require medical attention.
Used in chemical industry.

Fluorosulphonic acid. Liquid; low inflammability. See acids.
Used in chemical industry.

Formaldehyde. Gas/solution or suspension; high inflammability; irritant to eyes, nose and throat; irritates or burns skin. o Treatment after inhalation: remove from exposure, rest, keep warm; seek medical attention in severe cases; o after exposure to eyes: irrigate thoroughly with water; seek medical attention

in severe cases; o after exposure to skin: irrigate thoroughly with water.
Disinfectants and fumigants; plastics, rubbers and resins.
TLV 2ppm.

Formalin. See formaldehyde.

Formic acid. Liquid; high inflammability; irritant to eyes, nose and throat; irritates or burns skin. o Treatment after inhalation: remove from exposure, rest, keep warm; o after exposure to eyes: irrigate thoroughly with water; seek medical attention in severe cases; o after exposure to skin: drench with water and apply magnesia/glycerol paste; burns require medical attention.
Used in chemical industry; plastics, rubbers and resins; printing and dyestuffs; textiles and paper; metal industry and metal plating.
TLV 5ppm.

Fuming sulphuric acid. See oleum.

Furfural. Liquid; high inflammability; irritant to eyes, nose and throat; irritates or burns skin: prolonged exposure may lead to liver and/or kidney damage; interferes with nervous system. o Treatment after inhalation: remove from exposure, rest, keep warm; o after exposure to eyes: irrigate thorough with water; seek medical attention in severe cases; o after exposure to skin; drench with water, then wash with soap and water.
Used in chemical industry; lacquers, varnishes and adhesives; paints; plastics, rubbers and resins; printing and dyestuffs.
TLV 5ppm.

2-furaldehyde. See furfural.

Furs. Imported furs may carry anthrax. See section on industrial disease.
Fur trade, warehouses.

Gammexane. See benzene hexachloride.

Genkleen. See trichloroethane.

Genoxide. See hydrogen peroxide.

Gesarol. DDT.

Glacial acetic acid. Liquid; high inflammability; see acids

Glycol monobutyl ether. See butyl cellosolve.

Greenbank. See alkalis.
Used in chemical industry.

Halowax. Solid; low inflammability; skin sensitizer; dermatitis on prolonged exposure; prolonged exposure may also lead to liver and/or kidney damage. o Treatment after exposure to skin: drench with water, then wash with soap and water.
Thermal and/or electrical insulation; greases and lubricants.
TLV 0.2mg/cu.m.

Harvesan. See mercury compounds. Pesticides and herbicides.

Hay. Spores from mouldy hay can cause 'Farmer's Lung' – see section on industrial diseases.

Hexachlorobenzene. Solid; low inflammability. See chlorinated hydrocarbons.
Used in chemical industry; disinfectants and fumigants; explosives; stabilisers.

Hexachlorocyclohexane. See benzene hexachloride.

Hexachloroethane. Liquid; nonflammable; narcotic; vapour may cause dizziness; nausea and headache; prolonged exposure may lead to liver and/or kidney damage.
o Treatment after inhalation: remove from exposure, rest, keep warm; seek medical attention in severe cases; o after

exposure to eyes: irrigate thoroughly with water; seek medical attention in severe cases.
Used in chemical industry.
TLV 1ppm.

Hexachloronaphthalene. See halowax.

Hexamethylene tetramine. Solid; low inflammability; skin sensitizer; irritates or burns skin; dermatitis on prolonged exposure. o Treatment after exposure to eyes: irrigate thoroughly with water; seek medical attention in severe cases; o after exposure to skin: drench with water, then wash with soap and water.
Plastics, rubbers and resins.

Hexamine. See hexamethylene tetramine.

Hexo. See alkalis. Cleaning agents.

Hides. Imported hides may carry anthrax spores. See section on industrial diseases.
Docks, warehouses, tanning.

Hydrazine. Liquid, solution or suspension; low inflammability; irritant to eyes, nose and throat; skin sensitizer; dermatitis on prolonged exposure; irritates or burns skin; possible carcinogen (may cause cancer). o Treatment after exposure to eyes: irrigate thoroughly with water; seek medical attention in severe cases; o after exposure to skin: irrigate thoroughly with water.
Fuels and propellants.
TLV 1ppm.

Hydrobromic acid. Solution or suspension; nonflammable; See acids.
Used in chemical industry.

Hydrochloric acid. Solution or suspension; nonflammable; see acids.
Found extensively throughout industry.

Hydrocyanic acid. See hydrogen cyanide.

Hydrofluoric acid. Solution; nonflammable; irritant to eyes, nose and throat; irritates or burns skin. o Treatment after inhalation: remove from exposure, rest, keep warm; seek medical attention without delay; o after exposure to eyes: irrigate thoroughly with water; seek medical attention without delay; o after exposure to skin: wash with water for at least 15 minutes; seek medical attention without delay; drench with water and apply magnesia/glycerol paste.
Glass industry, stone cleaning, printed circuits.

Hydrogen chloride. Gas; nonflammable; irritant to eyes, nose and throat; irritates or burns skin. o Treatment after inhalation: remove from exposure, rest, keep warm; seek medical attention in severe cases; o after exposure to eyes: irrigate thoroughly with water; seek medical attention in severe cases; o after exposure to skin: drench with water and apply magnesia/ glycerol paste; burns require medical attention.
Found extensively throughout industry.
TLV 5ppm.

Hydrogen cyanide. Gas/liquid; high inflammability; vapour may cause dizziness, nausea, headache; unconsciousness; vomiting and stomach pains; paralysis. o Treatment after inhalation: remove from exposure, rest, keep warm; break amyl nitrite capsule for inhalation; seek medical attention without delay; o after exposure to eyes: irrigate thoroughly with water: seek medical attention in severe cases; o after exposure to skin: irrigate thoroughly with water.

Used in chemical industry; disinfectants and fumigants; pesticides and herbicides. TLV 10ppm.

Hydrogen peroxide. Liquid, solution or suspension; explosive – strong oxidizing agent; spontaneous ignition is possible on contact with other substances; irritant to eyes, nose and throat; irritates or burns skin. o Treatment after exposure to eyes: irrigate thoroughly with water; seek medical attention in severe cases; o after exposure to skin: irrigate thoroughly with water; burns and blisters must receive medical attention.
Fuels and propellants.
TLV 1ppm.

Hydrogen sulphide. Gas; high inflammability; irritant to eyes, nose and throat; may cause dizziness, nausea and headache. o Treatment after inhalation: remove from exposure, rest, keep warm; seek medical attention in severe cases.
Found extensively throughout industry; used in chemical industry; plastics, rubbers and resins, viscose rayon manufacture; analytical work; sewerage.
TLV 10ppm.

Hydroquinone. Solid; low inflammability; skin sensitizer; dermatitis on prolonged exposure; vapour may cause dizziness, nausea and headache. o Treatment after inhalation: remove from exposure, rest, keep warm; o after exposure to eyes: irrigate thoroughly with water; seek medical attention in severe cases; o after exposure to skin: drench with water, then

wash with soap and water.
Stabilisers.
TLV 2mg/cu.m.

4-hydroxy-4-methyl pentan-2-one. See diacetone alcohol.

Hydroxy naphthalenes. See naphthols.

α-hydroxytoluene. See benzyl alcohol.

Hylene. See isocyanates.

Iodine. Solid, suspension or solution; nonflammable; irritant to eyes, nose and throat; irritates or burns skin. o Treatment after inhalation: remove from exposure, rest, keep warm; o after exposure to eyes: irrigate thoroughly with water; seek medical attention in severe cases; o after exposure to skin: bathe in dilute sodium thiosulphate solution.
Used in chemical industry; pharmaceuticals and medicinals; printing and dyestuffs; detergents and soaps.
TLV 0.1ppm.

Iodomethane. See methyl iodide.

Isobutyl methyl ketone. See methyl isobutyl ketone.

Isocon. See isocyanates.

Isocyanates (see also di-isocyanates). Liquid, solid; high inflammability – nonflamable; irritant to eyes, nose and throat; skin sensitizer; dermatitis on prolonged exposure; asthmatic reaction. o Treatment after inhalation: remove from exposure, rest, keep warm; seek medical attention in severe cases; o after exposure to eyes: irrigate thoroughly with water; seek medical attention in severe cases; o after exposure to skin: drench with water, then wash with soap and water.
Used in chemical industry; plastics; paints; lacquers; thermal insulation.

Isophorone. Liquid; high inflammability; irritant to eyes, nose and throat; irritates or burns skin. o Treatment after inhalation: remove from exposure, rest, keep warm; o after exposure to eyes: irrigate thoroughly with water; seek medical attention in severe cases; o after exposure to skin: drench with water, then wash with soap and water. Solvent – found throughout industry; plastics, rubbers and resins. TLV 10ppm.

Isoprene. Liquid; high inflammability: irritant to eyes, nose and throat; narcotic; irritates or burns skin; o Treatment after inhalation: remove from exposure, rest, keep warm; o after exposure to eyes: irrigate thoroughly with water; seek medical attention in severe cases; o after exposure to skin: drench with water, then wash with soap and water. Plastics, rubbers and resins.

Isopropyl benzene. See cumene.

Isopropyl ether. Liquid; high inflammability; irritant to eyes, nose and throat; narcotic; irritates or burns skin. o Treatment after inhalation: remove from exposure, rest, keep warm; o after exposure to eyes: irrigate thoroughly with water; seek medical attention in severe cases; o after exposure to skin: drench with water, then wash with soap and water. Solvent – found throughout industry; petroleum and oil. TLV 250ppm.

Kacynoids. See cyanides.

Kaydox. See chlorinated hydrocarbons.

Kypchlor. See chlorinated hydrocarbons. Pesticides and herbicides.

Lead and compounds. Solid, liquid; nonflammable – high inflammability; vapour may cause dizziness, nausea and headache; interferes with nervous system; blood poison; vomiting and stomach pains; lead poisoning is one of the commonest of occupational diseases. Paints; petroleum and oil; printing and dyestuffs; metal industry and metal plating; scrap metal; battery manufacture. For full details see Section 5, Disease. TLV (inorganic compounds, fumes and dusts) 0.15 mg/cu.m.

Lead tetraethyl. See tetraethyl lead.

Leytosan. See mercury compounds. Pesticides and herbicides.

Lindane. See benzene hexachloride. TLV 0.5 mg/cu.m.

Lorexame. See benzene hexachloride.

Lunasan. See mercury compounds.

Lunevale. See mercury compounds.

Magenta. Controlled substance under Carcinogenic Substances Regulations 1967.

Malathion. Solid/solution or suspension; low inflammability; skin sensitizer; dermatitis on prolonged exposure; interferes with nervous system; paralysis. o Treatment after inhalation: remove from exposure, rest, keep warm; seek medical attention in severe cases; o after exposure to eyes: irrigate thoroughly with water; seek medical attention in severe cases; o after exposure to skin: drench with water, then wash with soap and water. Pesticides. TLV 10mg/cu.m.

N

Manganese and compounds.
Solid; strong oxidity agents –
spontaneous ignition is possible on contact with other
substances; low inflamma-
bility – nonflammable; interferes with nervous system;
loss of co-ordination, 'manganism'; causes acute lung
condition (pneumonitis) in
permanganate manufacture.
Textiles and paper; metal industry and metal plating;
welding and hard-facing;
glass industry.
TLV 5mg/cu.m.

MDI – see isocyanates.

MEK. See methyl ethyl ketone.

Mercury. Very toxic liquid
metal; nonflammable; mainly
chronic effects: attacks nervous system – tremor and
withdrawn behaviour on long
exposure; prolonged exposure
may also lead to liver and/or
kidney damage. o Treatment
after inhalation: remove from
exposure, rest, keep warm;
seek medical attention in severe cases; o after exposure to
eyes: irrigate thoroughly with
water; seek medical attention
in severe cases; o after exposure to skin: irrigate thoroughly with water.
Found extensively throughout
industry; chemicals; plastics;
thermometers, mercury
switches. Described more
fully in text.
TLV 0.05mg/cu.m.

Mercury compounds. Solid;
nonflammable – low inflammability. More acutely poisonous than the metal; also
serious long term effects.
Organic compounds among
the most toxic of all substances. Treatment as above.
Disinfectants and fumigants;
pharmaceuticals and medi-
cinals; pesticides, fungicides
(particularly seed dressings);
explosives; pigments. Describ-

ed more fully in text.
TLV 0.01mg/cu.m.

Mesityl oxide. Liquid; high inflammability; irritant to eyes,
nose and throat; irritates or
burns skin; prolonged exposure may lead to liver and/or
kidney damage. o Treatment
after inhalation: remove from
exposure, rest, keep warm;
o after exposure to eyes: irrigate thoroughly with water;
seek medical attention in severe cases; o after exposure to
skin: drench with water, then
wash with soap and water.
Solvent – found throughout
industry; plastics, rubbers and
resins.
TLV 25ppm.

Methacrylic acid. Liquid,
solid; high inflammability;
irritant to eyes, nose and
throat; irritates or burns skin.
o Treatment after inhalation:
remove from exposure, rest,
keep warm; o after exposure
to eyes: irrigate thoroughly
with water; seek medical attention in severe cases; o after
exposure to skin: irrigate
thoroughly with water.
Plastics, rubbers and resins.

Methoxychlor. Solid; low in-
flammability; see DDT.
Pesticides and herbicides.
TLV 10mg/cu.m.

Methyl acetate. Liquid; high
inflammability; see acetates.
o Treatment after inhalation:
remove from exposure, rest,
keep warm; seek medical attention in severe cases; o after
exposure to eyes: irrigate
thoroughly with water; seek
medical attention in severe
cases; o after exposure to
skin: drench with water, then
wash with soap and water.
Solvent – found throughout
industry; lacquers, varnishes
and adhesives; paints; plastics, rubbers and resins.
TLV 200ppm.

β-methyl acrolein. See crotonaldehyde.

Methyl acrylate. Liquid; high
inflammability; see acrylates.
o Treatment after inhalation:
remove from exposure, rest,
keep warm; o after exposure
to eyes: irrigate thoroughly
with water; seek medical attention in severe cases; o after
exposure to skin: drench with
water, then wash with soap
and water.
Plastics, rubbers and resins.
TLV 10ppm.

Methylamine. Gas, solution or
suspension; high inflammability. See amines.
TLV 10ppm.

Methyl amyl alcohol. See
methyl isobutyl carbinol.
TLV 25ppm.

'N-methyl aniline. Liquid; high
inflammability; see aniline.
Pharmaceuticals, and medicinals; plastics, rubbers and
resins; printing and dyestuffs.

O-methyl aniline. See O-toluidine.

Methyl benzene. Same as
toluene.

Methyl bromide. Liquid, gas;
easily penetrates clothing,
skin; high inflammability;
irritant to eyes, nose and
throat; irritates or burns skin;
may cause dizziness, nausea
and headache; vomiting and
stomach pains. o Treatment
after inhalation: remove from
exposure, rest, keep warm;
seek medical attention in severe cases; o after exposure to
eyes: irrigate thoroughly with
water; seek medical attention
in severe cases; o after exposure to skin: drench with
water, then wash with soap
and water; burns and blisters
must receive medical attention.
Used in chemical industry;
pesticides and herbicides;
used in fire extinguishers –

this type should not be kept
or used indoors.
TLV 15ppm.

2-methylbuta-1,3-diene. See
isoprene.

Methyl butyl ketones. Liquid;
high inflammability; irritant
to eyes, nose and throat; narcotic; irritates or burns skin.
o Treatment after inhalation:
remove from exposure, rest,
keep warm; o after exposure
to eyes: irrigate thoroughly
with water; seek medical attention in severe cases.
Solvent – found throughout
industry; lacquers, varnishes
and adhesives.
TLV 100ppm.

Methyl carbitol. See carbitol.

Methyl cellosolve. Liquid; high
inflammability; blood poison.
o Treatment after inhalation:
remove from exposure, rest,
keep warm; o after exposure
to eyes: irrigate thoroughly
with water; seek medical attention in severe cases; o after
exposure to skin: irrigate
thoroughly with water.
Solvent – used throughout industry; lacquers, varnishes
and adhesives.
TLV 25ppm.

Methyl chloride. Gas; high inflammability; narcotic; may
cause dizziness, nausea and
headache; prolonged expo-
sure may lead to liver and/or
kidney damage; interferes
with nervous system. o Treatment after inhalation: remove
from exposure, rest, keep
warm; seek medical attention
in severe cases.
Pharmaceuticals and medi-
cinals; refrigeration.
TLV 100ppm.

Methyl chloroform. See trichloroethane.

Methyl cyclohexanol. Liquid;
high inflammability. See
cyclohexanol.
Chemical industry. TLV 50ppm

Methyl cyclohexanone. Liquid, high inflammability. See cyclohexanone.
Chemical industry.

Methylene chloride. See dichloromethane.

Methyl ethyl ketone. Liquid; high inflammability; irritant to eyes, nose and throat; irritates or burns skin. o Treatment after inhalation: remove from exposure, rest, keep warm; o after exposure to eyes: irrigate thoroughly with water; seek medical attention in severe cases; o after exposure to skin: drench with water, then wash with soap and water.
Solvent – found throughout industry; lacquers, varnishes and adhesives; plastics, rubbers and resins.
TLV 200ppm.

Methyl iodide. Liquid; high inflammability; irritant to eyes, nose and throat; irritates or burns skin; vapour may cause dizziness, nausea and headache. o Treatment after inhalation: remove from exposure, rest, keep warm; seek medical attention in severe cases; o after exposure to eyes: irrigate thoroughly with water; seek medical attention in severe cases; o after exposure to skin: drench with water, then wash with soap and water.
Used in chemical industry.
TLV 5ppm.

Methyl isobutyl carbinol. Liquid; high inflammability; irritant to eyes, nose and throat; irritates or burns skin. o Treatment after inhalation: remove from exposure, rest, keep warm; o after exposure to eyes: irrigate thoroughly with water; seek medical attention in severe cases; o after exposure to skin: drench with water, then wash with soap

and water.
Solvent – found throughout industry; used in cosmetics industry; lacquers, varnishes and adhesives. TLV 25ppm.

Methyl isobutyl ketone. Liquid; high inflammability; irritant to eyes, nose and throat; narcotic; irritates or burns skin. o Treatment after inhalation: remove from exposure, rest, keep warm; o after exposure to eyes: irrigate thoroughly with water; seek medical attention in severe cases; o after exposure to skin: drench with water, then wash with soap and water.
Solvent – found throughout industry; lacquers, varnishes and adhesives; plastics, rubbers and resins.
TLV 100ppm.

Methyl isocyanate. Liquid; high inflammability; irritant to eyes, nose and throat; irritates or burns skin. o Treatment after inhalation: remove from exposure, rest, keep warm; seek medical attention in severe cases; o after exposure to eyes: irrigate thoroughly with water; seek medical attention in severe cases; o after exposure to skin: drench with water, then wash with soap and water.
Used in chemical industry.
TLV 0.02ppm.

Methyl isopropyl ketone. See methyl isobutyl ketone.

Methyl methacrylate. Liquid; high inflammability; irritant to eyes, nose and throat. o Treatment after inhalation: remove from exposure, rest, keep warm; o after exposure to eyes: irrigate thoroughly with water; seek medical attention in severe cases; o after exposure to skin: drench with water, then wash with soap and water.
Plastics, rubbers and resins.

TLV 100ppm.

4-methyl-3-penten-2-one. See mesityl oxide.

Methylated naphthalene. Solid; low inflammability; see naphthalene.

Methyl sulphate. See dimethyl sulphate.

M.I.B.K. See methyl isobutyl ketone.

Mica. Solid; nonflammable; can cause silicosis; no short term effects on exposure; see section on industrial diseases. Thermal and/or electrical insulation; plastics, rubbers and resins.

Monochlorobenzene. Liquid; high inflammability. See chlorinated hydrocarbons.

Monochloroethylene. See vinyl chloride.

Monochlorhydrin. Liquid; high inflammability; narcotic; prolonged exposure may lead to liver and/or kidney damage. o Treatment after inhalation: remove from exposure, rest, keep warm; o after exposure to eyes: irrigate thoroughly with water; seek medical attention in severe cases; o after exposure to skin: drench with water, then wash with soap and water. Printing and dyestuffs; textiles and paper; explosives.

Monsanto penta. See pentachlorophenol.

Murcocide. See mercury compounds.

Murcolite. See mercury compounds.

Murcurite. See mercury compounds.

Murfixtan. See mercury compounds.

Muriatic acid. See hydrochloric acid.

Naphtha. Liquid; high inflammability; narcotic; see benzene (not blood or cancer risk).

Solvent – found throughout industry; paints; plastics, rubbers and resins. TLV 100ppm.

Naphthols. Solid; low inflammability; irritant to eyes, nose and throat; skin sensitizer; dermatitis on prolonged exposure; irritates or burns skin; prolonged exposure may lead to liver and/or kidney damage. o Treatment after inhalation: remove from exposure, rest, keep warm; seek medical attention in severe cases; o after exposure to eyes: irrigate thoroughly with water; seek medical attention in severe cases; o after exposure to skin: irrigate thoroughly with water; swab with glycerol for 10 minutes. Pharmaceuticals and medicinals.

α-naphthylamine. Bladder carcinogen. Use controlled under the Carcinogenic Substances Regulations 1967. Sealed plants only.

β-naphthylamine. Powerful bladder carcinogen. Use prohibited under the Carcinogenic Substances Regulations 1967.

Nickel carbonyl (production of nickel by Mond process). Very toxic. Liquid; explosive; irritant to eyes, nose and throat; possible carcinogen (may cause cancer). o Treatment after inhalation: remove from exposure, rest, keep warm; seek medical attention in severe cases. Metal industry. TLV 0.001ppm.

Nicotine. Solid, solution or suspension; low inflammability; vapour may cause dizziness, nausea and headache; vomiting and stomach pains; mental disturbances. o Treatment after exposure to eyes: irrigate thoroughly with

water; seek medical attention in severe cases; o after exposure to skin: drench with water, then wash with soap and water.
Pesticide.
TLV 0.5mg/cu.m.

Nitramine. See tetryl.

Nitrating acid. See nitric and sulphuric acids.

Nitric acid. See acids. Strong oxidising agent – organic substances can burst into flames on contact; gives off nitrogen dioxide.
Found extensively throughout industry. See Section 5, Disease.
TLV 2ppm.

Nitroanilines. Solid; low inflammability. See aniline.
Printing and dyestuffs.
TLV (p-nitroaniline) 1ppm.

Nitrobenzene. Liquid; high inflammability; irritant to eyes, nose and throat; irritates or burns skin; vapour may cause dizziness, nausea and headache; unconsciousness; blood poison; vomiting and stomach pains. o Treatment after inhalation: remove from exposure, rest, keep warm; seek medical attention in severe cases; o exposure to eyes: irrigate thoroughly with water; seek medical attention in severe cases; o after exposure to skin: drench with water, then wash with soap and water.
Used in cosmetics industry; printing and dyestuffs; shoe polish; explosives.
TLV 1ppm.

Nitrodiphenyl. Solid; low inflammability; powerful bladder carcinogen; the use of this substance is prohibited in the UK by the Carcinogenic Substances Regulations 1967.

Nitrophenols. Solid; low inflammability; see phenol.
Printing and dyestuffs; analytical work.

Nitropropane. Liquid; high inflammability; irritant to eyes, nose and throat; prolonged exposure may lead to liver and/or kidney damage. o Treatment after inhalation: remove from exposure, rest, keep warm; o after exposure to eyes: irrigate thoroughly with water; seek medical attention in severe cases; o after exposure to skin: drench with water, then wash with soap and water.
Solvent – used throughout industry; plastics, rubbers and resins.
TLV 25ppm.

Nitrosamines. Liquid, solid; low inflammability – high inflammability; possible carcinogens; no short term effects on exposure.
Used in chemical industry.

N-nitrosodimethylamine. Powerful carcinogen. Don't work in same place as it unless process is completely sealed and every safeguard against exposure built in.

Nitrotoluenes. Liquid, solid; low inflammability – high inflammability; see nitrobenzene.
Printing and dyestuffs; explosives. TLV 5ppm.

Nitrous oxides, 'nitrous fumes'. See nitric acid.
Fertiliser manufacture; welding fumes; metal pickling; anywhere that nitric acid is used.
TLV (nitrogen dioxide) 5ppm.

'Octa klor'. See chlordane.

Octalene. See aldrin.

'Octalox'. See dieldrin.

Oil of mirbane. See nitrobenzene.

Oil of vitriol. See sulphuric acid.

Oleum. Liquid; nonflammable; see acids.
Used in chemical industry,

Orthophosphoric acid. Solid, solution or suspension; non-flammable; see acids.
Used in chemical industry.

Ortho-tolidine. Causes bladder cancer. Controlled substance under the Carcinogenic Substances Regulations 1967.

Oxalic acid. Highly toxic. Solid; low inflammability; irritates or burns skin; prolonged exposure may lead to liver and/or kidney damage. o Treatment after inhalation: remove from exposure, rest, keep warm; seek medical attention in severe cases; o after exposure to eyes: irrigate thoroughly with water; seek medical attention in severe cases; o after exposure to skin: irrigate thoroughly with water.
Used in chemical industry; printing and dyestuffs; cleaning agents. TLV 1mg/cu.m.

Oxalates. Solid; low inflammability; see oxalic acid.

Oxzone. See hydrogen per-oxide.

Ozone. Very highly toxic. Gas; explosive; nonflammable; strong oxidizing agent – spontaneous ignition is possible on contact with other substances; irritant to eyes, nose and throat; lung tissue; may cause nausea and headache. o Treatment after inhalation: remove from exposure, rest, keep warm; seek medical attention in severe cases.
Disinfectants and fumigants; petroleum and oil; textiles and paper; given off in arc welding. TLV 0.1ppm.

Paraquat. Liquid, solid or solution; systemic poison for which there is no known antidote; should be handled with great care especially concentrated liquids.
TLV 0.5mg/cu.m. Herbicide.

Parathion. Liquid, solution or suspension; low inflammability; penetrates skin; interferes with nervous system; vapour may cause dizziness, nausea and headache; unconsciousness; sweating. o Treatment after inhalation: remove from exposure, rest, keep warm; seek medical attention in severe cases; o after exposure to eyes: irrigate thoroughly with water; seek medical attention in severe cases; o after exposure to skin: drench with water, then wash with soap and water.
Pesticides.
TLV 0.1mg/cu.m.

Paris Green. See arsenic.

Pentaborane. Liquid; high inflammability; see boron hydrides.
TLV 0.005ppm.

Pentachlorethane. Liquid; low inflammability; irritant to eyes, nose and throat; vapour may cause dizziness, nausea and headache; prolonged exposure may lead to liver and/or kidney damage; interferes with nervous system; unconsciousness; blood poison. o Treatment after inhalation: remove from exposure, rest, keep warm; seek medical attention in severe cases; o after exposure to eyes: irrigate thoroughly with water; seek medical attention in severe cases; o after exposure to skin: drench with water, then wash with soap and water.
Solvent – found throughout industry.

Pentalin. See pentachloroethane.

Pentane-2,4-dione. See acetyl acetone.

Pentachlorphenol. Solid; low inflammability; irritant to eyes, nose and throat; skin sensitizer; dermatitis on prolonged exposure; uncon-

sciousness. o Treatment after inhalation: remove from exposure, rest, keep warm; seek medical attention in severe cases; o after exposure to eyes: irrigate thoroughly with water; seek medical attention in severe cases; o after exposure to skin: drench with water, then wash with soap and water.
Pesticides and herbicides. TLV 0.5mg/cu.m.

Pentyl acetate. Liquid; high inflammability; see amyl acetates.

Perchlorates. Solid; explosive; strong oxidizing agents – spontaneous ignition is possible on contact with other substances; irritant to eyes, nose and throat; irritates or burns skin; o Treatment after exposure to eyes: irrigate thoroughly with water; seek medical attention in severe cases; o after exposure to skin: irrigate thoroughly with water.
Used in chemical industry; analytical work.

Perchloric acid. Liquid; explosive; strong oxidity agent – spontaneous ignition is possible on contact with other substances; see acids.
Used in chemical industry; analytical work.

Perchloroethylene. See tetrachloroethylene.
Dry cleaning, degreasing. TLV 100ppm.

Peroxyl. See hydrogen peroxide.

Phelam. See mercury compounds.

Phenols. Solid/liquid (melts at 41degC); low inflammability; irritant to eyes, nose and throat; skin sensitizer; dermatitis on prolonged exposure; irritates or burns skin; vapour may cause dizziness, nausea and headache; prolonged ex-

posure may lead to liver and/or kidney damage. o Treatment after inhalation: remove from exposure, rest, keep warm; seek medical attention in severe cases; o after exposure to eyes: irrigate thoroughly with water for at least 10 minutes; seek medical attention in severe cases; o after exposure to skin: remove splashed clothing; irrigate thoroughly with water; swab with glycerol or polyethylene glycol for 10 minutes (this treatment must be applied immediately).
Used in chemical industry; disinfectants and fumigants; plastics, particularly bakelite manufacture, rubbers and resins. TLV 5ppm.

Phenyl ethylene. See styrene.

Phenyl hydrazine (and hydrochloride). Liquid, solid; high inflammability; irritant to eyes, nose and throat; skin sensitizer; dermatitis on prolonged exposure; vapour may cause dizziness, nausea and headache; prolonged exposure may lead to liver and/or kidney damage; blood poison. o Treatment after inhalation: remove from exposure, rest, keep warm; seek medical attention in severe cases; o after exposure to eyes: irrigate thoroughly with water; seek medical attention in severe cases; o after exposure to skin: drench with water, then wash with soap and water.
Used in chemical industry; pharmaceuticals and medicinals; printing and dyestuffs. TLV 5ppm.

Phosgene. Very toxic. Gas; nonflammable; easily breathed – hence its use as a war gas; interferes with nervous system; inflammation of lungs. o Treatment after inhalation: remove from exposure, rest, keep warm; seek medical attention without delay; o after exposure to eyes: irrigate thoroughly with water; seek medical attention in severe cases; o after exposure to skin: drench with water, then wash with soap and water. Printing and dyestuffs; metal industry and metal plating; given off when some degreasing agents are thermally decomposed notably chlorinated hydrocarbons. TLV 0.1ppm.

Phosphine. Gas; high inflammability; may cause dizziness, nausea and headache; interferes with nervous system; inflammation of lungs. o Treatment after inhalation: remove from exposure, rest, keep warm; seek medical attention in severe cases. Used in chemical industry; metal industry and metal plating; machining of spheroidal graphite iron. TLV 0.3ppm.

Phosphoric acid. Liquid; nonflammable; see acids. Used in chemical industry. TLV 1mg/cu.m.

Phosphoric oxide. See phosphorus pentoxide.

Phosphorus oxychloride. Liquid; nonflammable; irritant to eyes, nose and throat; irritates or burns skin; inflammation of lungs. o Treatment after inhalation: remove from exposure, rest, keep warm; seek medical attention in severe cases; o after exposure to eyes: irrigate thoroughly with water; seek medical attention in severe cases; o after exposure to skin: drench with water and apply magnesia/glycerol paste; burns require medical attention. Used in chemical industry.

Phosphorus pentachloride. Solid; nonflammable; irritant to eyes, nose and throat; irritates or burns skin; inflammation of lungs. o Treatment after inhalation: remove from exposure, rest, keep warm; seek medical attention in severe cases; o after exposure to eyes: irrigate thoroughly with water; seek medical attention in severe cases; o after exposure to skin: drench with water and apply magnesia/glycerol paste; burns must receive medical attention. Used in chemical industry. TLV 1mg/cu.m.

Phosphorus pentoxide. Solid; nonflammable; irritant to eyes, nose and throat; irritates or burns skin. o Treatment after inhalation: remove from exposure, rest, keep warm; seek medical attention in severe cases; o after exposure to eyes: irrigate thoroughly with water, seek medical attention; o after exposure to skin: drench with water and apply magnesia/glycerol paste; burns must receive medical attention. Used in chemical industry.

Phosphorus trichloride. Liquid; nonflammable; irritant to eyes, nose and throat; irritates or burns skin; inflammation of lungs. o Treatment after inhalation: remove from exposure, rest, keep warm; seek medical attention in severe cases; o after exposure to eyes: irrigate thoroughly with water; seek medical attention in severe cases; o after exposure to skin: drench with water and apply magnesia/glycerol paste; burns must receive medical attention. Used in chemical industry. TLV 0.5ppm.

Phosphoryl chloride. See phosphorus oxychloride.

Picric acid. Solid; explosive; skin sensitizer; dermatitis on prolonged exposure; vapour may cause dizziness, nausea and headache; vomiting and stomach pains. o Treatment after inhalation: remove from exposure, rest, keep warm; get medical attention; after exposure to eyes: irrigate thoroughly with water; seek medical attention in severe cases; o after exposure to skin: irrigate thoroughly with water.
Disinfectants and fumigants; pharmaceuticals and medicinals; printing and dyestuffs; explosives.
TLV 0.1mg/cu.m.

Pimelic ketone. See cyclohexanone.

Piperazine. Solid; low inflammability; irritant to eyes, nose and throat; irritates or burns skin; sensitizer. o Treatment after inhalation: remove from exposure, rest, keep warm; o after exposure to eyes: irrigate thoroughly with water; seek medical attention in severe cases; o after exposure to skin: irrigate thoroughly with water.
Pharmaceuticals and medicinals.

Polyurethane. Solid, liquid; highly inflammable; see isocyanates, and, particularly, TDI (used in manufacture). See hydrogen cyanide and carbon monoxide (given off when polyurethane foam burns). Foams must not be stored in large quantities. See Index for other references.

Potassium cyanide. Solid; nonflammable; see cyanides.

Potassium dichromate. Solid; strong oxidizing agent – spontaneous ignition is possible on contact with other substances. See chromates.

Potassium fluoride. Solid; non-flammable; see fluorides.

Potassium hydrogen fluoride. Solid; nonflammable. See fluorides.

Potassium hydrogen sulphate. Solid; nonflammable; irritant to eyes, nose and throat; irritates or burns skin. o Treatment after exposure to eyes: irrigate thoroughly with water; seek medical attention in severe cases; o after exposure to skin: drench with water, then wash with soap and water. Food additive.

Potassium hydroxide. Solid, suspension or solution; nonflammable; irritant to eyes, nose and throat; irritates or burns skin. o Treatment after exposure to eyes: irrigate thoroughly with water; seek medical attention in severe cases; o after exposure to skin: drench with water, then wash with soap and water. Found extensively throughout industry; pharmaceuticals and medicinals; printing and dyestuffs; metal industry and metal plating; detergents and soaps; analytical work.

Potassium perchlorate. Solid; strong oxidizing agent – spontaneous ignition is possible on contact with other substances. See perchlorates.

Propanol (propyl alcohol). Liquid; high inflammability; narcotic. o Treatment after inhalation: remove from exposure, rest, keep warm; after exposure to eyes: irrigate thoroughly; after exposure to skin: drench and wash with soap and water. Solvent used throughout industry. TLV 200ppm.

Propargyl bromide. See 3-bromopropyne.

Propiolactone. Liquid: high inflammability; irritates or burns skin; possible carcinogen (may cause cancer).

○ Treatment after exposure to eyes: irrigate thoroughly with water; seek medical attention in severe cases; ○ after exposure to skin: drench with water, then wash with soap and water.
Used in chemical industry; plastics, rubbers and resins.

β-propiolactone. Powerful carcinogen. Don't work in same place unless process is completely sealed and all possible safeguards built in.

Propionaldehyde. Liquid; high inflammability; irritant to eyes, nose and throat. ○ Treatment after inhalation: remove from exposure, rest, keep warm; ○ after exposure to eyes: irrigate thoroughly with water; seek medical attention in severe cases.
Used in chemical industry; cosmetics industry; food additive; lacquers, varnishes and adhesives; plastics, rubbers and resins.

Propionic acid. Liquid; high inflammability. See acids.

Propyl amines. Liquid; high inflammability. See amines.

Propyl cyanide. See butyronitrile.

Propylene dichloride. Liquid; high inflammability; one of the most toxic chlorohydrocarbons; irritates or burns skin; prolonged exposure may lead to liver and/or kidney damage. ○ Treatment after inhalation: remove from exposure, rest, keep warm; seek medical attention in severe cases; ○ after exposure to eyes: irrigate thoroughly with water; seek medical attention in severe cases; ○ after exposure to skin: drench with water, then wash with soap and water.
Solvent – found throughout industry; used in chemical industry; disinfectants and fumigants; cleaning agents.

TLV 75ppm.
Prussite. See cyanogen.
PTFE. See teflon.
Purochem. See tin compounds.
Pyridine. Liquid; high inflammability; irritant to eyes, nose and throat; skin sensitizer; dermatitis on prolonged exposure; irritates or burns skin; vapour may cause dizziness, nausea and headache; interferes with nervous system; vomiting and stomach pains. ○ Treatment after inhalation: remove from exposure, rest, keep warm; ○ after exposure to eyes: irrigate thoroughly with water; seek medical attention in severe cases; ○ after exposure to skin: irrigate thoroughly with water.
Solvent – found throughout industry; paints; plastics, rubbers and resins; explosives.
TLV 5ppm.

Quartz. See silica; causes silicosis – see Section 5, Disease.
Quicksilver. See mercury.
Quinol. See hydroquinone.
Quinone. See benzoquinone.
TLV 0.1ppm.

Resorcinol. Solid; low inflammability; see phenols. Disinfectants, printing and dyestuffs; analytical work.

Sextol. See cyclohexanol.
Sextone. See cyclohexanone.
Selenium compounds. eg hydrogen selenide. Gas, solid; generally low inflammability; irritant to eyes, nose and throat; skin sensitizers; dermatitis on prolonged exposure; irritates or burns skin; inflammation of lungs. ○ Treatment after inhalation: remove from exposure, rest, keep warm; ○ after exposure to eyes: irrigate thoroughly with water; seek medical attention in severe cases;

o after exposure to skin: drench with water, then wash with soap and water.

Paints; metal industry and metal plating; glass industry; stabilisers.

TLV 0.2mg/cu.m.

Silica (fine powder). Solid; nonflammable; can cause silicosis; no short term effects on exposure. Mining; quarrying; foundries; potteries; in manufacture of scouring powders.

Slate. See silica.

Sodamide. Solid; low inflammability; irritant to eyes, nose and throat; irritates or burns skin. o Treatment after inhalation: remove from exposure, rest, keep warm; o after exposure to eyes: irrigate thoroughly with water; seek medical attention in severe cases; o after exposure to skin: irrigate thoroughly with water. Used in chemical industry.

Sodium amide. See sodamide.

Sodium azide. Solid; nonflammable; irritant to eyes, nose and throat; irritates or burns skin. o Treatment after exposure to eyes: irrigate thoroughly with water; seek medical attention in severe cases; o after exposure to skin: drench with water, then wash with soap and water. Explosives.

Sodium chlorate. Solid; nonflammable; strong oxidizing agent – spontaneous ignition is possible on contact with other substances (eg when solution dries on grass in the sun); irritant to eyes, nose and throat; irritates or burns skin; vapour may cause dizziness, nausea and headache; prolonged exposure may lead to liver and/or kidney damage; vomiting and stomach pains. o Treatment after exposure to eyes: irrigate thoroughly with water; seek medical at-

tention in severe cases; o after exposure to skin: irrigate thoroughly with water. Pharmaceuticals and medicinals; herbicides (common weedkiller); explosives.

Sodium cyanide. Solid; nonflammable; see cyanides.

Sodium dichromate. Solid; nonflammable; strong oxidizing agent – spontaneous ignition is possible on contact with other substances; see chromates.

Sodium fluoride. Solid; nonflammable; see fluorides.

Sodium hydrogen sulphate. Solid; nonflammable; see acids.

Sodium hydroxide. Solid, solution or suspension; nonflammable; irritant to eyes, nose and throat; irritates or burns skin. o Treatment after exposure to eyes: irrigate thoroughly with water; seek medical attention; o after exposure to skin; irrigate thoroughly with water; seek medical attention

Found extensively throughout industry; petroleum and oil; plastics, rubbers and resins; textiles and paper; cleaning agents. TLV 2mg/cu.m.

Sodium hypochlorite. Solution or suspension; nonflammable; irritant to eyes, nose and throat; irritates or burns skin. o Treatment after exposure to eyes: irrigate thoroughly with water; seek medical attention in severe cases; o after exposure to skin: irrigate thoroughly with water. Used in chemical industry; disinfectants and fumigants, bleach.

Sodium peroxide. Solid; nonflammable; strong oxidizing agent – spontaneous ignition is possible on contact with other substances; irritant to eyes, nose and throat; irritates or

burns skin. o Treatment after inhalation: remove from exposure, rest, keep warm; o after exposure to eyes: irrigate thoroughly with water; seek medical attention in severe cases; o after exposure to skin: drench with water, then wash with soap and water.
Used in chemical industry.

Solunaptol. See phenol.

Solvesso. See benzene.

Stanclere. See tin compounds.

Stannic compounds. See tin compounds.

Stannicide. See tin compounds.

Stannous compounds. See tin compounds.

Stilbine. See antimony and tin compounds.
TLV 0.1ppm.

Styrene. Liquid; high inflammability; irritant to eyes, nose and throat; narcotic; irritates or burns skin. o Treatment after inhalation: remove from exposure, rest, keep warm; o after exposure to eyes: irrigate thoroughly with water; seek medical attention in severe cases; o after exposure to skin: drench with water, then wash with soap and water.
Used in chemical industry; plastics, rubbers and resins. Large amounts of vapour often given off in glass fibre reinforced plastic moulding.
TLV 100ppm.

Sulphonic acids. Solid, solution or suspension; low inflammability; see acids.

Sulphuretted hydrogen. See hydrogen sulphide.

Sulphur chlorides. Gas, liquid; low inflammability; irritant to eyes, nose and throat; irritates or burns skin. o Treatment after inhalation: remove from exposure, rest, keep warm; seek medical attention in severe cases; o after exposure to eyes: irrigate thoroughly with water; seek medical attention

in severe cases; o after exposure to skin: drench with water and apply magnesia/glycerol paste; burns must receive medical attention.
Plastics, rubbers and resins; pesticides and herbicides; textiles and paper.

Sulphur dioxide. Gas; nonflammable; irritant to eyes, nose and throat; irritates or burns skin. o Treatment after inhalation: remove from exposure, rest, keep warm; seek medical attention in severe cases; o after exposure to eyes: irrigate thoroughly with water; seek medical attention in severe cases.
Found throughout industry; food additive; textiles and paper; refrigeration; metal industry and metal plating; common atmospheric pollutant.
TLV 5ppm.

Sulphur fluorides. Gas, liquid; nonflammable; irritant to eyes, nose and throat; irritates or burns skin. o Treatment after inhalation: remove from exposure, rest, keep warm; seek medical attention in severe cases; o after exposure to eyes: irrigate thoroughly with water; seek medical attention in severe cases; o after exposure to skin: drench with water and apply magnesia/glycerol paste. Burns require medical attention.
Thermal and/or electrical insulation.
TLV (sulphur pentafluoride) 0.025ppm.

Sulphuric acid. Liquid; nonflammable. See acids.
TLV 1mg/cu.m.

Sulphur trioxide. Gas; nonflammable; irritant to eyes, nose and throat; irritates or burns skin. o Treatment after inhalation: remove from exposure, rest, keep warm; seek medical attention in severe cases; o after exposure to eyes: irrigate thoroughly with water; seek medical attention in severe cases.

Used in chemical industry.

'Suntobane'. See DDT.

Suprasec. See isocyanates.

Synthite. See formaldehyde.

Tar and pitch. Solid, liquid; low inflammability; fumes irritate eyes, nose and throat; burns from hot tar are main short-term risk; may cause skin cancer on prolonged exposure; keep skin and clothes clean. Watch for warts on skin.

Found extensively throughout industry; particularly construction, patent fuels.

TDI. See toluene di-isocyanate.

TEDP (tetraethyldithionopyrophospate). Liquid; low inflammability; interferes with nervous system. o Treatment after inhalation: remove from exposure, rest, keep warm; after exposure to eyes: irrigate thoroughly with water; seek medical attention in severe cases; o after exposure to skin: drench with water, then wash with soap and water. Pesticides and herbicides. TLV 0.2mg/cu.m.

Teflon. Solid; nonflammable; thermal decomposition products irritate eyes, nose and throat, cause 'polymer fume fever' – see Section 5, Disease. Long term effects not known. o Treatment after inhalation: remove from exposure, rest, keep warm; seek medical attention in severe cases. 'Non-stick' plastics.

Tellurium and compounds. Gas, solid; generally low inflammability; vapour may cause dizziness, nausea and headache; vomiting and stomach pains. o Treatment after

inhalation: remove from exposure, rest, keep warm; seek medical attention in severe cases; o after exposure to eyes: irrigate thoroughly with water; seek medical attention in severe cases; o after exposure to skin: drench with water, then wash with soap and water.

Plastics, rubbers and resins; metal industry and metal plating; glass industry. TLV 0.1mg/cu.m.

Tetrachloroethane. Liquid, easily absorbed through skin; low inflammability; narcotic; vapour may cause dizziness, nausea, and headache; prolonged exposure may lead to liver and/or kidney damage. o Treatment after inhalation: remove from exposure, rest, keep warm; seek medical attention in severe cases; o after exposure to eyes: irrigate thoroughly with water; seek medical attention in severe cases.

Solvent – found throughout industry. TLV 5ppm.

Tetrachloroethylene. Liquid; nonflammable; irritant to eyes, nose and throat; narcotic; vapour may cause dizziness, nausea and headache. o Treatment after inhalation: remove from exposure, rest, keep warm; o after exposure to eyes: irrigate thoroughly with water; seek medical attention in severe cases; o after exposure to skin: drench with water, then wash with soap and water.

Solvent – used throughout industry; detergents and soaps; cleaning agents. TLV 100ppm.

Tetraethyl lead. Liquid – easily penetrates skin; high inflammability; vapour may cause dizziness, nausea and headache; interferes with nervous system; mental disturbances. o Treatment after inhalation: remove from exposure, rest, keep warm; o after exposure to eyes: irrigate thoroughly with water; seek medical attention in severe cases; o after exposure to skin: drench with water, then wash with soap and water. Petroleum additive: workers in garages may unknowingly get exposure from petrol on skin. TLV 0.1mg/cu.m.

Tetraethyl-O-silicate. See ethyl silicate.

Tetraethyl pyrophosphate (TEPP). Liquid – penetrates skin; low inflammability; interferes with nervous system; paralyisis. o Treatment after inhalation: remove from exposure, rest, keep warm; o after exposure to eyes: irrigate thoroughly with water; seek medical attention in severe cases; o after exposure to skin: drench with water, then wash with soap and water. Pesticides and herbicides.

Tetrahydrofuran. Liquid; high inflammability; irritant to eyes, nose and throat; narcotic; blood poison. o Treatment after inhalation: remove from exposure, rest, keep warm; o after exposure to eyes: irrigate thoroughly with water; seek medical attention in severe cases; o after exposure to skin: drench with water, then wash with soap and water. Solvent – found throughout industry.

Tetrahydronaphthalene. See tetralin.

Tetralin. Liquid; high inflammability; irritant to eyes, nose and throat; narcotic; irritates or burns skin; prolonged exposure may lead to liver and/or kidney damage. o Treat-

ment after inhalation: remove from exposure, rest, keep warm; seek medical attention in severe cases; o after exposure to eyes: irrigate thoroughly with water; seek medical attention in severe cases; o after exposure to skin: drench with water, then wash with soap and water. Solvent – found throughout industry; paints; plastics, rubbers and resins; cleaning agents.

Tetramethyl lead. See tetraethyl lead. TLV 0.150 mg/cu.m.

Tetranitromethane. Liquid; explosive; irritant to eyes, nose and throat; prolonged exposure may lead to liver and/or kidney damage; inflammation of lungs. o Treatment after inhalation: remove from exposure, rest, keep warm; seek medical attention in severe cases; o after exposure to eyes: irrigate thoroughly with water; seek medical attention in severe cases; o after exposure to skin: drench with water, then wash with soap and water. Explosives. TLV 1ppm.

Tetryl. Solid; explosive; irritant to eyes, nose and throat; skin sensitizer; dermatitis on prolonged exposure; vapour may cause dizziness, nausea and headache. o Treatment after inhalation: remove from exposure, rest, keep warm; seek medical attention in severe cases; o after exposure to eyes: irrigate thoroughly with water; seek medical attention in severe cases; o after exposure to skin: drench with water, then wash with soap and water. Explosives.

Thionyl chloride. Liquid; nonflammable; irritant to eyes, nose and throat; irritates or burns skin. o Treatment after

inhalation: remove from exposure, rest, keep warm; seek medical attention in severe cases; o after exposure to eyes: irrigate thoroughly with water; seek medical attion in severe cases; o after exposure to skin: drench with water and apply magnesia/glycerol paste; burns must receive medical attention.
Used in chemical industry.

Tin compounds. Gas, solid; generally low inflammability; skin sensitizer; dermatitis on prolonged exposure; irritates or burns skin; prolonged exposure may lead to liver and/or kidney damage; inflammation of lungs. o Treatment after exposure to eyes: irrigate thoroughly with water; seek medical attention in severe cases; o after exposure to skin: drench with water, then wash with soap and water; rashes require medical attention.
Used in chemical industry; pesticides and herbicides; stabilisers.
TLV (organic compounds) 0.1mg/cu.m.
TLV (inorganic compounds) 2mg/cu.m.

Tolidene. Solid; low inflammability; irritates eyes, nose and throat; irritates or burns skin; possible carcinogen (may cause cancer). o Treatment after inhalation: remove from exposure, rest, keep warm; seek medical attention in severe cases; o after exposure to eyes: irrigate thoroughly with water; seek medical attention in severe cases; o after exposure to skin: drench with water, then wash with soap and water.
Printing and dyestuffs.

Toluene. Liquid; high inflammability; see benzene (not blood or cancer risk).

Solvent – used throughout industry; paints, 'thinners', plastics, rubbers and resins. TLV 100ppm. (Your nose loses its ability to warn you of toluene in the air.)

O-toluidine. Liquid; high inflammability; irritant to eyes, nose and throat; vapour may cause dizziness, nausea and headache; prolonged exposure may lead to liver and/or kidney damage; interferes with nervous system; possible carcinogen. o Treatment after inhalation: remove from exsure, rest, keep warm; o after exposure to eyes: irrigate thoroughly with water; seek medical attention in severe cases; o after exposure to skin: drench with water, then wash with soap and water.
Printing and dyestuffs.
TLV 5ppm.

Toluene di-isocyanate (TDI). Liquid. Highly toxic. Highly inflammable. Irritates eyes, nose and throat; small concentrations can cause permanent asthmatic condition; skin sensitizer, causing dermatitis on prolonged exposure.
o Treatment after inhalation: remove from exposure, rest, keep warm; o after exposure to eyes: irrigate thoroughly with water; o after exposure to skin: drench with water, then wash with soap and water. Get immediate medical attention after any exposure.
Plastics, rubbers and resins, particularly manufacture of polyurethane foams, paints and lacquers, 'wet-look' garments. All processes should be sealed and continuous monitoring instruments installed. Paints should be safe with good ventilation, providing they are not sprayed.
TLV 0.02ppm.

Toluol. Same as toluene.

Toxaphene. Solid; low inflammability; irritates or burns skin; prolonged exposure may lead to liver and/or kidney damage; interferes with nervous system. o Treatment after exposure to eyes: irrigate thoroughly with water; seek medical attention in severe cases; o after exposure to skin: drench with water, then wash with soap and water. Pesticides and herbicides.

Tributylphosphate. Liquid; low inflammability; interferes with nervous system. o Treatment after inhalation: remove from exposure, rest, keep warm; o after exposure to eyes: irrigate thoroughly with water; seek medical attention in severe cases; o after exposure to skin: drench with water, then wash with soap and water. Plastics, rubbers and resins. TLV 5mg/cu.m.

Trichloroacetic acid. Solid; low inflammability; see acids. Used in chemical industry; analytical work.

Trichloroethane. Liquid; low inflammability; narcotic; irritates or burns skin. o Treatment after inhalation: remove from exposure, rest, keep warm; o after exposure to eyes: irrigate thoroughly with water; seek medical attention in severe cases; o after exposure to skin: drench with water, then wash with soap and water. Solvent – one of the safest – found throughout industry; used in chemical industry; plastics, rubbers and resins; cleaning agents; see phosgene.

Trichloroethylene. Liquid; low inflammability; irritant to eyes, nose and throat; vapour may cause dizziness, nausea and headache; unconsciousness. o Treatment after inhalation: remove from exposure, rest, keep warm; o after exposure to eyes: irrigate thoroughly with water; seek medical attention in severe cases. Solvent – found throughout industry; paints plastics, rubbers and resins; see phosgene. TLV 100ppm.

Trichlorophenol. Solid; low inflammability; skin sensitizer; prolonged exposure can cause dermatitis and can lead to liver and/or kidney damage; inflammation of lungs. o Treatment after exposure to eyes: irrigate thoroughly with water; seek medical attention in severe cases; o after exposure to skin: irrigate thoroughly with water; swab with glycerol for 10 minutes. Disinfectants and fumigants; pharmaceuticals and medicinals.

Triethylamine. Liquid; high inflammability; see amines. TLV 25ppm.

'Trike'. See trichloroethylene.

Trinitrophenol. See picric acid.

Trinitrotoluene. (TNT) Solid; explosive; skin sensitizer; dermatitis on prolonged exposure; prolonged exposure also may lead to liver damage; blood poison. o Treatment after exposure to eyes: irrigate thoroughly with water; seek medical attention in severe cases; o after exposure to skin: drench with water, then wash with soap and water. Explosives. TLV 1.5mg/cu.m.

Triorthocresyl phosphate, (TOCP). Highly toxic oily liquid; low inflammability; vapour may cause dizziness, nausea and headache; interferes with nervous system – paralysis; vomiting and stomach pains. o Treatment after exposure to eyes: irrigate thoroughly with water; o after exposure to skin: drench with water, then wash with soap and water. Get medical attention for any exposure. Lacquers, varnishes and adhesives; plastics, rubbers and resins. Used as an additive in lubricating and hydraulic oils. TLV 0.1mg/cu.m.

Trioxifol. See cellosolve.

Tripwite. See hydrogen peroxide.

Tritolyl phosphate. See triorthoscresyl phosphate.

Truzone. See hydrogen peroxide.

T-stuff. See hydrogen peroxide.

Turpentine. Liquid; high inflammability; irritant to eyes, nose and throat; skin sensitizer; dermatitis on prolonged exposure; irritates skin; prolonged exposure also may lead to liver and/or kidney damage. o Treatment after inhalation: remove from exposure, rest, keep warm; o after exposure to eyes: irrigate thoroughly with water, seek medical attention in severe cases; o after exposure to skin: drench with water, then wash with soap and water. Solvent – found throughout industry; lacquers, varnishes and adhesives; paints; printing and dyestuffs. TLV 100ppm.

Urethane. See ethyl carbamate.

Vanadium and compounds. Solid; generally noninflammable; inflammation of lungs. o Treatment after inhalation: remove from exposure,, rest, keep warm; o after exposure to eyes: irrigate thoroughly with water; seek medical attention in severe cases; o after exposure to skin: seek medical attention in severe cases.

Used in chemical industry; metal industry and metal plating; contained in soot, oil-fired flues and in carbon deposits in engines. TLV (dust) 0.5mg/cu.m (fume) 0.05mg./cu.m.

Velsicol 1068. See chlordane.

Vinyl acetate. Liquid; high inflammability; see acetates. Plastics, rubbers and resins. TLV 10ppm.

Vinyl carbinol. See allyl alcohol.

Vinyl chloride. Gas; high inflammability; narcotic; irritates or burns skin; prolonged exposure may lead to liver and/or kidney damage. o Treatment after inhalation: remove from exposure, rest, keep warm; o after exposure to skin: burns and blisters must receive medical attention. Used in chemical industry; plastics, rubbers and resins. TLV 200ppm.

Vinyl cyanide. See acrylonitrile.

Vinyl ethylene. See butadiene.

Walchem. See formaldehyde.

Xylenes. Liquid; high inflammability; narcotic; anaesthetic; can cause blood, liver and kidney damage. See benzene. Solvent – found throughout industry; paint spraying; printing; plastics, rubber and resins. TLV 100ppm.

Xylenols. Solid, liquid; low inflammability; see phenol. Pharmaceuticals and medicinals; plastics, rubbers and resins; printing and dyestuffs.

Xylidine. Solid, liquid; high inflammability; see aniline. Used in chemical industry; printing and dyestuffs. TLV 5ppm.

Xylols. See xylenes.

Index

Chemicals that appear only in the Directory of Toxic Substances are not included in the Index.

Page numbers in bold indicate the main entry.